Heart Disease in Paediatrics

Third Edition

S.C. Jordan, MD, FRCP
Consultant Cardiologist,
Bristol Royal Infirmary

Olive Scott, MD, FRCP
Consultant Paediatric Cardiologist,
Leeds Regional Thoracic Centre,
Killingbeck Hospital, Leeds

Butterworths
London   Boston   Singapore   Sydney   Toronto   Wellington

PART OF REED INTERNATIONAL P.L.C.

First published 1973
Second edition 1981
Third edition 1989

EAST GLAMORGAN GENERAL HOSPITAL

CHURCH VILLAGE, near PONTYPRIDD

© Butterworth & Co. (Publishers) Ltd 1989

British Library Cataloguing in Publication Data

Jordan, S.C. (Stephen Christopher)
    Heart disease in paediatrics. - 3rd.ed.
    1. Children. Heart. Diseases
    I. Title   II. Scott, Olive, *1924-*
    618.92'12

    ISBN 0-407-19942-X

Library of Congress Cataloging in Publication Data

Jordan, S. C. (Stephen Christopher)
    Heart disease in paediatrics / S.C. Jordan,
    Olive Scott. -- 3rd ed.
        p.   cm.
    Includes bibliographies and index.
    ISBN 0-407-19942-X
    1. Heart--Diseases. 2. Pediatric cardiology. I. Scott, Olive.
    II. Title
    [DNLM: 1. Heart Diseases--in infancy & childhood.
    WS 290 J82h]
    RJ421.J67 1989
    618.92'12--dc19
    DNLM/DLC
    for Library of Congress   88-39637
                                                               CIP

Photoset by Butterworths Litho Preparation Department
Printed in Great Britain at the University Press, Cambridge

Preface to the third edition

There has been great progress in the diagnosis and management of congenital heart disease since the second edition of this book eight years ago and the third edition has been almost completely rewritten.

New non-invasive techniques are described in detail and illustrated. The use of Doppler echocardiography to provide haemodynamic information and the use of Doppler colour flow imaging to produce a picture resembling an angiocardiogram are explained. The lesions in which these techniques have replaced invasive investigation (with great benefit to the patient) are indicated.

Interestingly, as the number of diagnostic cardiac catheterizations has declined, the number of therapeutic catheterizations has increased. Interventional cardiology is now established and the various procedures of balloon valvuloplasty and angioplasty are described in a special section, as well as being appraised under the lesions for which they are used.

Up-to-date information is given about the risks, prevention and recurrence of congenital heart disease and the need for genetic counselling is indicated. This is particularly important now that patients who have been operated on are having children of their own. The use of fetal echocardiography to diagnose structural heart lesions and fetal arrhythmias is described and advised for all mothers whose babies are particularly at risk.

A new chapter is devoted to the prevention of heart disease in adult life and the risk factors which operate in childhood. The chapter on social problems has been expanded to give more information about education, exercise, immunization, travel, life insurance, psychological problems and the value of Parents' Associations.

New attitudes to the treatment of heart failure are discussed; the increased use of prostaglandins is described and their value assessed. New developments in surgery are described together with heart and heart–lung transplantation.

The authors have been fortunate in obtaining the help of Dr L. M. Gerlis (a cardiac pathologist) to illustrate this edition. Previous diagrams have been redrawn to produce greater clarity and new ones have been added. Line drawings help the reader to interpret the echocardiograms which replace many of the angiocardiograms. We thank Dr Neil Wilson and Dr John Gibbs of Killingbeck Hospital for some of the echocardiograms.

The aim of the book has not changed. It is not intended as a comprehensive work. The authors have tried to keep the book simple and practical and to give up-to-date information to paediatricians, cardiologists who occasionally see children, general practitioners, community paediatricians, nurses and technicians.

The principles of management remain unchanged – early referral, early investigation, and, when necessary, early treatment, so that the child grows up with as few secondary effects from his heart lesion as possible and can enjoy a normal or near-normal life.

S.C.J.
O.S.

Preface to the first edition

This book does not aim to be a comprehensive work on all aspects of paediatric cardiology. It is intended for the paediatrician and others who look after children to use as an introduction to paediatric cardiology and to provide up-to-date knowledge of the methods of diagnosis and treatment, particularly of congenital heart disease. The approach is essentially a practical one. It indicates to what extent the clinical signs and symptoms, assisted by radiological and electrocardiographic findings, can indicate the diagnosis, and when further investigation by cardiac catheterization and angiography will be required.

The two authors, one a paediatrician with cardiological training and one a cardiologist with special experience in paediatric cardiology, have slightly different views on some of the subjects, so that the text has been a result of the two approaches. In a book of this size it has not been possible or desirable to discuss in detail some of the more controversial aspects of paediatric cardiology, and indeed views on such topics as early corrective surgery in infancy are changing rapidly at the moment. This should not deter the paediatrician, as the same principles apply with regard to referral of patients for further investigation and treatment.

Few paediatricians will be directly concerned with cardiac catheterization, but decisions regarding surgery are frequently influenced by the results of this investigation and a section has therefore been included on the technique and interpretation.

One of the most striking changes in paediatric cardiology in recent years has been the increasing interest in the management of the newborn infant with heart disease and a special chapter has been included, which presents a scheme to simplify diagnosis in this difficult group of patients.

S.C.J.
O.S.

Contents

Part 1

General cardiology

Chapter 1

Incidence, aetiology and recurrence of congenital heart disease

Incidence

Congenital heart disease is the commonest single group of congenital abnormalities, accounting for about 30% of the total. The incidence is at least 8/1000 live births. There are eight common lesions which account for about 80% of all cases. They are, in descending order to prevalence, ventricular septal defect, patent ductus arteriosus, atrial septal defect, tetralogy of Fallot, pulmonary stenosis, coarctation of the aorta, aortic stenosis and transposition of the great arteries. The remaining 20% or so is made up of a variety of more rare and complex lesions. Figures for the prevalence of the various lesions vary in different regions and are dependent on the time at which they are assessed. Table 1.1 gives the incidence in Bristol in different years and includes lesions with an incidence of 1% or more of the total.

Table 1.1 Bristol congenital heart disease register 1966–87. Incidence of lesions comprising more than 1% of total

Lesion	1966–76	1977–87	1966–87
Ventricular septal defect	29.4	36.1	33.3
Atrial septal defect	9.4	8.2	8.7
Pulmonary stenosis	9.1	6.9	7.8
Patent ductus arteriosus	6.4	7.9	7.3
Coarctation	6.2	5.9	6.0
Aortic stenosis	5.4	5.7	5.6
Tetralogy of Fallot	6.2	4.6	5.3
Transposition	4.5	3.8	4.1
Atrioventricular septal defect	2.7	3.6	3.2
Pulmonary atresia	3.0	2.6	2.8
Primitive ventricle	—	2.2	1.9
Tricuspid atresia	1.2	1.5	1.4
Mitral regurgitation	1.3	1.4	1.4
Aortic atresia	1.1	1.4	1.3
Hypertrophic cardiomyopathy	1.2	1.3	1.3
Total anomalous pulmonary venous connection	1.3	1.2	1.2
Ebstein's anomaly	1.2	—	1.0
Total	89.6	94.3	93.6

Aetiology

The first question parents ask when they realize that their child has a heart defect is, 'What caused it?' Unfortunately, we are still unable to answer this question in the majority of patients. Only a minority of cases run in families. The most likely explanation is that there is a genetic susceptibility for the mother to have a baby with congenital heart disease, but it only actually happens if some environmental hazard occurs at the appropriate time during her pregnancy. Nora and Nora (1983) have constructed a timetable for teratogenic activity to occur to produce the various lesions. This of course depends on the time when the various parts of the heart are forming. For truncus arteriosus to occur, the most sensitive vulnerable period is between 18 and 29 days' gestation, for atrioventricular defects between 18 and 33 days, and for ventricular septal defect between 18 and 39 days. The vulnerable period is longer – 18–50 days – in atrial septal defect and semilunar valve abnormalities. In patent ductus and coarctation of the aorta it is 18–60 days. This gives a guide in looking for a possible teratogenic factor at a particular time in pregnancy. The problem is that the mother may not have realized that she was pregnant when the teratogenic insult occurred.

Inheritance

Hypertrophic obstructive cardiomyopathy, sometimes atrial septal defect and supravalvar aortic stenosis all behave as autosomal dominant traits. Marfan's syndrome is an autosomal dominant disorder in which there is cardiac involvement; Pyeritz, Brinker and Varghese (1979) estimate that nearly all patients have echocardiographic evidence of aortic dilatation or mitral valve prolapse or both. Idiopathic mitral valve prolapse appears to be inherited in an autosomal dominant mode with variable expressivity (Devereux and Brown, 1983). The Holt–Oram syndrome is caused by an autosomal gene with dominant inheritance but there is variable expression in the limb anomalies; about one-half of patients have cardiac anomalies, most commonly atrial and ventricular septal defects. At least 10% of patients with Noonan's syndrome (a phenocopy of Turner's syndrome) have been shown to have dominant inheritance and the figure may be higher than that. One-half of patients with Noonan's syndrome have a heart lesion, most commonly dysplastic pulmonary valves (see pages 138, 326).

Chromosomal aberrations

About 6–10% of all patients with congenital heart disease have some chromosomal aberration (Hoffman and Christianson, 1978). On the other hand, about 30% of newborn infants with various chromosomal aberrations have congenital heart disease. The incidence in trisomy 13 is as high as 90% and in trisomy 18, 80%. The commonest heart lesions in chromosomal aberrations are septal defects and patent ductus arteriosus. About 40% of patients with Down's syndrome have congenital heart disease (Roussay *et al.*, 1978) and at least 40% of these have atrioventricular defects (Park *et al.*, 1977). (A quarter of all patients with atrioventricular defects have Down's syndrome (Greenwood and Nadas, 1976).) Ventricular septal defects, tetralogy of Fallot and patent ductus (in descending order of prevalence) also occur in Down's syndrome. Twenty per cent of patients with Turner's syndrome have coarctation of the aorta or aortic stenosis or both.

Environmental factors

There is much more concern now in identifying environmental factors in the hope of preventing exposures to them during early pregnancy. Drugs, infections and maternal illnesses have all been implicated.

Drugs
The drugs which may cause cardiovascular anomalies are listed below, together with the most common lesions produced.

Alcohol	Transposition of great arteries; Ventricular and atrial septal defects; Patent ductus arteriosus
Amphetamines	Transposition of great arteries; Ventricular and atrial septal defects; Patent ductus arteriosus
Phenytoin	Pulmonary and aortic stenosis; Coarction of the aorta; Patent ductus arteriosus
Lithium	Particularly Ebstein's abnormality of the tricuspid valve
Sex hormones (oestrogens and progestogens)	Transposition of great arteries; Tetralogy of Fallot; Ventricular septal defect

Infections
Rubella has been most implicated but other viruses, particularly cytomegalovirus and herpes virus, have been found to be teratogenic (Blattner *et al.*, 1973). The association of the mumps virus with endocardial fibroelastosis has not been proven (Chen, Thompson and Rose, 1971).

Maternal conditions
Diabetes mellitus in the mother carries a 5% risk of structural heart disease in the fetus (Rowland, Hubbell and Nadas, 1973). A form of hypertrophic cardiomyopathy also occurs in these infants but this resolves with time and can be seen to do so on echocardiographic studies. Meticulous control of the diabetes is thought to reduce the risks of malformations (Miller *et al.*, 1981). Systemic lupus erythematosus carries a risk of complete heart block in the fetus (Scott *et al.*, 1983).

Twin studies

Monozygotic twins have double the incidence of heart defects compared with single pregnancies (Burn and Corney, 1984). The monozygotic process itself is liable to cause heart defects, perhaps associated with altered haemodynamics *in utero*. The possibility of one twin being affected or both of them is equally common.

Multifactorial inheritance

To summarize, the most readily acceptable theory for the genetic basis of congenital heart disease is the multifactorial hypothesis. This suggests that the genetic material concerned with the normal development of the heart is carried on a number of genes and that abnormalities of these genes may not in themselves be enough to cause cardiac abnormalities, but in the presence of other environmental factors the genes predispose to the occurrence of such defects. In other words there is a genetic susceptibility to develop congenital heart disease if the appropriate environmental hazard occurs. Furthermore, the environmental hazard must occur during a narrow sensitive period of pregnancy between the second and ninth weeks.

Greater effort must be made to find the particular environmental hazards which may interact with the genetic predisposition to cause cardiac anomalies. There has already been a fall in the number of patients presenting with the rubella syndrome – and the thalidomide syndrome no longer occurs. Doctors must be aware of the effects of alcohol, lithium, amphetamines, anticonvulsants and sex hormone drugs and try to prevent them being taken during the vulnerable period of pregnancy. There must be careful records from mothers of babies with heart disease to try to identify new teratogens. Sometimes there is a brisk rise in the frequency of a particular heart lesion in the newborn and a possible teratogen operating 7 or 8 months earlier must be sought.

If an uncommon abnormality suddenly increases in frequency it is much more likely to be noticed (e.g. the increase of cases of Ebstein's malformation associated with lithium) than if it is a common abnormality such as a ventricular septal defect. Some agents may not be harmful to the general population but affect certain groups with some genetic predisposition to cardiovascular malformations. It is well to remember that substances which are teratogenic in animals are not necessarily so in man.

Research in identifying genetic risks is progressing and there is hope for better prevention in the future.

Recurrence in family

If one sibling in a family has congenital heart disease, the risks of another child being affected varies in individual lesions and is in the region of 1–3%. Nora and Nora (1978) have combined the data in various series to give a figure for the overall risk. Table 1.2 summarizes their findings. There is a high degree of concordance in that two siblings usually have the same lesion or one of its components (e.g. pulmonary stenosis or ventricular septal defect occurs in siblings of patients with tetralogy of Fallot).

Now that children with congenital heart disease survive to have children of their own it is important to know the risks of their children being affected. It is important first to determine whether any of the known teratogens exist such as phenytoin or rubella or whether the mother has diabetes, is an alcoholic or smokes heavily, as these will increase the risks. A family history of heart disease will also increase the risks as will the presence of known syndromes such as Noonan's and Holt–Oram. The results of various studies are widely different. Emmanuel et al. (1983) found an incidence of 10% of heart defects in the offspring of mothers with atrioventricular defects. Rose et al. (1985) found an overall recurrence risk of affected offspring of 8.8%. Dennis and Warren (1981) studied the recurrence in the offspring of patients with ventricular septal defects and right ventricular outflow tract obstruction or combination of the two, and found a recurrence rate of only 3.4%. Czeizel et al. (1982) found an incidence of 4.9% in the offspring of patients who had had surgery for congenital heart disease. Whittemore, Hobbins and Engle (1982) found an incidence in offspring of 16% but there may be a bias because they focused on more

Table 1.2 Recurrence risks if one child has congenital heart disease

Anomaly	Combined suggested risk (%)
Ventricular septal defect	3.0
Patent ductus arteriosus	3.0
Atrial septal defect	2.5
Tetralogy of Fallot	2.5
Pulmonary stenosis Coarction of aorta Aortic stenosis Transposition Atrioventricular defects	2.0
Tricuspid atresia Ebstein's anomaly Truncus arteriosus Pulmonary atresia	1.0
Hypoplastic left heart	2.0

Table 1.3 Recurrence in offspring if one parent has congenital heart defect (After Nora and Nora, 1983)

Anomaly	Combined suggested risk (%)
Ventricular septal defect	4.0
Patent ductus arteriosus	4.0
Atrial septal defect	2.5
Tetralogy of Fallot	4.0
Pulmonary stenosis	3.5
Coarctation of aorta	2.0
Aortic stenosis	4.0

severe cases. Nora and Nora (1978) have combined the various studies and suggested figures for the risk of recurrence. Table 1.3 summarizes these. More prospective studies are needed but it seems clear that the risk to the offspring of a parent with congenital heart disease is greater than the risk to the siblings of an affected child.

Fetal echocardiography

A service is now becoming available in major centres to provide fetal echocardiography, particularly for mothers who already have one child with a heart lesion or have congenital heart disease themselves. Great progress has been made in this field and by the eighteenth week of fetal life most major heart defects can be identified. Mothers should therefore be offered this service. Allen (1986) found that in over 2500 pregnancies studied, no major false positive diagnosis was made. Some minor defects were overlooked and it may be impossible to avoid this; nevertheless, the prognosis in all such minor lesions is good. Coarctation of the aorta, which is an important defect, is still difficult to diagnose but the use of Doppler studies is improving results (see page 122).

If no abnormality is seen, the mother can be reassured that the heart is normal or any defect present is mild. If there is a serious inoperable abnormality then abortion can be discussed. Problems arise, however, when a heart lesion is found in which operation offers good results. If the mother can face the problem and is given adequate support, then arrangements can be made for delivery to take place near a major centre for paediatric cardiology so that immediate help is available and investigation and treatment can be carried out promptly when necessary. When Allen (1986) studied the outcome of 81 predictions of serious congenital heart disease, she found that nearly half the parents chose termination of pregnancy because of severe heart disease; intra-uterine death occurred in 16 and neonatal death in 22. There were only 4 survivors.

Bibliography and references

Aetiology

Allen, L. D. (1986) Fetal echocardiography. In *Topics in Circulations* Vol. 1.2. pp. 2–4

Blattner, W. A., Kirstenmacher, M. L., Tsai, S., *et al.* (1980) Clinical manifestations of familial 13:18 translocation. *Journal of Medical Genetics,* **17,** 373–379

Burn, J. and Corney, G. (1984) Congenital heart defects and twinning. *Acta Geneticae Medicae et Gemellologiae* **33,** 61–69

Chen, S., Thompson, M. W. and Rose, V. (1971) Endocardial fibroelastosis; familial studies with special reference to counselling. *Journal of Paediatrics* **79,** 385–392

Czeizel, A., Pornoi, A., Peterffy, E., *et al.* (1982) Studies of children of parents operated on for congenital cardiovascular malformations. *British Heart Journal,* **47,** 290–293

Dennis, N. R. and Warren, J. (1981) Risks to the offspring of patients with some common congenital heart defects. *Journal of Medical Genetics,* **18,** 8–16

Devereux, R. B. and Brown, W. T. (1983) Genetics of idiopathic mitral valve prolapse. In *Progress in Medical Genetics 5,* Saunders, Philadelphia, p. 147

Emmanuel, R., Somerville, J., Inns, A., *et al.* (1983) Evidence of congenital heart disease in the offspring of parents with atrioventricular defects. *British Heart Journal,* **49,** 144–147

Greenwood, R. D. and Nadas, A. S. (1976) The clinical course of cardiac disease in Down's syndrome. *Pediatrics, Springfield,* **58,** 893–897

Hoffman, J. I. E. and Christianson, R. (1978) Congenital heart disease in a cohort of 19 502 births with long-term follow-up. *American Journal of Cardiology,* **42,** 641–647

Miller, E., Hare, J. W., Cloherty, J. P., *et al.* (1981) Elevated maternal haemoglobin A in early pregnancy and major congenital anomalies in infants of diabetic mothers. *New England Journal of Medicine,* **304,** 1331–1334

Nora, J. J. and Nora, A. H. (1978) *Genetics and Counselling in Cardiovascular Diseases.* Charles C. Thomas, Springfield, Ill.

Nora, J. J. and Nora, A. H. (1983) Genetic epidemiology of congenital heart disease. In *Progress in Medical Genetics* Vol. 5 (eds A. G. Steinberg, A. G. Bearn, A. G. Motulsky *et al.*), Saunders, Philadelphia, p. 102

Park, S. C., Mathews, R. A., Zuberbuhler, J. B., *et al.* (1977) Down syndrome with congenital heart malformation. *American Journal of Disease in Children,* **131,** 29–33

Pyeritz, R. E., Brinker, J. A. and Varghese, P. J. (1979) Clinical and echocardiographic correlates in 127 young Marfan patients. *Clinical Research,* **27,** 196A

Rose, V., Gold, R. J. M., Lindsey, G., *et al.* (1985) A possible increase in the incidence of congenital heart defects among the offspring of affected parents. *Journal of the American College of Cardiology,* **6,** 376–382

Roussay, M., Duclaut, A. M., Almange, C., *et al.* (1978) Les cardiopathies congenitales des trisomiques 21. *Pediatrie,* **33,** 437–449

Rowland, T. W., Hubbell, J. P. and Nadas, A. S. (1973) Congenital heart disease in infants of diabetic mothers. *Journal of Pediatrics*, **83**, 815–820

Scott, J. S., Maddison, P. J., Taylor, P. V., *et al.* (1983) Connective-tissue disease, antibodies to ribonucleoprotein, and congenital heart block. *New England Journal of Medicine*, **309**, 209–212

Whittemore, R., Hobbins, J. C. and Engle, M. A. (1982) Pregnancy and its outcome in women with and without surgical treatment of congenital heart disease. *American Journal of Cardiology*, **50**, 361–370

The fetal circulation and the changes at birth in relation to congenital heart disease

The fetal circulation

To appreciate the haemodynamic effects of congenital heart lesions, there must be clear understanding of the fetal circulation and the changes which take place after birth to establish the normal, independent circulation. These changes influence the circulation in normal infants but are of profound importance in infants with congenital heart disease. *A congenital heart lesion is not a static condition; changes continue to take place throughout the patient's life, but the most significant of these occur at birth.*

In the fetus, blood comes from the placenta via the umbilical vein and is relatively well oxygenated ($Po_2 = 30$ mmHg). Half of this blood passes through the liver and the remainder bypasses the liver through the ductus venosus and continues up the inferior vena cava, which receives blood leaving the liver by the hepatic veins and blood returning from the lower half of the body of the fetus. Most of the inferior vena caval blood passes through the foramen ovale to the left atrium and so to the left ventricle, ascending aorta and coronary circulation. This ensures that blood of a high Po_2 enters the cerebral and coronary circulations. A small amount of inferior vena caval blood passes through the tricuspid valve into the right ventricle. Blood returning from the head and neck of the fetus enters the right atrium by the superior vena cava, is joined by coronary sinus blood and then enters the right ventricle and pulmonary artery (Figure 2.1). In the fetus only about 15% of the right ventricular blood enters the lungs, and the rest passes through the ductus arteriosus into the descending aorta where it is joined by blood from the ascending aorta. In the fetus the ductus arteriosus is as large as the aorta itself and pressures in the pulmonary artery and aorta are equal.

In the fetus there is a high pulmonary vascular resistance and the muscular pulmonary arteries are constricted and have a thick medial muscular layer.

After birth the following changes take place.
1. The pulmonary vascular resistance falls and the pulmonary blood flow increases.
2. The systemic vascular resistance rises.
3. The patent ductus arteriosus closes.
4. The foramen ovale closes.
5. The ductus venosus closes.

The initial fall in pulmonary vascular resistance at birth is associated with expansion of the lungs with air. The pulmonary arterial vasoconstriction ceases and there may

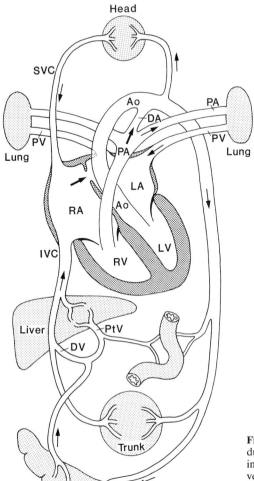

Figure 2.1 The fetal circulation. Ao, aorta; DA, ductus arteriosus; DV, ductus venosus; IVC inferior vena cava; LA, left atrium; LV, left ventricle; PA, pulmonary artery; PtV, portal vein; PV pulmonary vein; RA right atrium; RV, right ventricle; SVC, superior vena cava

be active dilatation of the vessels. The greatest fall in the pulmonary artery pressure takes place in the *first two to three days of life* and then there is a more gradual fall to normal adult levels by *two weeks of life* (Rudolph, 1970). The medial muscle layer of the small pulmonary arteries thins out in the first few days of life as these vessels dilate, and thereafter the histological changes in the pulmonary vessels follow the fall in the pulmonary artery pressure.

Once the low resistance placental circulation is removed at birth, the systemic resistance rises. While the ductus remains open, there is a preferential flow through it from the aorta to the lungs. In turn the pulmonary venous return is increased and there is increased flow to the left atrium and left ventricle. The ductus closes functionally within 10–15 hours of birth, so any flow through it lasts a relatively short time. If there is hypoxia of the fetal blood for any reason (for example, pulmonary disease) it will cause a rise in pulmonary artery pressure and favour a right-to-left shunt through the ductus. The administration of 100% oxygen causes the ductus to constrict. In normal mature infants the ductus closes permanently within two or three weeks of birth. The histological changes have been well described by Gittenberger-de-Groot (1979).

The foramen ovale closes functionally at birth. A shunt through it from the right atrium to the left may occur if the pulmonary artery and right ventricular pressures rise in response to hypoxia. Occasionally, a left-to-right shunt through the foramen may persist for some months if the flap covering it does not seal completely.

The importance of changes in the circulation after birth in relation to congenital heart disease has been clearly shown by Rudolph (1970).

The relevance of changes in the circulation at birth to congenital heart defects

Large communication between pulmonary and systemic circulations

Since the pulmonary vascular resistance falls rapidly in the first two or three days of life, it would be expected that a large communication between the pulmonary and systemic circulations, such as patent ductus arteriosus, ventricular septal defect and aortopulmonary window, would exert its greatest effect in the first days of life, due to a preferential flow of blood from the high resistance systemic circulation to the low resistance pulmonary circulation. This does not in fact happen.

It seems that when a large communication exists, the rate of fall of pulmonary vascular resistance proceeds more slowly; this delays the onset of symptoms and helps the circulation to adapt to the defect more gradually. The postnatal changes in the main pulmonary artery and its branches may also play a part in maintaining the pulmonary artery pressure at a higher level for a longer period. There is frequently a pressure drop between the main pulmonary artery and its branches, suggesting some stenosis, but as the infant grows this pressure difference disappears (Rudolph, 1970). All these lesions tend to produce left ventricular failure due to the high pulmonary flow which in turn leads to an increased pulmonary venous return and high left atrial pressure. The symptoms and signs of left ventricular failure in left-to-right shunts are rarely seen before 3–4 weeks of age. If lung disease is present, the left-to-right shunt may decrease because of the rise in pulmonary artery pressure and a right-to-left shunt through these defects may occur.

Heart lesions dependent on ductal patency

If the oxygenation of arterial blood after birth is inadequate the closure of the ductus may be delayed or prevented. The incidence of patent ductus arteriosus in individuals born and living at high altitude is greater than those born at sea level. In some congenital heart defects, babies can only survive if the ductus arteriosus remains patent. Such defects are pulmonary atresia and critical pulmonary stenosis; aortic atresia and critical aortic stenosis; severe coarctation of the aorta and transposition of the great arteries. Even though the normal constriction of the ductus depends on a rise in arterial oxygen concentration, the duct still constricts after birth in hypoxic babies and this may happen suddenly. Severe hypoxaemia and acidosis results, making the risks of any palliative surgery extremely high. The only way of helping these babies is to maintain the patency of the ductus with prostaglandins.

Pharmacological manipulation of the ductus arteriosus

Prostaglandins have been found in high concentrations in the area of the ductus and can be shown to play a part in the normal patency of the ductus prior to delivery (Olley and Coceani, 1979). It has been suggested that postnatal exposure of the duct to oxygen reduces the responsiveness of the duct to prostaglandins and it therefore closes. This discovery led to the possibility of pharmacological manipulation of the ductus (Olley and Coceani, 1979) and is one of the most important advances in paediatric cardiology.

Manipulation of the ductus has therefore been directed on the one hand to the use of E type prostaglandins to keep the duct open and on the other hand to the use of drug inhibition of prostaglandin synthesis to encourage ductus constriction. Indomethacin is the drug most widely used as a prostaglandin synthetase inhibitor, but is of value only in the premature infant (see page 78).

Silove (1986) recommends the use of prostaglandin E_2 which he found had fewer toxic effects than E_1. The toxic effects are probably dose-related and experience has shown that lower doses than those used initially are effective in keeping the ductus open. Apnoea and cardiovascular complications are much less with low doses although diarrhoea and fever still occur. Silove recommends PGE_2 0.03 µg/kg/min intravenously but a higher dose may be necessary for the first few hours. Treatment can be maintained using oral PGE_2 in a dose of 20–25 µg/kg hourly and the dose reduced after one week. Although treatment by the oral route can be continued, there have been reports of the ductus becoming friable and the pulmonary vascular smooth muscle being damaged. The sooner surgery can be undertaken after the child's condition has improved, the better.

Persistent patency of the ductus arteriosus in premature infants

In the premature infant there is delay in closure of the ductus and about 50% of infants under 1500 g in weight have patency of the ductus. The incidence is higher when there is associated hyaline membrane disease. In the premature infant there is a rapid fall in pulmonary vascular resistance which favours a left-to-right shunt. Cardiac failure commonly occurs if the duct is open in premature infants. If the infant can tolerate the heart failure and the latter responds to medical treatment, then the duct will eventually close – it rarely remains open for more than three months (Hallidie-Smith and Girling, 1971; Rudolph, 1977). The situation has changed now that more premature infants survive with ventilatory support (see page 77).

Obstruction of flow into or from the left ventricle (mitral atresia; aortic atresia; coarctation of aorta)

When there is severe obstruction to flow of blood from the left ventricle, the pressure in it rises and this results in a high left atrial pressure. The valvular action of the foramen ovale may then be overcome and it remains widely open with a resultant left-to-right shunt at atrial level. This left-to-right shunt, however, may be beneficial by reducing the left atrial pressure and lessening the severity of pulmonary oedema. Similarly, in mitral atresia the left atrial pressure rises and an open foramen ovale may be the only means by which pulmonary venous blood may enter the right side of the heart.

Obstruction of flow from the right atrium or right ventricle (tricuspid atresia; pulmonary atresia with intact ventricular septum)

The only way in which blood can reach the left side of the heart is by the open foramen ovale. A high right atrial pressure favours the foramen remaining open. Similarly, in total anomalous pulmonary venous drainage, the foramen ovale must remain open to permit blood to reach the left side of the heart.

Transposition of the great arteries

An open foramen ovale and a patent ductus arteriosus may be the only routes by which blood can shunt from the systemic to the pulmonary circulation and vice versa in transposition of the great arteries. If the left atrial pressure rises the foramen may close despite its patency being essential for life. Enlargement of the foramen ovale or the creation of an atrial septal defect has been effective in prolonging life in this lesion.

Total anomalous pulmonary venous drainage to the portal vein

The ductus venosus usually closes at birth but may remain open when the pulmonary veins all drain into the portal vein, thus making a free passage of blood into the inferior vena cava without going through the liver. When the ductus venosus closes, however, the blood in the anomalous vein has to pass through a high resistance circuit in the liver, the pressure in the anomalous pulmonary vein rises and pulmonary oedema results.

References

Fetal circulation

Gittenberger-de-Groot, A. (1979) Ductus arteriosus – histological observations in paediatric cardiology. In *Heart Disease in the Newborn*, Vol. 2 (eds M. J. Godman and R. M. Marquis), Churchill Livingstone, London

Hallidie-Smith, K. A. and Girling, D. J. (1971) Persistent ductus arteriosus in ill and premature babies. *Archives of Disease in Childhood*, **46**, 177–181

Olley, P. M. and Coceani, F. (1979) Mechanism of closure of the ductus arteriosus. In *Paediatric Cardiology*, Vol. 2 (eds M. J. Godman and R. M. Marquis), Churchill Livingstone, London, pp. 15–31

Rudolph, A. M. (1970) The changes in the circulation after birth. *Circulation*, **41**, 343–359

Rudolph, A.M. (1977) In *Paediatric Cardiology*, Vol. 47 (eds R. H. Anderson and E. A. Shinebourne), Churchill Livingstone, London, pp. 409–412

Silove, E. (1986) Pharmacological manipulation of the ductus arteriosus. *Archives of Disease in Childhood*, **61**, 827–829

Chapter 3

Normal haemodynamics: the generation of heart sounds and murmurs

Normal haemodynamics

It is important for the reader to be familiar with the normal physiology of the heart before he studies the abnormal.

The heart can be considered as two pumps connected in series by two systems of vessels. The pressure generated by the right ventricle drives the blood through the pulmonary circuit and the pressure generated by the left ventricle drives the blood through the systemic circuit.

In a normal heart the resistance to flow of blood imposed by the pulmonary circuit is low, but the resistance imposed by the systemic circuit, as soon as the adaptation following birth occurs, is much higher, being about ten times greater than the pulmonary resistance. The resistance in the systemic circuit varies under differing physiological conditions and during exercise it falls when the muscle vessels dilate to allow a greater flow of blood through them. The pulmonary resistance shows little variation except when there is hypoxia or acidaemia, both of which cause it to increase.

Cardiac output

The output of blood from the right and left ventricles must be the same in a healthy heart; this is simply termed the 'cardiac output' and is expressed in litres/minute. According to Starling's 'law of the heart', the force generated by the muscle fibres is a function of their resting length. In practice, the resting length depends upon the degree of filling of the ventricles, so that increased filling of the heart results in increased cardiac output. The contractile properties of the heart can be increased by drugs such as digoxin and isoprenaline and are reduced in heart failure.

Normal pressures and oxygen saturations

The normal resting values in childhood are shown in Figure 3.1. The state of the patient must be stable throughout the period of measurement. There is a variation in the oxygen values in the right atrium depending on the exact site of sampling. The figures given are average ones. If a sample is taken in the atrium near the mouth of the coronary sinus the value is low; if the sample is rather low down in the inferior vena cava the oxygen saturation may be high because it contains blood from the renal veins which have a high oxygen saturation. There must be a rise of

Systolic murmurs

Systolic murmurs have been classified by Leatham (1958) as follows:

1. Ejection systolic murmurs, caused by forward flow of blood through a normal or diseased semilunar valve, aortic or mitral.
2. Regurgitant murmurs, caused by retrograde flow of blood through an incompetent atrioventricular valve or through a ventricular septal defect.

Ejection murmurs show a diamond-shaped pattern on the phonocardiogram and end before the onset of the second sound. They are heard in aortic stenosis and pulmonary stenosis when blood is flowing though a narrowed orifice. A similar, though softer, type of murmur occurs when there is an increased flow of blood through a normal semilunar valve, as occurs through the pulmonary valve in atrial septal defect. Murmurs due to aortic stenosis are rather shorter than those due to pulmonary stenosis.

Regurgitant murmurs usually last throughout systole (pansystolic) and are plateau-shaped on the phonocardiogram. In an uncomplicated ventricular septal defect there is a gradient between the left and right ventricles throughout systole. In free mitral regurgitation there is a gradient between the left ventricle and left atrium throughout systole. Early systolic murmurs are heard in very small ventricular septal defects, late systolic murmurs in very mild mitral regurgitation.

Diastolic murmurs

Diastolic murmurs occur when the semilunar valves are incompetent, when the atrioventricular valves are narrowed, or when they are normal but there is an increased volume of blood flow through them. The murmur of aortic regurgitation has a high pitch and is soft and often difficult to hear. It is best heard down the left sternal edge when the patient sits forward and holds his breath in expiration. The murmur of pulmonary incompetence associated with a high pulmonary artery pressure (Graham Steell murmur) is indistinguishable from it. The murmur of pulmonary incompetence when there is a low pulmonary artery pressure is lower pitched.

The diastolic murmurs of mitral stenosis are low pitched and rumbling, and best heard when the patient turns onto the left side. The murmur due to increased flow through the mitral valve with ventricular septal defects and patent ductus arteriosus is short and low pitched. The diastolic murmur due to increased flow through the tricuspid valve is softer, increases with inspiration and is best heard in the erect posture after exericise. It is heard rather sooner after the second sound than the mitral diastolic flow murmur.

Continuous murmurs

Continuous murmurs are heard when blood flows between two parts of the circulation with a gradient in diastole and systole. The usual cause is a patent ductus arteriosus (see page 73).

The various types of murmur are illustrated diagrammatically in Figure 3.2.

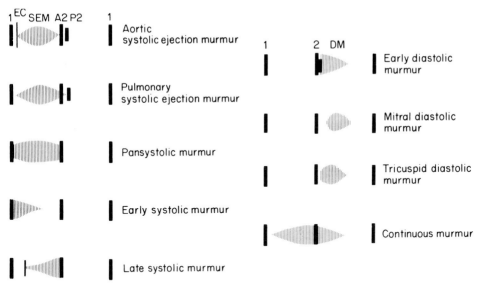

Figure 3.2 Types of murmur. 1, first sound; 2, second sound; EC, ejection click; SEM, systolic ejection murmur; A2 and P2, aortic and pulmonary components of second heart sound; DM, diastolic murmur

Innocent murmurs

The terms 'benign', 'functional' and 'physiological' are also used to describe innocent murmurs. 'Innocent' seems the most satisfactory term because it is best understood by the child or his parents. The term is used to describe murmurs which occur in patients who have no abnormality of the heart. It is very important that doctors appreciate the innocence of these murmurs and that parents are reassured that their child's heart is normal and the child's activities are not unnecessarily restricted. If there is any doubt the child should be referred to a cardiologist.

The frequency with which innocent murmurs are heard varies, but they are often accentuated by factors which produce tachycardia – fever, excitement and exercise – and disappear when the heart rate slows. They often vary with respiration, disappearing with inspiration, and are affected by changes in posture. Innocent murmurs may occur in systole or be continuous. A diastolic murmur by itself is never innocent.

Three main types of innocent systolic murmur are recognized in childhood.

Vibratory murmur

The character and pitch of the vibratory murmur are very like the buzzing of a bee. It is very short and occurs in mid-systole. It is less obvious when the patient sits up and extends his neck, and often disappears when he sits with his hands behind him and arches his back. It is commonest under the age of 10 years and usually disappears at puberty (Figure 3.3).

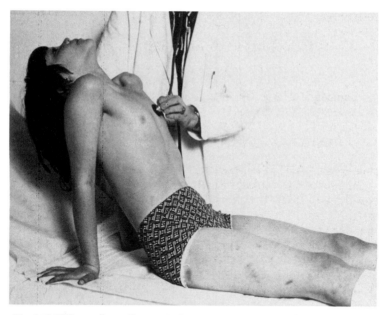

Figure 3.3 Vibratory systolic murmur is markedly reduced or disappears when patient sits up with neck extended

Pulmonary systolic murmur

The pulmonary systolic murmur is a soft, blowing, ejection systolic murmur occupying the early part of systole, heard in the second left interspace close to the sternum and conducted upwards to the infraclavicular region. The differential diagnosis is a mild degree of pulmonary stenosis, but the second sound is normally split when the murmur is innocent and the electrocardiogram and radiograph are quite normal. It is commonest in older children and adolescents.

Venous hum

A venous hum, due to blood cascading into the great veins, is a blowing, continuous murmur best heard in the supraclavicular fossa but often quite loud below the clavicles. The hum is abolished or greatly diminished when the internal jugular vein on the same side as the murmur is compressed, when the patient turns his head from the side to a midline position and when he lies down flat or performs the Valsalva manoeuvre.

Blood pressure

This used to be a difficult measurement in children because of determining accurate end-points in a restless child. More sophisticated equipment has made it easier but it is still essential to use the correct width and length of cuff. Steinfeld *et al.* (1978) did much to clarify this. They conclude that the cuff bladder should be as follows:

1. *Width*. This should cover 75% of the upper arm. It is better for the cuff to be too wide than too narrow;
2. *Length*. The bladder should completely encircle the upper arm; overlap does not matter.

The Korotkoff sounds can be enhanced by using an ultrasonic Doppler device which gives a clear signal indicating the systolic pressure. One must be careful, however, to keep the sensor over the artery which may be difficult in a restless child. The newly developed method using the oscillometric principle gives accurate systolic, diastolic and mean arterial pressures but the correct size of cuff is still essential.

If sophisticated equipment is not available, the flush method is satisfactory even in restless infants. The pressure recorded is a little below the true systolic pressure. The correct size of cuff is applied and a crêpe bandage is wrapped firmly around the hand and forearm. The cuff is inflated to a level above the expected systolic pressure and the bandage removed. The skin appears blanched. The sphygmomanometer pressure is then lowered 5 mmHg at a time, slowly, and the skin observed. A reading is made when the skin shows a pink flush. This method is valuable in coarctation of the aorta in infants when the absolute systolic pressure is not so important but it is important to know whether there is a difference between the arms and legs.

The Dynamap oscillometric unit is now being used increasingly. It has the advantage that the cuff can be placed on the infant's arm and attached to the machine, then subsequent readings can be made without disturbing the child. As long as the machines are serviced regularly, they give very accurate results.

In older children recordings should be made with the child sitting and his arm supported. If a mercury manometer is being used the observer's eyes should be at the centre of the scale to avoid parallax. The systolic reading should be made as soon as the Korotkoff sounds appear and the distolic reading when all sounds disappear.

Values of blood pressure in normal infants and children are given in Chapter 21.

References

Heart murmurs

Leatham, Aubrey (1958) Auscultation of the heart. *Lancet*, **2,** 757

Blood pressure

Steinfeld, L., Dimich, I., Reder, R., *et al.* (1978) Sphygmomanometry in the pediatric patient. *Journal of Pediatrics*, **92,** 934–938

Chapter 4

Cardiac investigations

Radiology

A radiograph of the heart and lungs in congenital heart disease is only of value if the film fulfils strict criteria.

1. It must be straight.
2. It must be taken during full inspiration.
3. It must be of the correct penetration for accurate assessment of the vascularity of the lungs.

A posteroanterior film should be taken initially and lateral or oblique views can then be added as indicated. In children over 6 months of age the posteroanterior film is taken with the patient erect at a tube distance of 6 feet. In children under 6 months of age the film is taken with the patient lying down and is an anteroposterior one with a tube distance of 5 feet.

Heart size and shape

The size of the heart is best estimated by measuring the cardiothoracic diameter, i.e. the ratio of the transverse diameter of the heart to the greatest *internal* diameter of the chest. A line is drawn down the centre of the film and the distance from this central line to the furthest point on the right heart border, added to the distance from the central line to the furthest point on the left heart border, gives the transverse cardiac diameter (Figure 4.1). If the cardiothoracic ratio is less than 0.5, the heart is not enlarged overall.

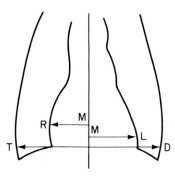

Figure 4.1 Measurement of cardiothoracic ratio. The cardiac diameter is the sum of M–R and M–L, the distances of the right and left cardiac borders from the midline. The thoracic diameter (TD) is the greatest diameter inside the ribs

The heart chambers and great vessels should than be assessed. The reader must be familiar with the normal heart before he can assess the abnormal. The right heart border is made up of the superior vena cava above, and the right atrium below, and the inferior vena cava is seen below the right atrium (Figure 4.2). On the left heart border the aorta, pulmonary artery and left ventricular outlines are seen. The main pulmonary artery is straight or slightly convex. The left atrial appendage lies below the pulmonary artery but normally merges imperceptibly with the left ventricular border.

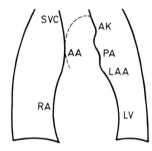

Figure 4.2 Normal cardiac silhouette. AA, ascending aorta; AK, aortic knuckle; LAA, left atrial appendage; LV, left ventricle; PA, pulmonary artery; RA, right atrium; SVC, superior vena cava

Details about the enlargement of the heart chambers and great vessels are given under individual lesions and a table of common heart shapes in infancy is given on pages 236–237. Figure 4.3 shows the enlargements of various structures for comparison one with another. In the posteroanterior film, when there is enlargement of the right ventricle the cardiac apex is tilted upwards and has a small radius of curvature; when the left ventricle is enlarged the apex points downwards and has a larger radius. The size of the ventricles cannot be assessed accurately, however, a posteroanterior film and a lateral film are necessary for this. An enlarged right ventricle is seen bulging anteriorly. An enlarged left ventricle bulges posteriorly over the vertebral bodies.

Vascularity of the lungs

An assessment of lung vascularity is of great importance in the diagnosis of congenital heart disease. When it is increased, there must be a left-to-right shunt, resulting in an excessive flow of blood to the lungs. When it is decreased, there must be some obstruction to the flow of blood into the lungs.

The hilar vessels should be noted on the right and left side. The left hilum is more difficult to assess because of the overlying pulmonary trunk. The pulmonary arteries branch like a tree, producing a definite vascular pattern. The assessment of minor changes in pulmonary vascularity is difficult and it may only be possible to say that the vascularity is *not* increased or *not* decreased — comments which nevertheless are helpful in diagnosis when used in conjunction with clinical findings and electrocardiograms.

Bronchial arteries

The bronchial arteries frequently enlarge in congenital heart lesions, particularly when there is a diminished flow to the lungs by the normal route through the pulmonary artery. These vessels, however, do not show the free, tree-like

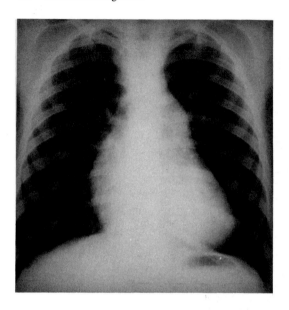

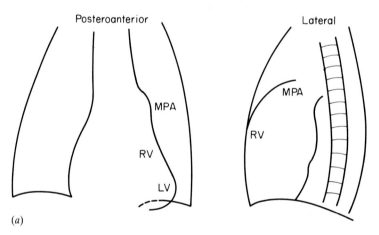

(a)

Figure 4.3 Radiological signs of ventricular enlargement, with line drawings in posteroanterior and lateral projections. Ao, aorta; LA, left atrium; LV, left ventricle; MPA, main pulmonary artery; RV, right ventricle; (a) Right ventricular enlargement (severe pulmonary stenosis)

branching of pulmonary arteries and appear as more uniform 'blobs' throughout the lungs. The bronchial supply is sometimes excessive and the lung fields appear well vascularized without a prominent pulmonary artery being seen. We can then infer that there is severe pulmonary stenosis or atresia.

Pulmonary venous congestion

Differentiation of pulmonary venous congestion from increased pulmonary vascularity is important. In the former the lungs have a hazy appearance and the

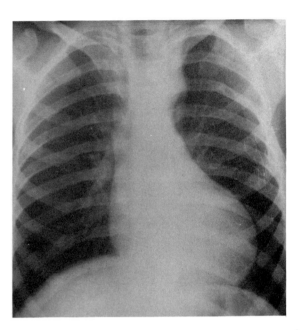

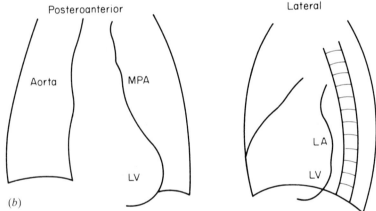

Figure 4.3 (*b*) Left ventricular enlargement (aortic stenosis and coarctation)

shadowing is diffuse, the hilar shadows are prominent but indistinct and smudgy. It is seen in lesions causing obstruction to flow on the left side of the heart. Such obstruction may be at any level from the pulmonary veins to the aorta.

Enlargement of the thymus gland

In infancy a large thymus often makes interpretation of the heart shape difficult. The thymus can assume many guises. There may be a broad pedicle, or a sail-shaped shadow or an apparently large globular heart (Figure 4.4). A lateral view often helps by showing that the shadow is in the upper anterior mediastinum but sometimes it merges with the heart shadow and one cannot be certain that it is the thymus from radiographic evidence alone. The absence of symptoms and signs of congenital heart disease, however, and the normal electrocardiogram support the opinion that the thymus gland is enlarged and repeat radiography some six or twelve months later shows that the shadow has become smaller or disappeared.

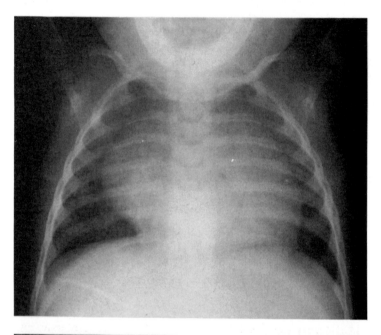

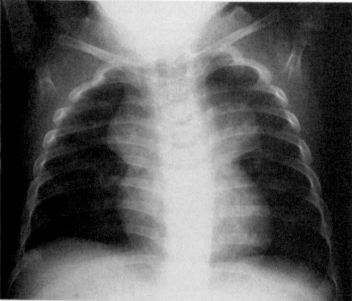

Figure 4.4 Variations in thymic enlargement in infancy

Tracheobronchial anatomy

In suitably penetrated radiographs, the trachea, the right and left main bronchi and their first branches can be seen. The trachea normally enters the chest to the right of the midline, displaced by the left-sided aortic arch. Deviation of the trachea to the left suggests a right-sided aortic arch, and study of the mediastinal shadows on either side of the translucency of the trachea often allows the conclusion that the paratracheal shadow on one side is too narrow to provide room for the aorta, which is then, by implication on the opposite side.

Study of the bronchial anatomy provides valuable clues to the atrial situs in patients with complex abnormalities, particularly those with abnormal situs (see Chapter 12), since the atrial situs almost invariably follows the situs of the lungs (liver and stomach positions are less reliable). The normal right lung has a more vertical main bronchus than the left and the distance from the carina to its first (eparterial) bronchus is shorter. It is usually possible, by comparing the two sides, to determine which side has the anatomically right lung, and the right atrium can then be expected to be on that side. In some instances, when the situs is ambiguous, both lungs have similar anatomy. This is most commonly that of the normal right lung and is seen in association with midline liver and absent spleen. Bilateral 'left' lungs are extremely rare. There are tables of respective angles and lengths to the first bronchial division which allow absolute recognition of bronchial anatomy.

Abdominal viscera

The upper part of the abdomen is visible on the chest radiograph and the observer should note the position of the stomach and liver. The gas bubble of the stomach is usually clearly visible on the left side and the liver edge is seen running obliquely upwards and to the left. In dextrocardia the stomach may be on the right side, and in cases associated with cyanosis and asplenia the horizontal border of a midline liver may be noted.

Skeletal structures

The vertebrae and ribs should be examined carefully. Rib notching may be seen in children with coarctation and, rarely, from enlarged collateral pulmonary ateries in pulmonary atresia. Slipper vertebrae and hemivertebrae are sometimes seen as associated congenital abnormalities.

Fluoroscopy

Fluoroscopy is rarely used now in the diagnosis of congenital heart disease. The increased radiation involved and the marginal help it gives make it unjustifiable, except occasionally in identifying paracardiac shadows such as pericardial cysts or pericardial effusions.

Barium swallow

Occasionally, a barium swallow is used to confirm left atrial enlargement and to show the presence of coarctation of the aorta, aberrant arteries or a vascular ring.

Electrocardiography

Special training and experience are required to produce good electrocardiograms from restless infants and children. In infants it is easier to make the recording when the child is taking a feed or sucking a dummy and they are often happier sitting on their mother's knee than lying on a couch. Technicians need time to win the child's confidence.

Direct-writing machines are the most practical. The paper should be at least 5 cm wide and it is useful to be able to record at 50 mm/s as well as 25 mm/s. Movements are common in infants and deflect the tracing off the paper, so a machine with an automatic self-centring device is valuable.

Electrode positions

The epidermis in infants and children is thin and skin resistances are lower than in adults. It is sufficient to wipe the skin with a dry swab and apply a little jelly before positioning the electrode. The limb electrodes may be placed on the upper arms or thighs rather than wrists and ankles if it is more convenient. In children it is necessary to record further leads from the right chest, V_3R or V_4R, in addition to the usual precordial leads. If they are not recorded, right ventricular hypertrophy and atrial hypertrophy may be missed. The standard and unipolar limb leads are the same as in adults. If the patient has dextrocardia then leads V_6R to V_1 must be recorded.

Recording

Records are made at a paper speed of 25 mm/s and the machine must be standardized so that a current of 1 mV produces a deflection of 10 mm. (Each small square on the paper is 1 mm^2.) If the QRS complexes are tall, the standardization can be halved so that 1 mV produces a deflection of 5 mm and the trace can then be accommodated on the paper.

Interpretation

Electrocardiograms are often bewildering to paediatricians and yet they are of great help in the diagnosis of congenital heart disease. In a few lesions such as tricuspid atresia and endocardial cushion defects they are diagnostic. In conditions such as ventricular septal defects, the electrocardiogram gives useful information about the haemodynamic state, and in lesions like pulmonary stenosis it is valuable in assessing the severity of the lesion and the need for further investigation. The more the electrocardiogram is studied the greater help it may be, but it is proposed here to summarize the findings which will help the paediatrician most in making the diagnosis, assessing its severity and deciding when to refer the patient to a cardiologist. An electrocardiogram should always be performed when the patient is first seen. Changes in the electrocardiogram as the patient grows may be very valuable in making decisions about investigations with a view to surgery or in supporting the impression that the lesion is improving with growth, as may happen sometimes in ventricular septal defect.

Deflections of the electrocardiogram (Figure 4.5)

The P wave

P waves in children and infants are of shorter duration than in adults, and the initial (right atrial) and terminal (left atrial) components are less well separated. The P wave duration in infancy is between 0.04 and 0.07 s and gradually increases with age to between 0.06 and 0.1 s in adolescence. The tallest P waves are usually seen in standard lead 2, V_4R and V_1, and 2.5 mm (0.25 mV) is the upper limit of normal.

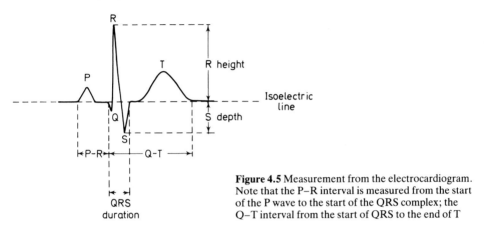

Figure 4.5 Measurement from the electrocardiogram. Note that the P–R interval is measured from the start of the P wave to the start of the QRS complex; the Q–T interval from the start of QRS to the end of T

Atrial hypertrophy

Right atrial hypertrophy produces spiked P waves over 2.5 mm in leads 2 and V_1 or V_4R. In infancy left and right atrial hypertrophy may be difficult to distinguish, but in leads V_4R and V_1 left atrial hypertrophy may produce a large negative component to the P wave (Figure 4.6). Right atrial hypertrophy is seen in severe pulmonary stenosis, pulmonary atresia and tricuspid atresia. Left atrial hypertro-

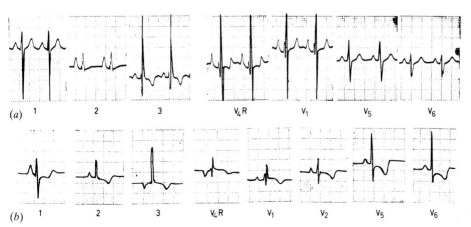

Figure 4.6 (*a*) Right and (*b*) left atrial hypertrophy. Note that the shape of the P wave in leads 1 and 2 is similar in both tracings and also that the deep, wide, negative P wave of left atrial hypertrophy seen in V_4R would have been missed if this lead had been omitted. Tracing (*a*) from a 10-year-old boy with severe Fallot's tetralogy; tracing (*b*) from a 12-year-old girl with congestive cardiomyopathy

phy is seen with mitral valve disease, left ventricular obstruction and primary myocardial disease affecting the left ventricle.

Besides demonstrating left and right atrial hypertrophy, the P waves may show an abnormal pattern, indicating that the atria are being activated by an anomalous pacemaker.

The QRS complex

The duration of the normal QRS complex is between 0.06 and 0.08 s and varies little with actual age within the paediatric span. Prolongation of the QRS duration may be due to ventricular hypertrophy, bundle branch block (or lesser degrees of intraventricular conduction delay), electrolyte abnormalities (high serum potassium), metabolic diseases (hypothyroidism) or drugs (digitalis).

The Q wave is due to depolarization of the interventricular septum (from the left side of the heart to the right). In children, Q waves are normally present in leads 2, 3, aVF, V_5 and V_6. Large Q waves occur in these leads when there is hypertrophy of the septum in left ventricular hypertrophy or biventricular hypertrophy. Q waves in other leads are rare in childhood but may occur with anomalous coronary arteries, hypertrophic obstructive cardiomyopathy and L-transposition of the great arteries. In the latter condition the ventricular septum is depolarized in a direction opposite to normal and Q waves occur in leads V_4R and V_1 instead of V_5 and V_6. The normal Q wave usually measures between 2 and 3 mm, and values greater than 4 mm are abnormal.

R and S waves. The sizes of the R and S waves in the various leads of the electrocardiogram are determined by the thickness of the ventricular wall. Detection of early right or left ventricular hypertrophy is accomplished by recognizing that these voltages lie outside the normal range for the patient's age (Table 4.1). More precise data on percentiles for various QRS measurements based on computer analysis of data are available (Davignon *et al.*, 1980).

Table 4.1 Normal voltages (mm = 0.1 mV) in precordial leads

	V_4R R	V_1		V_5 R	V_6	
		R	S		R	S
Birth	8 (4–12)	12 (5–20)	10 (0–20)	9 (2–20)	5 (1–13)	6 (0–15)
6 months	5 (2–7)	11 (3–17)	10 (1–25)	20 (10–28)	14 (5–25)	3 (0–10)
1 year	4 (0–7)	9 (2–16)	10 (1–12)	20 (5–30)	14 (5–25)	3 (0–7)
10 years	2.5 (0–6)	5 (1–12)	10 (1–25)	20 (5–40)	16 (5–30)	2 (0–5)

Figures in parentheses indicate the normal range.

QRS axis

The electrical axis of the heart is the direction of the maximum electrical force during depolarization. Its approximate value can be derived from the QRS complexes in two or more leads. The usual method is to employ leads 1 and 2, but an easier method uses lead 1 and aVF (Figure 4.7). The normal QRS axis at birth

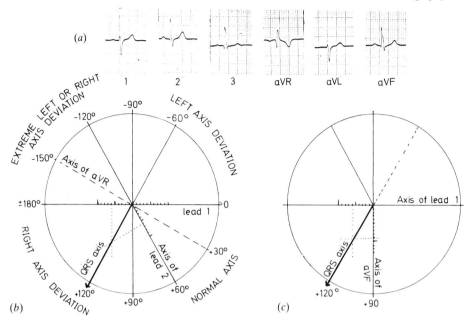

Figure 4.7 Calculation of the QRS axis (in the frontal plane), (*b*) Using leads 1 and 2. Measure the height of R in lead 1 (2 mm) and subtract the depth of S (8 mm). Plot the answer (−6) along the axis of lead 1, which is horizontal (0 degrees) in arbitrary units. In lead 2, R−S=9−3=+6 which is plotted on the axis of lead 2, which is at 60 degrees. Drop perpendiculars from these axes and the line from the origin through the intersection is the electrical axis. (*c*) The same calculation, using aVF instead of lead 2. This has the advantage that it is at right-angles to lead 1, but the result of R−S (10−3=7) has to be multiplied by a factor, 1.3, to allow for the fact that aVF is an augmented unipolar lead and not, like lead 1, a bipolar lead. (A rough method is to look for a lead where R and S are nearly equal, in this case aVR. The axis will be at right-angles to the axis of that lead, and it will be clear from examining one other lead in which direction it points)

averages +135 degrees (+60 to +180 degrees) and changes gradually to +60 (+10 to +100 degrees) at 1 year and more slowly to +65 (+30 to +90 degrees) at 10 years. Right axis deviation is usually due to right ventricular hypertrophy, but left axis deviation is usually not due to left ventricular hypertrophy but to some intereference with the conduction tissue in the left ventricle (as in ventricular septal defects or atrioventricular canal defects). The reason for the paradox is that whereas the free wall of the right ventricle lies to the right of the left ventricle, the free wall of the left ventricle lies posteriorly. Left axis deviation is a feature of endocardial cushion defects and of tricuspid atresia.

Unless otherwise specified the electrical axis is that in the frontal plane, and is derived from the standard or unipolar leads. Using the chest leads (usually V_2 and V_5) it is possible similarly to calculate the horizontal plane axis. Usually the transition zone between right and left ventricles, where there are equal R and S waves, is at lead V_3. Clockwise rotation is indicated by an S wave greater than R in V_4 and anticlockwise rotation by an R wave greater than S in V_2. Clockwise rotation is caused by enlargement of the right atrium or right ventricle. Anticlockwise rotation is seldom seen alone, and, if it is, usually represents a change in overall position of the heart (as in collapse of the right lower lobe, or left pneumothorax).

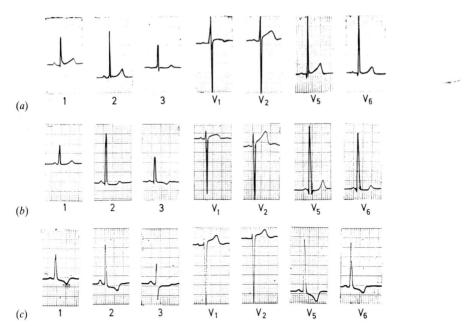

Figure 4.8 Left ventricular hypertrophy. (*a*) Mild. (*b*) Moderate. (*c*) Severe. All three tracings are from patients with aortic stenosis

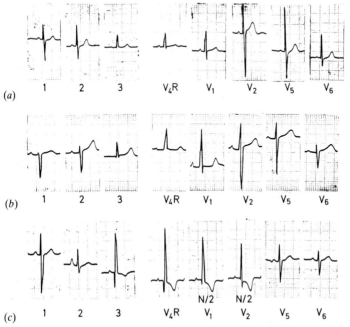

Figure 4.9 Right ventricular hypertrophy. (*a*) Mild. (*b*) Moderate. (*c*) Severe. All three tracings are from patients with pulmonary stenosis of different degrees

Criteria of left ventricular hypertrophy (LVH) (Figure 4.8)

1. Tall R waves in V_5 and V_6 and deep S waves in V_1. Figures for individual leads outside normal limits for age, or the sum of S in V_1 and R in V_5 or V_6 (whichever is the larger) of more than 40 mm (over 1 year) or more than 30 mm under 1 year (mild LVH). (When the main bulk of the left ventricle lies posteriorly, deep S waves are seen in V_1 but V_5 and V_6 do not show large R waves. When the left ventricle lies more anteriorly and to the left, R in V_5 and V_6 is tall, but S in V_1 not so deep. The use of the sum of S in V_1 and R in V_5 or V_6 to some extent overcomes the effect of variations in position.)
2. Any of the criteria in (1) plus either prolongation of QRS duration beyond normal limits for age, or flattening of T waves in V_5 and V_6 (moderate LVH).
3. Criteria of (1) and (2) plus T wave inversion in V_5 and V_6 (severe LVH). Left bundle branch block may also occur with severe left ventricular hypertrophy, but this is rare in childhood.

Left ventricular hypertrophy occurs in aortic stenosis and aortic regurgitation, coarctation of the aorta, moderate sized ventricular septal defect, patent ductus and mitral regurgitation. It is also seen in systemic hypertension, and in both congestive and obstructive cardiomyopathy.

Criteria of right ventricular hypertrophy (RVH) (Figure 4.9)

1. Frontal plane QRS axis to right of normal limits for age *or* R waves in V_4R or V_1 greater than normal *or* (over the age of 12 months) R wave greater than S in V_1.
2. S in V_6 greater than normal for age (15 mm in first week, 10 mm from 1 to 24 weeks, 7 mm from 6 to 12 months, 5 mm above 1 year).
3. Large R waves in V_4R or V_1 plus prolongation of QRS duration (moderate RVH), usually with reduced R waves in V_5 or V_6.
4. Upright T waves in V_4R and V_1 after the age of 3 days, with R wave greater than S in V_1 (moderate RVH).
5. Tall R waves in V_4R and V_1 widening of QRS beyond 0.09 s and deep T wave inversion in V_4R and V_1 (severe RVH). In severe right ventricular hypertrophy the right ventricle frequently extends as far as V_5 or V_6. T wave inversion in these leads does not therefore indicate associated left ventricular hypertrophy.

In addition to these criteria, right ventricular hypertrophy may simulate right bundle branch block. The distinction is difficult without resource to vectorcardiography. Pre-excitation (Wolff–Parkinson–White syndrome) may simulate right ventricular hypertrophy.

Right ventricular hypertrophy occurs in pulmonary stenosis and pulmonary hypertension, in Fallot's tetralogy and in transposition of the great arteries.

Biventricular hypertrophy (Figure 4.10)

Moderate or severe hypertrophy of one ventricle usually results in an apparent diminution of the electrical activity of the other ventricle. For this reason coexisting hypertrophy of both ventricles is difficult to diagnose. The following criteria are the most helpful.

1. Tall R waves and deep S waves in leads V_3 and V_4 (total R+S over 50 mm at any age).

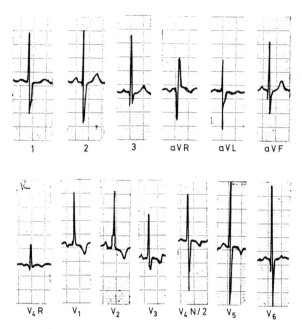

Figure 4.10 Biventricular hypertrophy. The R wave in V_1 is 18 mm, indicating right ventricular hypertrophy, but R in V_6 is 25 mm, which is just within normal limits. In V_4 (which is recorded at half normal sensitivity) RS measures 70 mm, indicating that there is biventricular hypertrophy. The q wave in V_6 is 5 mm, which is also suggestive. From a 3-year-old girl with a large ventricular septal defect and hyperdynamic pulmonary hypertension

2. Left ventricular hypertrophy plus a wide or bifid R wave in V_4R or V_1 over 8 mm in height.
3. Right ventricular hypertrophy plus T wave inversion in V_{5-6} (T upright in V_{1-2}) or q waves 3 mm or more in V_{5-6}.
4. Criteria for right ventricular hypertrophy and left ventricular hypertrophy satisfied.

Suggestive features are also deep q waves in leads V_5 and V_6 (due to septal hypertrophy) and the presence of moderate or marked hypertrophy of one ventricle together with normal activity of the other.

Q–T
The Q–T interval is measured from the earliest portion of the QRS complex to the end of the T wave. It is affected both by heart rate and by age, being longest in older children with slow rates. The normal range is from 0.2 s at birth to 0.4 s in adolescence.

An increased Q–T interval is seen in myocarditis, hypothyroidism, hypothermia and hypocalcaemia; a short Q–T in hypokalaemia.

A long Q–T interval may be familial and sometimes associated with deafness (Lange–Nielsen syndrome). Sudden death may occur due to ventricular arrhythmias (pages 286–287).

T waves

The normal T wave should measure about one-quarter to one-third of the magnitude of the R wave in leads with predominant R waves. After the first 3 days of life the T wave is inverted in V_4R and V_1 and usually inverted in V_2 and V_3 in early childhood. The age at which the T waves become upright in V_2 and V_3 varies from 5 to 15 years, and usually the T waves go through a biphasic or 'dimpled' pattern, rather than becoming flat, in the intermediate period. Inverted T waves are also seen normally in aVR and, when the heart is in a vertical position, in aVL. When the heart is horizontally inclined, T is also inverted in lead 3. Inverted T waves in other leads may be due to ventricular hypertrophy, myocardial disease, pericarditis and severe hypothyroidism. Flat T waves are seen in myocarditis and hypothyroidism. Abnormally tall T waves are seen in hyperkalaemia.

Specific electrocardiographic diagnosis

A few electrocardiographic patterns are suggestive of certain lesions:

Prolongation of P–R interval is seen in Ebstein's anomaly and atrioventricular septal defects. Complete atrioventricular block may occur as an isolated abnormality and is seen in corrected transposition, some forms of primitive ventricle and occasionally following surgery for atrioventricular septal defects, tetralogy of Fallot and transposition (Mustard operation).

Right bundle branch block pattern suggests atrial septal defect or Ebstein's anomaly. It is also seen following ventriculotomy for repair of tetralogy of Fallot or ventricular septal defect.

Left axis deviation between 0 and −90 degrees suggests atrioventricular septal defect, or in a cyanosed child tricuspid atresia. Extreme left axis deviation (−90 to −180 degrees) suggests complete atrioventricular septal defect or double outlet right ventricle.

Right atrial hypertrophy and the absence of the usual right ventricular dominance in cyanotic lesions suggests a hypoplastic right ventricle. If the axis is between 0 and +90 degrees pulmonary atresia with intact interventricular septum is likely; if between 0 and −90 degrees, tricuspid atresia.

Absence of right ventricular hypertrophy in a cyanosed patient with signs of pulmonary hypertension (who otherwise appears to have the Eisenmenger syndrome) suggests a primitive ventricle of left ventricular type, rather than a large ventricular septal defect.

Presence of q waves in anterior precordial leads (V_1 and V_4R) suggests either right atrial enlargement or corrected transposition.

Deep T wave inversion in left ventricular leads (V_{5-6}) in a heart with no murmur suggests primary myocardial disease (cardiomyopathy or endocardial fibroelastosis). Deep Q waves in the absence of ventricular hypertrophy suggest hypertrophic cardiomyopathy or anomalous coronary artery.

Echocardiography

Introduction

The study of the heart by ultrasound or echocardiography, first introduced in 1952 and gradually refined and added to, has become the most important diagnostic investigation in paediatric cardiology. The technique is painless and safe and can therefore be repeated as often as required to follow changes in a child's cardiac condition and to monitor the effects of medical and surgical treatment.

The aim of an echocardiographic study is to determine the anatomy of the heart, including identifying all chambers and valves and their connections, assessing the function of each component, detecting abnormal features such as septal defects, to look at the normal flow through valves and to detect abnormal flow such as valvar regurgitation or left-to-right shunts. An experienced echocardiographer with a quiet patient can check on the normal parts of the heart in just a few minutes and then concentrate on the abnormalities suspected clinically or shown by this quick check.

Three different methods of study are employed, usually with apparatus contained in a single machine. These are termed cross-sectional (or two-dimensional) echocardiography, M-mode and Doppler. Other methods or modifications are sometimes used in specific instances.

Cross-sectional echocardiography

Cross-sectional studies provide a two-dimensional picture of the heart. A transducer placed over the heart has either a single crystal which is caused to rotate in an arc or a phased array of crystals which point in slightly different angles and are activated in sequence to build up a picture of the structures which lie under the skin. These pictures can be viewed as they are produced, recorded on a videotape or 'frozen' as single pictures for photography. Many different cross-sections can be taken using different positions and angulations of the transducer. It is important to carry out a series of views in a logical way to avoid missing details of anatomy.

Subcostal four-chamber view (Figure 4.11(a))
With the transducer directed more backwards than upwards, this gives an excellent four-chamber view, including the interatrial septum. The inlet portion of the interventricular septum is well seen so that this is the best view for atrioventricular defects and some ventricular septal defects. By angulating the transducer more upwards than backwards the aortic valve and subaortic ventricular septal defects can be seen.

Long-axis parasternal view (Figure 4.11(b, c))
The transducer is placed in the fourth left intercostal space as close as possible to the sternum and pointing along a line from the apex to the aortic area. This gives a view of the left ventricle, interventricular septum, mitral and aortic valves and left atrium, and is used for studying mitral and aortic valves, left ventricular hypertrophy and function and sites of entry of pulmonary veins into the left atrium. Ventricular septal defects and over-riding of the aorta can also be seen in this plane.

Short-axis parasternal view (Figure 4.11(d))
The transducer is placed in the fourth left intercostal space, as for the long-axis view, but rotated through 90 degrees. This normally shows the aortic valve in cross section (as a circle), and the right ventricle wrapped round it anteriorly with the tricuspid valve inferiorly and the pulmonary valve and pulmonary artery superiorly. The right atrium, interatrial septum and part of the left atrium are seen behind the aortic valve. This view is used particularly for studying the right heart, and the structure of the aortic valve. It is often possible to see the bifurcation of the pulmonary artery and the region of the ductus arteriosus, but a similar view one intercostal space higher often shows these structures better.

Apical four-chamber view (Figure 4.11(e))
For this view the patient needs to be turned to the left to bring the apex of the heart nearer the chest wall, and the transducer is placed over the cardiac apex (usually in the fourth or fifth left interspace just inside the anterior axillary line). This shows the apices of the two ventricles, mitral and tricuspid valves and the two atria. By a slight change in angulation, the aortic valve can also be brought into view.

Suprasternal view (Figure 4.11(f))
The patient lies flat with the neck somewhat extended and the transducer is placed in the suprasternal notch, angled caudally. With the line of imaging backwards and slightly to the left the aortic arch is shown. With a more sagittal plane the superior vena cava and the two brachiocephalic (innominate) veins are shown.

Although these are the main views, the operator will change the positions and angulations according to what is seen. For this and other reasons, the best person to understand the results is the operator (or those actually viewing the ultrasound pictures as they are produced) and his or her technique will be adapted to solve the particular problem. Thus, most echocardiographic examinations are carried out by the paediatric cardiologist or by a technician with a specialized knowledge of paediatric cardiology.

M-mode echocardiography

This was the first form of echocardiography to be applied to the heart, since the equipment is somewhat simpler than for cross-sectional echocardiography. The 'M' stands for motion, and the technique allows the motion of different parts of the heart to be studied. In practice nowadays the same transducer is used as for cross-sectional echocardiography, but the transducer element remains stationary, or in a phased array only one crystal is used. This produces echoes from a narrow (typically about one square centimetre or less) core of tissue below the transducer, and these echoes are displayed as a series of continuous lines representing the movements of the parts of the heart during the cardiac cycle. An electrocardiogram is displayed simultaneously to help identify the parts of the cardiac cycle. By altering the position and angulation of the transducer, different parts of the heart can be studied (Figure 4.12). The technique is particularly useful for studying valve movement and left ventricular function. Normal patterns of the different valves are known and the presence and degree of, for example, mitral valve obstruction can be estimated.

Contrast echocardiography

Cross-sectional and M-mode echocardiograms normally show up the cardiac structures, but the blood in the heart does not produce echoes. However, the blood can be made echogenic for a short period by injecting saline (preferably shaken briefly to produce microbubbles) or radiographic contrast medium into a peripheral vein. In this way the passage of blood through the right heart can be demonstrated and right-to-left shunting detected. The blood containing the microbubbles shows a 'snow-storm' effect, which can be imaged by either cross-sectional or M-mode methods. Since it involves setting up an intravenous cannula the technique is not strictly non-invasive as other echocardiographic methods, and is not widely used.

Figure 4.11 Cross-sectional echocardiography. Normal views. AA, aortic arch; AO, aorta; AV, aortic valve; DA, descending aorta; IA, innominate artery; LA, left atrium; LCC, left common carotid artery; LPA, left pulmonary artery; LSA, left subclavian artery; LV, left ventricle; MPA, main pulmonary artery; MV, mitral valve; PM, papillary muscle; RA, right atrium; RPA, right pulmonary artery; RV, right ventricle; TV, tricuspid valve

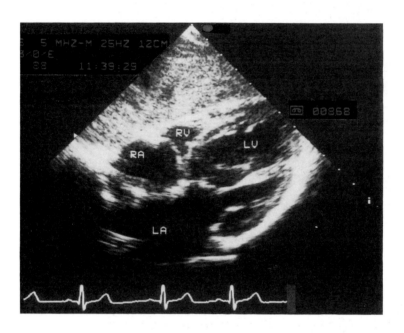

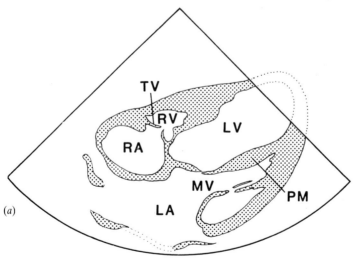

Figure 4.11 (*a*) Subcostal four-chamber view

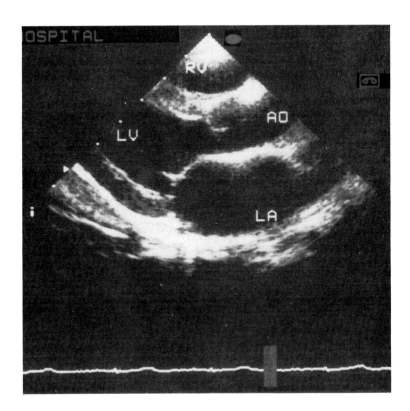

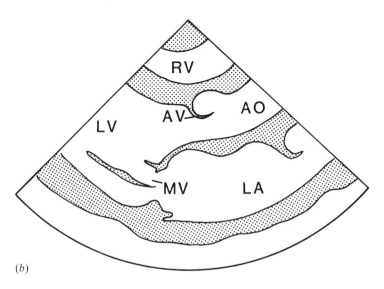

(b)

Figure 4.11 (b) Parasternal long-axis view in end-systole

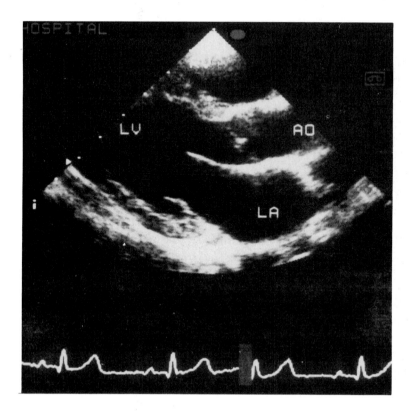

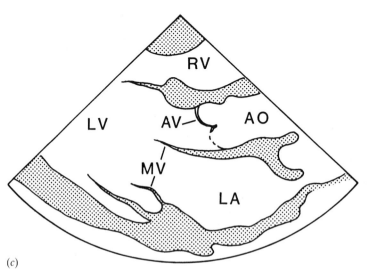

(c)

Figure 4.11 (c) Parasternal long-axis view in diastole

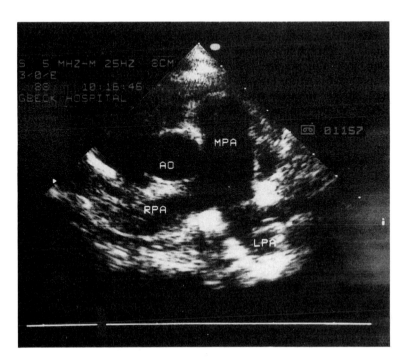

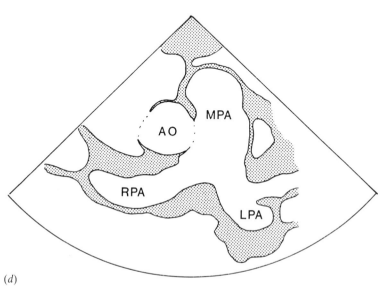

(*d*)

Figure 4.11 (*d*) Parasternal short-axis view (angulated to show main pulmonary artery and branches)

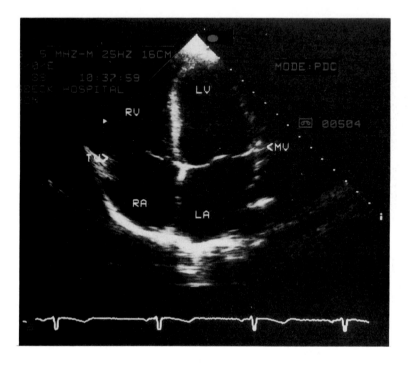

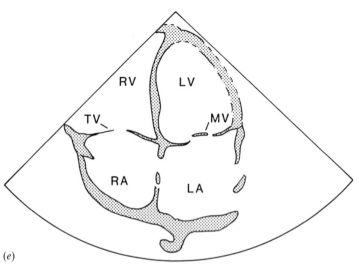

(e)

Figure 4.11 (e) Apical four-chamber view

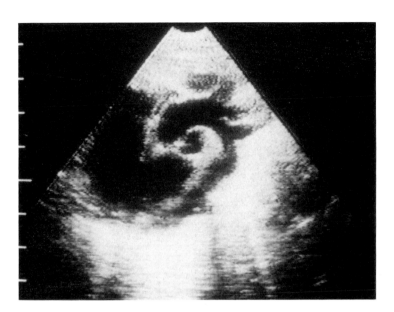

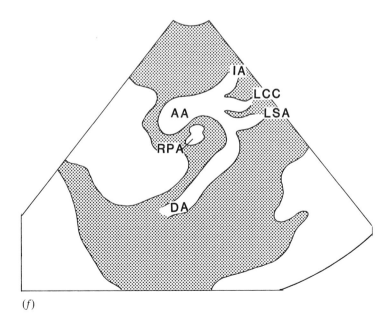

(f)

Figure 4.11 (f) Normal aortic arch from suprasternal notch

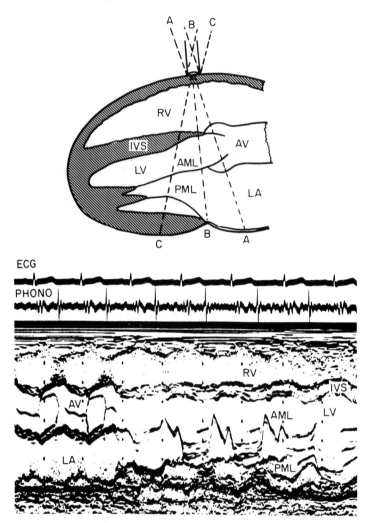

Figure 4.12 M-mode scan. As the transducer is angled from position A through B to C the corresponding parts of the heart are displayed. AML, anterior mitral valve leaflet; AV, aortic valve; IVS, interventricular septum; LA, left atrium; LV, left ventricle; PML, posterior mitral valve leaflet; RV, right ventricle

Doppler echocardiography

The principle described by Doppler was that moving objects altered the frequency (or wavelength) of sound waves which they reflected. In echocardiography this was first used to detect movement of blood and, more recently, to measure flow rates, since the amount of alteration of the reflected frequency is proportional to the velocity. Coupled with another important physical principle this has also allowed calculation of flow gradients across valves, since blood must flow with a greater velocity through a narrow orifice than an obstructed one. The simple formula used is:

$$\text{gradient} = (\text{maximum velocity})^2 \times 4$$

Although a machine recording only Doppler flow signals can be used, one which combines Doppler and cross-sectional methods is most useful as this allows accurate localization of the Doppler path.

Two methods of transmitting and receiving the Doppler pulse are used.

Continuous-wave Doppler uses two transducers mounted side-by-side, one for transmitting and one for receiving a continuous signal. The signal path is indicated by a line on the cross-sectional image and the operator can vary its position. This will demonstrate the velocities of flow at all parts of the signal path, and these are displayed as a 'spectral' record. Generally it is the maximum velocity that is required, e.g. through the pulmonary valve, and this technique allows very high velocities, up to 5 m/s (the typical velocity through a severely stenotic aortic or pulmonary valve, equivalent to a gradient of 100 mmHg, from the above formula).

Pulsed-wave Doppler allows the operator to select not only the direction but also the depth at which the velocity is measured. It does this by looking at each pulse of ultrasound individually and analysing the signal according to the time at which it gets back to the transducer, since signals reflected from deeper structures will arrive back at the transducer later than those from structures nearer the transducer. In practice the signal is 'gated' so that only signals reflected from a predetermined depth are analysed. The operator sees on the cross-sectional image a line indicating the direction and a cross or other marker showing the depth which is being investigated (Figure 4.13). This allows very accurate localization of flow, e.g. through a ventricular septal defect, but for technical reasons high-velocity signals are difficult to display and therefore measurement of large gradients is better carried out with the continuous-wave technique.

Colour-coded Doppler flow imaging

A recent sophistication allows both conventional cross-sectional echoes and Doppler flow patterns to be simultaneously shown, the anatomical picture in black and white and the flow in different colours, e.g. blue indicating flow away from the transducer and orange towards it (see Plates 1 and 2, between pages 54 and 55). The technique is valuable for demonstrating abnormal flow, such as valvular regurgitation or through a ventricular septal defect, but is less useful for making actual measurements of flow. The fact that flow is shown as and where it occurs has led to it being called the 'ultrasound angiogram' as the appearances are comparable to those of cine-angiography.

Areas of turbulent flow within the heart are immediately shown, and then the area under question can be studied by continuous-wave Doppler to allow actual measurements of flow velocity. Jets of flow in unusual directions, such as from muscular ventricular septal defects, can more readily be visualized, and this allows the angle between the jet direction to be estimated and the appropriate correction to be made to the calculated velocity.

In congenital heart disease the technique has proved useful in detecting partial and complete anomalous venous drainage, in showing the shunting in atrioventricular septal defects and in detecting flow through the ductus arteriosus or Blalock shunts.

In the operating theatre the transducer (inside a suitable sterile sheath) can be placed on the heart following surgery to check for residual problems such as additional ventricular septal defects, and an intra-oesophageal transducer is also available which can, in particular, show the left atrium and left ventricle better than

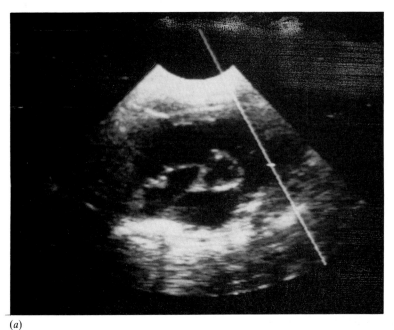

(a)

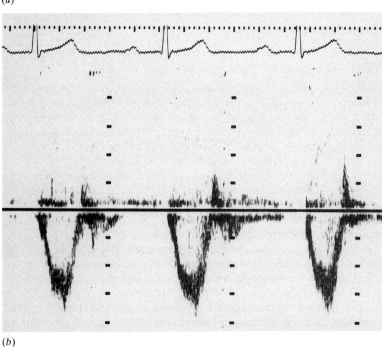

(b)

Figure 4.13 Recording flow by pulsed Doppler technique. (a) Positioning of direction of sampling beam (long line) and sampling depth (short marker) in the pulmonary artery. (b) Flow recorded at that point. The systolic signal is below the base line, indicating flow away from the transducer and has an 'open' appearance indicating laminar non-turbulent flow. The marks are at 0.2 m/s intervals so that maximum flow is about 0.7 m/s

in other views. Its main use is in showing mitral regurgitation, particularly that around prosthetic valves, so that it is more commonly used in adults.

Overall, the main advantage of colour-coded Doppler flow imaging is the speed with which normal and abnormal patterns of flow can be shown. Its main limitation is that the information is qualitative, so that it needs to be combined with conventional pulsed or continuous-wave measurements to allow estimation of flow velocities and gradients.

Fetal echocardiography (see pages 7, 8 and 345)

Interpretation

Most ultrasound machines now incorporate sophisticated electronics which will carry out measurements and calculations of the images automatically. Most echocardiographers, however, like to record the basic data in addition and, like any investigation, the results must be regarded as only a part of the assessment of an individual patient, rather than diagnostic in their own right.

To sum up, echocardiography and Doppler echocardiography can now be used to:

1. Make an anatomical diagnosis of a lesion;
2. Assess myocardial function;
3. Measure valve gradients;
4. Measure blood flows and shunts;
5. Monitor the function of prosthetic valves;
6. Monitor surgical results;
7. Make serial studies during the patient's life;
8. Diagnose pericardial effusion;
9. Show vegetations associated with endocarditis.

The increasing amount of information from echocardiography has resulted in a brisk fall in the number of cardiac catheterizations performed. A complete study with Doppler calculations is time-consuming and needs cooperation by the patient. It may take from 20 to 40 min and sedation is required in some small children. Chloral hydrate in a dose of 50–100 mg/kg is usually adequate.

Magnetic resonance imaging

The newest type of imaging to be applied to cardiology is magnetic resonance imaging. This technique depends on the fact that strong magnetic fields affect protons in any substance, causing them to align themselves along the lines of magnetic force. Both when the force is applied and when it is switched off the movements of the protons generate electromagnetic waves which can be detected at a distance as electrical currents and these currents are then computer processed to produce pictures which reflect the proton density. Water, which occurs in all body tissues, is the most abundant source of protons, but all tissues contain hydrogen and produce different density patterns. In addition, and most valuable from the cardiac imaging standpoint, moving blood produces different images from static tissues and this allows indication of both direction and velocity of flow (Figure 4.14).

The possibilities of this new technique are still only being explored, but it is now possible to obtain gated pictures showing clearly the walls of the heart and blood vessels allowing pictures of complex anomalies to be produced. This is particularly

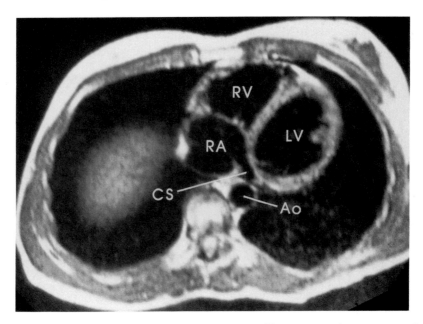

Figure 4.14 (*a*) Magnetic resonance image showing normal heart structure in transverse section. Ao, aorta; CS, coronary sinus; LV, left ventricle; RA, right atrium; RV, right ventricle

valuable in older children and adults where ultrasound and angiographic imaging are less easy than in small children, and to show blood vessel patterns in the lungs, where ultrasound is not possible. The detection of flow is now a standard technique, but its use in measuring flow and gradients has still to be evaluated.

Cardiac catheterization

Once the ultimate in cardiac diagnosis, cardiac catheterization is now required in only a minority of patients with heart problems. This is mainly due to the refinement in echocardiography, but also to a better understanding of physical signs, radiographs and electrocardiograms. Anatomical diagnosis of intracardiac anatomy can usually be made at least as reliably by cross-sectional echocardiography, and Doppler echocardiography provides evidence of flow and gradients. However, intracardiac pressures and flows cannot be estimated as accurately with echocardiography as with direct measurement and some parts of the circulation, in particular the intrapulmonary vessels, are not accessible to echocardiographic imaging.

In general cardiac catheterization will be advised in the following situations:

1. When there is an intracardiac communication diagnosed clinically or by echocardiography and there is reason to believe that there is pulmonary hypertension. Since operability depends, amongst other things, on the level of pulmonary vascular resistance, this needs to be measured by cardiac catheterization.

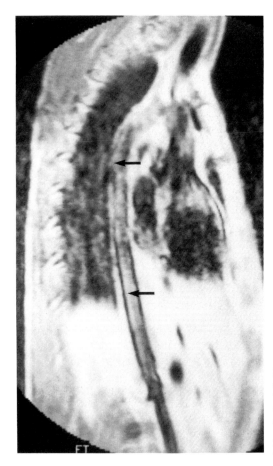

Figure 4.14 (*b*) Magnetic resonance image showing flow in aorta (sagittal section). In the first part of the descending aorta flow is mildly turbulent (upper arrow). In the abdominal aorta it is laminar (lower arrow)

Figures 4.14 (*a*) (*b*) by courtesy of Bristol MRI trustees

2. Where echocardiography has shown multiple ventricular septal defects or a defect in the muscular septum, since angiography is better at demonstrating multiple defects.
3. Where the anatomy of the intrapulmonary arteries requires definition, as in pulmonary atresia without demonstrable central pulmonary arteries, or in peripheral pulmonary artery stenosis.
4. Where small vessel anatomy needs to be studied, e.g. coronary artery anomalies, or the anastomotic vessels in coarctation.
5. When, for technical reasons, it has been impossible to obtain adequate information by echocardiography. This does not include lack of patient cooperation, since it is better to sedate the child and repeat the echocardiogram.

Preparation

As much preliminary information as possible should be obtained, particularly by echocardiography. This not only reduces the time of the procedure, but also the amount of contrast medium required for angiography. (Excessive use of contrast medium, particularly those high in sodium, is an important cause of post-catheter morbidity.) The procedure is explained to the parents and to older patients. The small element of risk must be explained together with the reasons for requiring the catheter, emphasizing that the risks of treating the patient without adequate diagnostic information will be considerably greater than those of the actual test. Although simple procedures on fit children can be carried out on a day-patient basis, very few cardiac catheters fall into this category. In practice, the majority are carried out on sick infants who are already in-patients. In well children there is no need to perform any blood tests, but a chest radiograph and electrocardiogram will be performed unless these have been done recently as part of outpatient evaluation. Patients taking diuretics need to have electrolytes checked and digoxin is stopped 24 hours before catheterization to prevent the possibility of the digoxin making the heart more likely to arrhythmias.

Sedation and anaesthesia

Sedation or light general anaesthesia will be required for all children up to the age of about 14 years. For older children (over 1 year of age) about half the UK centres use pre-anaesthetic sedation followed by light general anaesthesia. The others use preoperative sedation which is topped-up, if required, by intravenous diazepam. However, it is generally unsatisfactory for the operator to have to control the sedation and observe for respiratory obstruction or apnoea. In infants (under 1 year of age) most centres now use light general anaesthesia with intubation and controlled ventilation. Anaesthesia also has the advantage that increased inspired oxygen can be used to avoid hypoxia, which not only is hazardous to the child but also has a marked effect on pulmonary vascular resistance (hyperoxia has very much less effect). Whichever method is used, as well as preventing the child being awake and upset, it is important that the condition remains stable throughout, since much of the investigation involves comparing pressures and saturations sequentially in different parts of the heart, and this cannot be achieved if the child's conscious state varies or if there are periods of hypoventilation and hypoxia.

Techniques

Most catheter investigations start with the insertion of a venous catheter into the femoral vein, using a percutaneous technique. The femoral vein, which lies immediately medial to the femoral artery pulse, is found using a suitable gauge needle; a flexible guide wire is inserted into the vein, the needle withdrawn and a dilator and sheath inserted into the vein. Finally, the guide wire and dilator are withdrawn and the catheter itself inserted into the sheath. Occasionally, for example when the inferior vena cava does not drain directly into the right atrium, the operator may elect to insert catheters into an arm vein or into the subclavian vein, percutaneously. In a small infant it may be difficult to find the femoral vein (especially when the femoral pulse cannot be felt) and a cut-down in the groin is used to expose and cannulate the long saphenous vein. The catheter can usually then be passed through the right heart into the pulmonary artery and its branches. If it is advanced right out into the peripheral pulmonary arteries as far as possible it will usually be found that the recorded pressure drops and alters its waveform to that of the left atrium. This 'wedged' pressure is frequently used instead of the left atrial pressure if the left atrium cannot be catheterized directly.

In infants it is often possible to enter the left side of the heart through the foramen ovale, or through a ventricular septal defect. If this is not possible, catheterization of the femoral artery is carried out in the same way as for the femoral vein, and catheters passed back into the aorta, left ventricle and usually the left atrium. Particularly in infants catheterization of the femoral artery leads to spasm and the pulse may be lost after the catheter is withdrawn. This does not lead to any immediate problems, but the leg may grow slightly less than the unaffected leg, which is clearly undesirable. For this reason arterial catheterization should only be carried out in small children when absolutely necessary. An alternative way into the left heart, suitable for children from about 3 years upwards is to use a special kit to puncture the interatrial septum from the venous route and advance a catheter into the left atrium and left ventricle (Brockenbrough technique).

Although clinical examination and echocardiography will have demonstrated where in the heart the problem lies, it is advisable to make a routine of pressure measurement and samples from every chamber entered. This not only allows the occasional additional lesion to be detected, but increases the amount of haemodynamic information and calculation that can be made.

Catheterization consists of a number of separate investigations. First, the passage of the catheter may indicate an abnormal communication or connection, as when a patent ductus arteriosus is crossed. Next it allows measurements of pressures within the heart and great vessels to be measured, and the taking of blood samples (normally about 0.1 ml each) enables the saturation of the blood to be determined. Since all the blood on the left side of the heart is 96–98% saturated, any reduction over the route pulmonary vein to left atrium to left ventricle to aorta indicates a right-to-left shunt. (It is clearly important to check that pulmonary vein blood is fully saturated, i.e. that the patient is not hypoxic due to respiratory disease or hypoventilation.) On the right side the saturation may be from 65 to 85%, but should normally be similar in right atrium, right ventricle, pulmonary artery and its main branches. (The superior vena cava blood is usually more highly saturated than that in the right atrium; inferior vena cava blood varies in its saturation according to whether sampling is from the renal vein stream (about 90% saturated), lower limbs (65–80%) or hepatic veins (40–50%).)

Angiocardiography

One of the main purposes of cardiac catheterization is to allow angiography to be performed, that is the injection of radio-opaque contrast medium into the heart. Its passage is then recorded on cine film, usually with two cameras running simultaneously showing two different views of the heart in two different planes. A different type of catheter which will allow rapid injection of contrast medium through a number of side holes is usually substituted for this part of the procedure. Earlier contrast media were highly hypertonic and contained a lot of sodium in ionized form, and this frequently led to aggravation of heart failure and even asystole. Newer media are less toxic, but can cause deterioration, especially in infants, so that the number of times an injection can be made is limited, usually to two or three separate injections. A pump injector is used and can be programmed to deliver the contrast medium at planned volume and speed. (Too fast an injection at high pressure causes arrhythmias and can perforate the heart; too slow an injection does not produce good enough contrast for adequate imaging.)

Digital subtraction angiography

Pictures obtained at angiography can be converted into digital information, and this allows the electronic manipulation of data. For example, a picture of the chest can be obtained before any contrast is injected and this picture is electronically stored and subtracted from pictures in which there is contrast inside the heart to eliminate unwanted images from ribs and vertebrae. An image in which contrast has reached the left atrium can be subtracted from a later one so that only the left ventricular part of the image is shown. In addition, measurements of contrast-filled chambers can be made and automatic calculation of ventricular size and ejection fraction made. Until recently the rather slow times for acquiring the data made the system more suitable for studying relatively immobile structures such as the aorta, but larger memories and more rapid acquisition now make study of all parts of the heart possible. Reduction in both contrast medium and radiographic exposure can be made, which are clearly beneficial to the child.

Risks and complications

The overall risk of death or permanent complications is small, about 5 per 1000 for infants and 2 per 1000 for older children. The main complications are:

1. Arrhythmias. Atrial and ventricular extrasystoles are always produced, when the inside of the heart is touched by the catheter tip. Atrial flutter and fibrillation may occur, particularly if the atria are stretched by increased pressure. They usually revert spontaneously to sinus rhythm but occasionally require a DC shock to restore sinus rhythm. Ventricular fibrillation is rare, but a defibrillator is always kept next to the catheter table and defibrillation can be carried out within 10 to 15 s, so that external cardiac compression is not usually required. Transient atrioventricular nodal block is common due to the catheter compressing the atrioventricular node or surrounding tissues. Nodal rhythm then supervenes which is usually at a safe rate. Normal conduction occurs within a few minutes of withdrawing the catheter from the heart. Asystole or extreme bradycardia may occur when there is poor cardiac output for any reason and may be precipitated by injection of contrast medium. It requires external cardiac compression, injection of isoprenaline or adrenaline and correction of any hypoxia or metabolic acidosis.

2. Cardiac perforation may occur through the atrial appendages or the outflow of the right ventricle. Provided it is recognized and the catheter withdrawn, no serious harm is produced but the patient must be carefully observed for the next 24 hours with serial echocardiograms to check for continuing bleeding into the pericardium.

3. Intramural injection of contrast medium may occur, particularly if high pressure injection through small catheters is used. In conscious patients this causes chest pain and in all patients there is elevation of the ST segments on the electrocardiogram. The dye is absorbed over the next few hours, but there is usually some bruising of the wall and sometimes temporary impairment of contractility.

4. Systemic embolism of air or clot is possible but can be avoided by scrupulous technique. However, permanent neurological damage is possible, although rare.

5. Pyrexia is common following the procedure, but actual infection is rare. (Most investigators do not cover the procedure with antibiotics as practice has shown a negligible incidence in infective endocartitis.) Blood culture should be taken if the

pyrexia persists for more than 4 hours and antibiotics given if the patient's condition warrants them.

6. Necrotizing enterocolitis is a real risk in neonates, particularly those with poor blood supply to the gut (coarctation or a generally low cardiac output). Contrast medium entering the descending aorta in high concentrations seems to be the precipitating factor and this should be avoided in susceptible infants.

Calculations

The measurements made allow further calculations to be made. To measure cardiac output (or in cases with intracardiac shunting, systemic and pulmonary blood flow) it is necessary to know the oxygen uptake from the lungs, which is assumed to be the same as the oxygen utilization by the body. Actual measurement is quite tedious and it is usual to estimate oxygen uptake from tables, relating it to the body surface area.

$$\text{Pulmonary blood flow} = \frac{\text{Pulmonary oxygen uptake}}{(\text{Pulmonary venous oxygen content} - \text{pulmonary artery oxygen content})}$$

$$\text{Systemic blood flow} = \frac{\text{Systemic oxygen uptake}}{(\text{Systemic arterial oxygen content} - \text{systemic venous oxygen content})}$$

It is useful to express the pulmonary blood flow as a ratio of the systemic flow (pulmonary to systemic flow ratio, P:S). In the normal heart the ratio is clearly 1:1.

In patients with a left-to-right shunt the ratio is greater than one, from 1.3:1 in a small ventricular septal defect to 6:1 in a large defect.

With right-to-left shunts the ratio will be less than 1, but roughly the same information can be conveyed by simply quoting the arterial oxygen saturation. However, in complex lesions with both total mixing and reduced pulmonary flow it may be useful to express the ratio as, for example, 0.7:1.

It is also useful to calculate the resistances in the pulmonary and systemic circuits (pulmonary vascular resistance, PVR, and systemic vascular resistance, SVR). It is possible to express these in scientific units but conventionally the figures used are obtained with the blood flow measured in litres per minute and the pressures in mmHg as suggested by Paul Wood and are called 'Wood units' or just 'units'.

$$\text{Pulmonary vascular resistance} = \frac{(\text{Pulmonary artery pressure} - \text{left atrial pressure})}{\text{Pulmonary blood flow}}$$

$$\text{Systemic vascular resistance} = \frac{(\text{Aortic pressure} - \text{right atrial pressure})}{\text{Systemic blood flow}}$$

The pulmonary to systemic vascular resistance can also be calculated. This is normally low, reflecting the low pulmonary resistance, typically 0.1 or lower.

Whilst the normal ratios of blood flow and resistance are similar in babies and older children the actual figures for flow and resistance vary according to size. To allow comparisons between children of different sizes or in the same child at different ages, it is usual to relate the absolute figures to body size, a process sometimes called indexing. The flows are divided by the body surface area and the resistances multipled by body surface area. (A small baby has a lower blood flow but higher vascular resistance.) A typical set of calculations would then be:

(Body surface area 0.5 m^2)
Pulmonary blood flow = 5.5 l/min = 11.0 l/min/m^2.
Systemic blood flow = 2.5 l/min = 5.0 l/min/m^2.
Pulmonary : systemic flow ratio 2.2:1
Pulmonary vascular resistance = 4.8 units = 2.4 units. m^2.
Systemic vascular resistance = 28 units = 14 units. m^2.
Pulmonary : systemic resistance ratio 0.17:1

(Note that after indexing the flow units are 'litres per minute per square metre' while the resistance units are described as 'units times square metre' or, as that is a little unwieldy, as units indexed.)

Interpretation

The information obtained by cardiac catheterization is only one of the factors considered in deciding on treatment of a child with cardiac disease. Although there are some 'rules of thumb', such as advising closure of ventricular septal defects with a pulmonary to systemic flow ratio greater than 2:1, the information needs to be studied in conjunction with the child's clinical condition, radiographs and echocardiograms. Detailed study of results and angiograms may show discrepancies which require further evaluation by further echocardiograms or echoes. Most units use the time immediately following the cardiac catheterization as a convenient time for discussions between cardiologists and cardiac surgeons to plan treatment.

Interventional cardiology

In 1966 Rashkind and Miller first introduced balloon atrial septostomy for early palliation in transposition of the great arteries. Since then large diameter polyethylene balloons have been constructed which are able to withstand high pressures and are yet small enough for percutaneous insertion. They maintain their size and shape at high inflation pressures and in the event of a rupture they tear longitudinally so that there is no difficulty in extracting them. These catheters are now being used to dilate stenotic valves, to relieve coarctation and re-coarctation of the aorta and to dilate obstructed caval pathways which may result from the Mustard operation. Attempts are also being made to dilate stenosed pulmonary arteries and veins. It is interesting to reflect that while the cardiac catheterization laboratory is less used for diagnostic purposes, it is now required for therapeutic purposes.

Atrial septostomy is safe and effective in the early palliation of transposition of the great arteries until 1 month of age but after that the tearing of the septum becomes increasingly difficult and inadequate. A 'blade septectomy' is therefore advised to cut the septum.

Balloon dilatation or valvuloplasty is now the treatment of choice in isolated pulmonary valve stenosis (see Chapter 8). The valve is often thin and pliable and obstruction is caused by the fusion of the valve cusps which can be torn by the

Plate 1 Colour-coded Doppler echocardiography in the normal heart. In all views flow of blood towards the transducer, which is upward, in orange and flow away, downward, is in blue. In the accompanying diagrams upward flow is shown by open arrows, corresponding to orange in the plates, and downwards flow, corresponding to blue in the plates, by closed arrows. Ao, aorta; LA, left atrium; LV, left ventricle; MPA, main pulmonary artery; RA, right atrium; RV, right ventricle

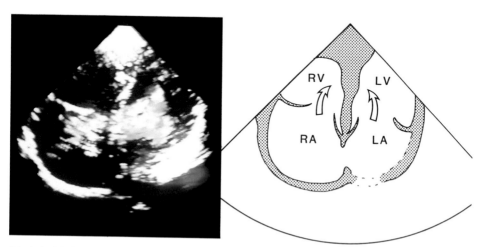

(*a*) Apical 4-chamber view in diastole showing flow through tricuspid and mitral valves

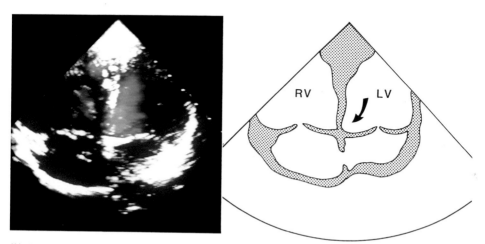

(*b*) Apical 4-chamber view in systole showing flow towards the aortic valve

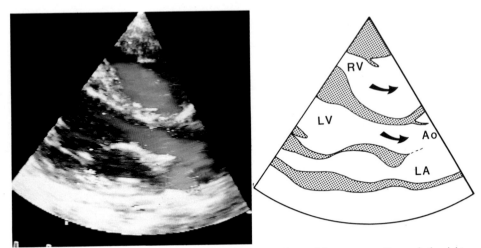

(c) Parasternal long-axis view in systole showing flow from left ventricle to aorta and towards the right ventricular outflow

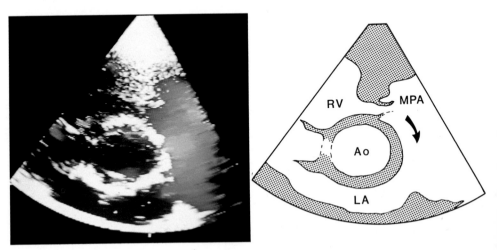

(d) Short-axis view in systole showing flow in the main pulmonary artery

Plate 2 Demonstration of ventricular septal defects (labelling as in Plate 1)

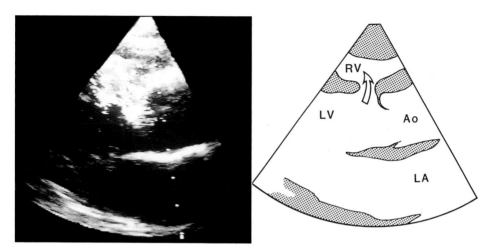

(*a*) Perimembranous defect

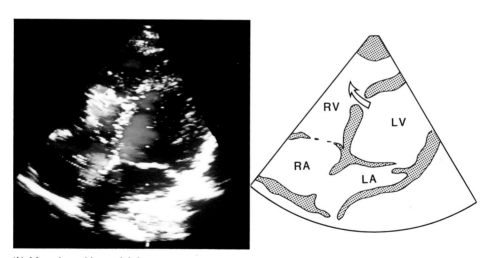

(*b*) Muscular, mid-septal defect

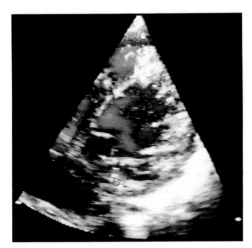 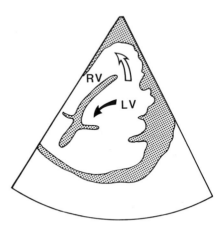

(c) Apical muscular defect

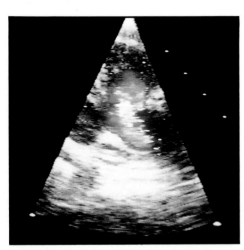 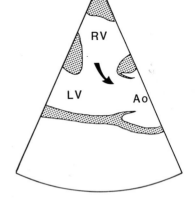

(d) Defect in tetralogy of Fallot showing right-to-left flow

inflated balloon. Pulmonary regurgitation is rare following the procedure but if it does occur it does not give rise to any problems in the low-pressure pulmonary circuit (see page 141).

Dilatation of a stenosed aortic valve is more difficult and the morbidity greater because the balloon catheter has to be introduced through an artery. If significant aortic regurgitation occurs it causes problems in the high-pressure systemic circulation. Furthermore, there is much more variation in the deformity of aortic valves than pulmonary ones (see page 109).

Dilatation of a re-coarctation which has followed an operation for coarctation is often effective and well worth trying. Dilatation of an untreated coarctation has been successful in children over 1 year of age but there is always the risk of aneurysm formation. The results in the newborn infants have not been successful so far.

Obstruction of the superior and inferior caval pathways may follow the Mustard operation for transposition of the great arteries. Re-operation carries a significant risk and it is always worthwhile trying to dilate the vein with a balloon catheter.

There are encouraging results of dilatation of stenosed branches of the pulmonary arteries which may occur as an isolated abnormality or may occur at the site of a previous Blalock–Taussig shunt.

A closed mitral valvotomy in rheumatic heart disease can be achieved using a balloon catheter passed through the atrial septum.

Therapeutic embolization is being tried for blocking unwanted aortopulmonary collateral vessels in pulmonary atresia and for blocking pulmonary arteriovenous malformations and coronary fistulae.

Detachable devices are being used in some centres to close patent ductus and atrial septal defects. The overall failure rate and complications of such devices, however, are in the region of 25%, so the procedure is not yet generally applied.

Myocardial biopsy

In some circumstances it is important to obtain information about the state of the myocardium. Echocardiography and angiocardiography can tell the cardiologist about the overall function, but the cause of impaired function remains uncertain. Examination of sections of myocardium by light and electron microscopy can be supplemented by staining for specific substances, such as glycogen, and for a range of enzymes. In some conditions the studies have become extremely specialized but once a biopsy has been obtained it can be sent to a laboratory specializing in myocardial disorders for an opinion.

The biopsy specimen is usually obtained by passing a bioptome by one or other venous route into the heart and using the small jaws on the end to remove a specimen from the right ventricular side of the interatrial septum. (The thickness of the septum makes it unlikely that any damage will be done, but care has to be taken to avoid removing the specimen from the free wall and producing perforation.) Cardiologists using the technique regularly pass the bioptome through a sheath placed percutaneously into the internal jugular vein, since this gives the most direct passage into the right ventricle. Those doing only an occasional biopsy usually opt for the more familiar approach from the femoral vein and use a curved sheath to direct the instrument into the right ventricle. It is assumed that any changes in the myocardium will be generalized, but if there is reason to believe that the left ventricle is more involved in a disease than the right it is possible to pass the bioptome into the left ventricle using trans-septal catheterization with a long sheath.

The procedure is used now for checking for evidence or rejection in transplanted hearts, to look for evidence of specific biochemical disorders, and in 'primary' myocardial disease (cardiomyopathy and endocardial fibroelastosis) to see whether there is active myocarditis which might benefit from steroid treatment.

The procedure has a small risk of perforation and ventricular arrhythmias and should only be used when there is a real likelihood that the findings will allow some form of effective treatment.

Bibliography

Bull, C. (1986) Interventional catheterisation in infants and children. *British Heart Journal*, **56**, 197–200

Cassels, D. E. and Ziegler, R. F. (eds) (1966) *Electrocardiography in Infants and Children*. Grune and Stratton, New York

Cohn, H. E., Freed, M. D., Hellenbrand, W. F., *et al.* (1985) Complications and mortality associated with cardiac catheterisation in infants under one year: a prospective study. *Pediatric Cardiology*, **6**, 123–31

Davignon, A., Rautaharju, P., Boisselle, E., *et al.* (1980) Normal ECG standards for infants and children. *Pediatric Cardiology*, **1**, 123

Goldberg, S. J. (1984) A review of pediatric Doppler echocardiography. *American Journal of Diseases in Children*, **138**, 1003–9

Grenadier, E., Oliveira, C., Allen, H. D., *et al.* (1984) Normal intracardiac and great vessel Doppler flow velocities in infants and children. *Journal of the American College of Cardiologists* **4**, 343–50

Liebman, J. (1968) In *Heart Disease in Infants, Children and Adolescents*, (eds Moss, A. J. and Adams, F. H.), Williams and Wilkins, Baltimore, p. 183

Leung, M. P., Mok, C. K., Lau, K. C., *et al.* (1986) The role of cross-sectional echocardiography and pulsed Doppler ultrasound in the management of neonates in whom congenital heart disease is suspected. *British Heart Journal*, **56**, 73–82

Rao, P. S. (1987) Transcatheter management of heart disease in infants and children. *Pediatric Review Communications*, **1**, 1–18

Scott, O. and Franklin, D. (1963) The electrocardiogram in the normal infant. *British Heart Journal*, **25**, 441

Wilson, N., Goldberg, S. J., Dickinson, D. F., *et al.* (1985) Normal intracardiac and great artery blood flow measurements by pulsed Doppler echocardiography. *British Heart Journal*, **53**, 451–8

Chapter 5

Cardiac surgery

About 60% of all children with congenital heart disease will require some form of surgery and it is therefore appropriate to consider some of the principles involved.

Two principles are paramount. The surgery should provide clear long-term benefit to the child which more than balances the risks of the procedure and it should be carried out at the time when the risk, related to benefit, is lowest. Sometimes parents press for early operation even when aware that the risks are greater and occasionally may demand surgery when little benefit is likely to result. In conditions such as transposition of the great arteries, where the natural history is very poor and the results of surgery generally very good, there is little doubt about the advice which should be given, but in a young child with a small ventricular septal defect it may be better to wait and see whether the defect closes or becomes tiny, especially as echocardiography now allows localization of the site of the defect and a better idea of those which are likely to close.

In general, the earlier the defect is corrected the quicker will heart size and function return to normal. Closure of an atrial septal defect in adult life seldom results in a normal sized heart, and a very hypertrophied ventricle of severe pulmonary or aortic stenosis may have irreversible fibrosis. Delay in operating on coarctation of the aorta can result in persistently raised blood pressure and the need to take treatment throughout life. This has, however, sometimes to be weighed against the rather higher mortality of open heart surgery under the age of a year, and the fact that any prosthetic conduits or valves will not grow as the child grows.

Types of operation

Operations are usually classed as corrective or palliative, although the distinction is often blurred. Some paediatricians prefer to define an intermediate class of 'extended palliation' to include treatment which, although not strictly corrective, is designed to provide life-long relief of symptoms. In addition, some corrective operations still require long-term restrictions or precautions, such as those to lessen the risk of infective endocarditis, or can give rise to late complications such as arrhythmias.

Palliative operations

These are used either in infants deemed too small for corrective surgery or in children with conditions not amenable to corrective surgery.

Systemic to pulmonary artery shunts

These are designed to increase pulmonary blood flow in conditions in which there is diminished flow and thereby reduce cyanosis. They may also be used to encourage growth of pulmonary arteries considered too small for corrective surgery.

1. *Classical Blalock–Taussig shunt* (Figure 5.1(a)) in which the subclavian artery is trans-sected and anastomosed to the corresponding pulmonary artery.
2. *Modified Blalock–Taussig shunt* (Figure 5.1(b)) where the subclavian artery is left intact and a Gore-Tex tube inserted between it and the pulmonary artery. This allows a larger anastomosis, but, since its length does not increase with growth, it may lead to tenting and obstruction of the pulmonary artery. The inside becomes lined with an endothelium which is only loosely attached to the wall and may 'peel' off causing obstruction, particularly if attempts are made to pass catheters into it.
3. *Central shunts* (Figure 5.1(c)) of Gore-Tex from the aorta to the main pulmonary artery or its right or left branches.

Other arterial shunts, between the ascending aorta and right pulmonary artery (Waterston shunt) or between the descending aorta and left pulmonary artery (Potts) have been used in the past but have now been abandoned because of complications.

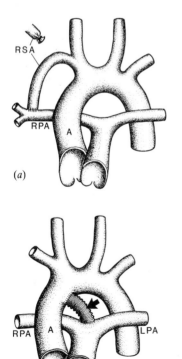

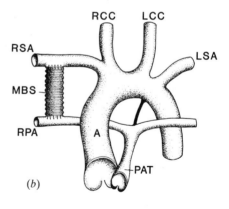

Figure 5.1 (*a*) Blalock–Taussig shunt. (*b*) Modified Blalock–Taussig shunt. (*c*) Central shunt. A, aorta; LCC, left common carotid artery; LSA, left subclavian artery; MBS, modified Blalock shunt; MPA, main pulmonary artery; PAT, pulmonary artery trunk; RCC, right common carotid artery; RPA, right pulmonary artery; RSA, right subclavian artery

Banding of the pulmonary artery

Infants with complex abnormalities associated with high pulmonary blood flow and pulmonary artery pressures at or near systemic levels may be helped by restricting the blood flow through the lungs. This is achieved by 'banding', that is tying a piece of tape around the pulmonary artery, tight enough to reduce the pressure beyond to approximately half that proximally (Figure 5.2). The Toronto group have devised a formula for the size, according to the baby's surface area and this is used as a guide when first positioning the band. Operation notes refer to a band being 1 or 2 mm below or above the Toronto formula.

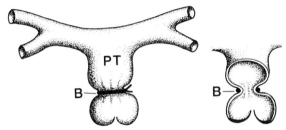

Figure 5.2 Banding (B) of pulmonary trunk (PT)

This procedure was at one time widely used to treat heart failure in infants with large ventricular septal defects, but has now been superseded by early operative closure, except in multiple defects. Its main use, however, is in complex lesions such as primitive ventricle without pulmonary stenosis.

Most palliative operations including shunts and banding of the pulmonary artery are carried out through a lateral thoracotomy. Banding is usually done from the left side while shunts can be done on either side. Following a shunt operation patients (including infants) usually return to the ward breathing spontaneously and require little in the way of supportive therapy. Following banding, because the lungs are usually tense and non-compliant, assisted ventilation is usually required for a few days.

Corrective operations

Corrective operations may be extracardiac, such as for patent ductus and coarctation, or intracardiac, which means using extracorporeal circulation (cardiopulmonary bypass). In the past simple intracardiac operations were done using just surface cooling (for small atrial septal defects which could be closed by a few sutures) or inflow occlusion in which the venae cavae were occluded for up to 90 s to allow the stenosed pulmonary valve to be incised. Nothing particular needs to be said at this stage about closed operations but the principles of cardiopulmonary bypass will be described.

Cardiopulmonary bypass

The technique which is almost universally used for intracardiac operations on infants and children is a combination of two techniques which were developed almost simultaneously to allow the surgeon to arrest the heart for surgical repair.

Total cardiopulmonary bypass drains the blood from the right side of the heart, oxygenates it and pumps it back at a pressure similar to the normal arterial pressure into the aorta (Figure 5.3). Provided that the aortic valve is competent the heart can be emptied of blood and intracardiac repair carried out. However, the beating heart does not provide good operation conditions and the more delicate parts of the repair require the heart to be temporarily arrested by cross-clamping the aorta below the aortic cannula so that ischaemic arrest occurs.

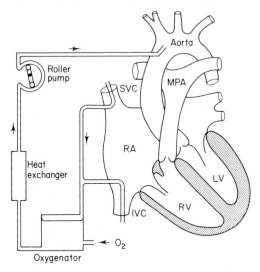

Figure 5.3 Total cardiopulmonary bypass. IVC, inferior vena cava; LV, left ventricle; MPA, main pulmonary artery; RA, right atrium; RV, right ventricle; SVC, superior vena cava

The other part of the currently used technique is to cool the patient's body, including the heart, by means of heat exchangers in the extracorporeal circuit. This enables the actual perfusion to be reduced and, if necessary, stopped for 10–20 min without risk of damage to the heart.

Currently, surgeons use the circuit shown in Figure 5.3, which includes both an oxygenator and a heat exchanger. After the cannulae have been inserted the patient is fully heparinized and the extracorporeal circulation is started up. The patient's blood is cooled over a period of about 30 min, the rest of the patient's body cooling at the same time. When the patient's nasopharyngeal temperature (the nearest measurable point to the brain) is down to about 20°C the aorta is cross-clamped and ice-cold Ringer's solution containing an excess of potassium is perfused via the root of the aorta into the coronary arteries. This cases immediate stopping of the heart and protects the myocardium from the results of ischaemia. The circulation to the rest of the body is continued so that brain damage in particular is avoided. The surgeon can then operate within the heart for 2–3 hours. When the repair is complete the patient is rewarmed back to normal temperatures and the heart takes over the pumping from the heart–lung machine which can then be stopped. Protamine is given to reverse the effects of the heparin and the cannulae removed.

A variation commonly used in infants is to carry out the first part of the initial cooling by applying ice-bags to the trunk and this extended surface cooling enables the temperature to be dropped to about 25°C. It shortens the total period of perfusion and also allows the lungs to continue to be perfused for part of the operation.

Effects of cardiopulmonary bypass

Although the aim of cardiopulmonary bypass is to protect the various organs of the body it is only partially successful. Even using the cold potassium cardioplegia technique described above, the cardiac muscle function is impaired, particularly if the period of arrest is over one hour. Electron microscopy indicates that all enzyme systems are impaired, but particularly the calcium handling inside the cell. This results in both impairment of contraction and, particularly in infants, impairment of relaxation so that high filling pressures are needed in the postoperative period. Some impairment of function may persist for some months, and may occasionally be permanent.

During cardiopulmonary bypass the lungs are not perfused and the production of surfactant rapidly ceases. This results in diminished lung compliance and the need for high ventilator pressures postoperatively. These changes last for up to 2 weeks and in the most severe forms the chest radiograph shows dense, uniform opacification of the lungs ('pump lung'). This is particularly likely in infants whose alveoli are smaller and therefore more reliant on surfactant to keep them open. Recent work with epoprostenol (prostacyclin) suggests that it may have a protective effect and use of this agent may become routine.

During its passage through the heart–lung machine the blood is subjected to a number of physiological insults. Although large amounts of heparin are used to prevent clotting, the platelets adhere to the various parts of the circuit so that by the end of the operation their number and effectiveness are considerably diminished. Infusions of platelets are frequently needed to prevent oozing of blood from operation sites. The red cells, too, become crenated and this reduces their deformability, which is an important factor allowing them to squeeze easily through narrow vessels. This may well be the cause of postoperative impairment in many organs including liver and kidneys. In addition, there may be some breakdown of red cells producing free haemoglobin, which has to be excreted by the kidneys.

During the operation it is usual to give a diuretic, such as frusemide, to encourage diuresis, partly to flush out any free haemoglobin filtered from the blood. When 5% dextrose is used as a diluent to the blood used to prime the extracorporeal circulation this also has a diuretic effect. Provided a good peripheral circulation is maintained the kidneys usually continue to excrete urine, but the control of sodium and potassium excretion is often impaired leading to electrolyte disturbances.

Obvious effects on cerebral function are rare, but detailed psychomotor testing has shown that minor degrees of impairment are common. (Most of the recent work has been on adults but older work showed that children were not immune.) Postoperative studies suggest that children who have had major cardiac surgery may be marginally poorer at learning than comparable children with no cardiac problem, but it is difficult to know what part other factors, such as more time off school or slower motor development, play.

Risks of open-heart surgery

It is still a popular misconception amongst both doctors and parents that cardiopulmonary bypass is in itself a risky procedure. In experienced hands, using the technique regularly, deaths due to the procedure itself are virtually unknown and the true risk for the most straightforward operations, such as closure of an atrial septal defect, is of order of 2 per 1000. The actual risks are more related to the condition itself and the ability of the surgeon to correct the abnormality. The reason why the overall mortality from open-heart surgery remains significant is that more complicated operations are now attempted at an earlier age and not all of them are actually corrective. Last decade's operation with 20% mortality may have become this decade's operation with 5% mortality but surgeons have added a new operation for a previously untreatable condition which currently has a 20% mortality.

Postoperative care

Following most extracardiac operations (for patent ductus, coarctation and shunts) and straightforward intracardiac operations such as closure of atrial or ventricular septal defect, the patient returns to the ward breathing spontaneously and requires little specific postoperative treatment. The exception is operations for banding of the pulmonary artery since these patients have stiff lungs and usually require assisted ventilation for a few days. More complex intracardiac operations such as for transposition of the great arteries require more intensive postoperative care including assisted ventilation and the use of inotropic agents such as dopamine. Even when such patients leave hospital they may need to take diuretics and digoxin for several weeks. The total convalescent period obviously varies according to the severity of the operation from a 7-day stay in hospital and 6 weeks in total off school for an atrial septal defect, to a week in intensive care followed by 2 weeks in hospital and a longer period off school for complex operations.

Antibiotics are given routinely (usually for 48 hours) to cover the perioperative risk of infective endocarditis and all patients require such cover for dental extractions for at least one year after surgery. A synthetic patch to a septal defect warrants two years and insertion of any other material or leaving any potential focus, such as minimal pulmonary stenosis, requires lifelong cover. (In particular this means that all patients who have had repair of tetralogy of Fallot will require such cover.) Prosthetic or tissue valves are particularly prone to troublesome infections and special regimes are necessary, usually a combination of intravenous antibiotics.

Long-term complications outside the cardiovascular system are rare. Cerebral damage has been virtually eliminated. Protracted intubation for ventilatory assistance occasionally leads to tracheal stenosis. Prolonged urinary catheterization, particularly in boys, may lead to urinary infection, phimosis and urethral stricture. Children often become withdrawn during the postoperative period and prolonged stay in an intensive care ward is often associated with psychological problems for months or even years.

Late results and complications of surgery

After successful surgery most children have a rapid period of growth and increased wellbeing; this is most striking in children who have previously had heart failure. Patients who have been cyanosed (tetralogy of Fallot) become pink immediately after surgery but the finger clubbing takes 6–9 months to regress. It is important to remember that when a Blalock–Taussig shunt has been performed the arm pulses on the affected side will be absent or markedly reduced. This does not happen after a Waterston operation. A Horner's syndrome is not uncommon after a shunt operation in small children and resolves after 2–3 months.

Residual murmurs

After closure of patent ductus, ventricular septal defect or atrial septal defect, the heart sounds should be normal and there are no murmurs. In other operations loosely described as 'curative' residual murmurs are common. Following pulmonary valvotomy for pulmonary stenosis, a soft systolic murmur is heard and often an early diastolic murmur of pulmonary incompetence owing to failure of the valve to close completely after it has been cut. Such systolic and diastolic murmurs are often impressive after correction of tetralogy of Fallot when a patch has been used to widen the pulmonary valve ring. Aortic valvotomy is frequently followed by systolic and early diastolic murmurs for the same reasons. It is important to stress that the persistence of murmurs does not mean that the operation has been unsuccessful.

Chest radiograph

The heart size gradually returns to normal after repair of ventricular septal defects, atrial septal defects and closure of patent ductus arteriosus. Where a patch has been inserted, e.g. in the right ventricular outflow tract in repair of tetralogy of Fallot, the heart shadow will appear larger on the radiograph and there will be a bulge on the upper left heart border. Also, after a shunt procedure the heart will increase in size and the lung fields show increased pulmonary blood flow.

Electrocardiogram

This may actually look worse after a right ventriculotomy as there is usually a complete right bundle branch block pattern. This is not associated with any symptoms in childhood. If, however, some of the branches of the left bundle are severed and the distal part of the bundle of His is damaged, the patient also shows left axis deviation on the electrocardiogram, and is at risk of complete heart block when healing and fibrosis occur. Such patients usually have transient complete heart block in the immediate postoperative period. If the heart block recurs a pacemaker is required and the parents must be warned to report any episodes of syncope or dizziness. It is uncommon now for injury to the sinus node to occur following repair of atrial septal defects but the sinus node may be injured during the Mustard operation for transposition of the great arteries. Nodal rhythm may result and this may become very slow and periods of sinus arrest occur. Sudden death may follow if a pacemaker is not inserted. Ambulatory electrocardiographic monitoring will help in showing periods of marked slowing or sinus arrest.

Ventricular extrasystoles and ventricular tachycardia may occur postoperatively when there has been severe left or right ventricular hypertrophy preoperatively, or when either ventricle has been incised, particularly if there have been multiple operations. Ventricular tachycardia always needs treatment, occasional ventricular extrasystoles can be ignored, but multifocal ones, or those occurring in runs of two or more, should be treated as indicated in Chapter 18. This complication might be avoided by earlier operation and surgical techniques designed to minimize trauma to ventricular muscle, such as closing venticular septal defects from the right atrium.

Infective endocarditis

This is possible following pulmonary or aortic valvotomy, repair of tetralogy of Fallot and most complex operations, but does not occur following successful repair of ventricular septal defect, atrial septal defect or patent ductus. The need to prevent this complication is one of the best reasons for long-term follow-up in patients with susceptible lesions.

Late deterioration

Patients who have had complex operations, particularly those in whom conduits or valves have been inserted, may show gradual or sudden deterioration. Shrinkage of the intracardiac patch following Mustard's operation leads to pulmonary oedema, and degeneration of conduits, particularly those with heterograft valves, leads to gradually increasing cardiac failure. Even though it may be inconvenient for patients and parents, it is essential for the cardiac team to follow such patients carefully, and in most cases indefinitely (with echocardiograms and, if necessary, further cardiac catheters). It is not known for how long conduits and prosthetic valves will remain satisfactory and serial studies by echocardiography are valuable in following the patient's progress.

Patients who have had operations involving valve replacement or insertion of conduits early in life will certainly require operations as they outgrow their implanted prostheses. Additionally, artificial valves seem particularly prone to clotting in young children, even when anticoagulants are given, and reoperation may be required urgently.

A particular problem is posed by the teenager who has already had several palliative operations for a severe but correctable abnormality (e.g. pulmonary atresia with ventricular septal defect). When the pericardial and both pleural cavities have been entered with resultant vascular adhesions, the risks of operation may be so high as to outweigh the possible benefits of a corrective operation.

Pre- and postoperative counselling

After the initial discovery that a child has a serious cardiac problem the admission to hospital and the operation itself are among the most stressful events in the parents' lives. Cardiologists, surgeons and nursing staff should be involved in discussions with parents (and with older children), preferably together as this avoids the possibility that the descriptions given by different people of the same planned treatment may appear to conflict. Following operation parents are understandably worried and will seek precise advice with regard to such things as schooling, level of exercise and susceptibility to intercurrent infection. Although parents and teachers may be wary of allowing the child to do 'too much' most children have no inhibitions about enjoying their new-found ability to do more.

Specific advice about precautions to lessen the risks of infective endocarditis should be given to parents and general practitioners also need advice about management and therapy and, in particular, the importance of not giving antibiotics for unexplained fever until infective endocarditis has been excluded.

Valve and conduit insertion

Leaking or severely stenotic valves present the paediatric cardiac surgeon with problems additional to those found in adult patients. First, very small sizes of artificial valves are simply not made, largely because it is technically impossible to obtain an adequate orifice in a valve with very small outside dimensions and also because the small numbers required do not make it economic to set up production. Secondly, the patient is growing and the valve will not grow with him, so that repeated operations would be necessary. A third point is that tissue valves (made from pig or calf periardium) degenerate very much faster in children so that serious dysfunction may be seen as early as a year following insertion. The theoretical objection that anticoagulant therapy, which is required for all mechanical valves, would be difficult in children has not proved to be a major obstacle.

Surgeons will therefore try very hard to treat valve lesions conservatively, even though this may leave a less than perfect result. Limited aortic valvotomy for aortic stenosis and partial repair of cleft mitral valve in atrioventricular septal defects are preferred to valve replacement. Even so, there is an occasional need for valve replacement, particularly when severe mitral or aortic regurgitation results from infective endocarditis. In the mitral position the valve usually employed is the Bjork–Shiley tilting disc prosthesis. In the aortic position some surgeons use homograft valves, which are rather more durable than animal tissue valves, or the Bjork–Shiley or Starr Edwards prostheses (Antunes, 1984; Schaff et al., 1984; Schahner et al., 1984). Anticoagulants are required for prosthetic valves and parents and medical attendants must be made aware that the control is affected by a wide range of drugs, including antibiotics. In addition, particular care must be taken to avoid infective endocarditis, and this involves intravenous antibiotics for dental extractions or similar procedures likely to produce a bacteraemia.

Artificial conduits may be used from the right ventricle to the pulmonary artery in a number of conditions in which there is pulmonary valve atresia or discontinuity between right ventricle and pulmonary artery as in complex forms of transposition. These may either be simple tubes of synthetic material (unvalved conduits) or may contain a valve, either in the form of the aortic homograft or a prosthetic or tissue valve sewn into the conduit. When a homograft is used, calcification occurs in the tube and base of the valve, but the cusps themselves are usually spared and continue to function. Synthetic conduits become lined with a 'peel' which may become detached or corrugated and cause obstruction. Prosthetic valves frequently become obstructed by clot or pannus and are best avoided (Meldrum-Hanna et al., 1986). Anticoagulants do not modify any of these degenerative processes and are not used. Patients with such conduits require careful follow-up with Doppler or catheter estimation of the degree of obstruction (Reeder et al., 1984), and replacement of the conduit when this becomes haemodynamically important. (Virtually all conduits produce a loud systolic murmur so that the presence of such a murmur is no guide to the development of stenosis.) Such conduits are also susceptible to infective endocarditis and the same precautions are required as for artificial valves.

Cardiac and cardiopulmonary transplantation

These operations, which currently offer a 50% chance of 3-year survival, should be regarded as palliative although, unlike other forms of palliation, they are unlikely to be followed by other, longer-term operations. In addition to the usual ethical problems of advising treatment with only a limited expectation for prolongation of survival, they entail further problems, both organizational and emotional.

Some centres practising cardiopulmonary or cardiac bypass do not consider it justifiable to operate on newborn babies with rapidly lethal conditions such as hypoplastic left heart syndrome, on the grounds that it is not ethically justifiable to prolong the life of a baby for a few years only to produce greater grief for the parents when he or she does finally die. Others feel that the wish of the parents to have life prolonged, if even for a few years should be respected. In addition, there is always the hope that new forms of immunosuppression will appear which will allow indefinite survival after transplantation.

One problem which affects the availability of transplants in children, even more than in adults, is the supply of donors. Infants and very small children are unlikely to be subjected to severe head injury leaving them with no cerebral or midbrain function and there is even greater reluctance on the part of parents to allow organs to be used for transplant. In cardiac transplants there is some leeway with regard to donor organ size, but in cardiopulmonary transplants the donor and recipient's chest sizes must match to within 10%, which imposes a very tight restriction on suitability.

In theory, any child who has an inoperable cardiac condition which has a short life expectation or important symptoms is a possible candidate for either cardiac or cardiopulmonary transplantation. In practice only a small number of conditions which are inoperable by conventional means are suitable for cardiac transplantation alone, but more are suitable for cardiopulmonary transplantation, having either severe pulmonary hypertension, as in the Eisenmenger syndrome, or having abnormal pulmonary arteries, as in pulmonary atresia with ventricular septal defect and complex pulmonary blood supply.

Currently, the majority of cardiac transplants in children have been performed for myocardial disorders (cardiomyopathy and endocardial fibroelastosis) or for variants of the hypoplastic left heart syndrome. Cardiopulmonary transplants have been mainly for Eisenmenger syndrome (although few in children), complex lesions such as primitive ventricle complicated by pulmonary hypertension, primary pulmonary hypertension or complex pulmonary atresia, as well as end-stage cystic fibrosis. Patients who have already had operations are likely to have a higher mortality from transplantation, but are sometimes deemed suitable.

Initial selection of patients with anatomically suitable lesions is usually made by paediatric cardiologists and most transplant centres then insist on a period of in-patient evaluation. This is necessary to ensure that patients (if old enough) and parents understand fully the expectations of any proposed operation and also the fairly rigorous programme of pre- and postoperative investigation and treatment which will be necessary.

Once selected as a potential recipient for transplant the child will have to wait for a suitable donor, which generally averages 3–6 months, so that there is effectively no place for emergency transplant operation except on the rare occasions when a patient is actually in the hospital when a donor heart becomes available. Currently matching for ABO compatibility only is used but, particularly for heart–lung transplants, matching for cytomegalovirus is attempted as implanting organs from someone who has had a cytomegalovirus infection (as shown by antibodies) into someone who has not, is likely to give rise to a severe infection in the recipient.

Cardiac transplantation

The heart is removed (in the hospital where the donor has been treated) aseptically through a median sternotomy after cooling the heart with a cardioplegic solution. The aorta and pulmonary artery are clamped and transected and then all but the posterior part of the two atria (including the right atrium around the venae cavae) is removed *en bloc*. The donor heart is packed in ice and transferred as quickly as possible (4 hours is the maximum allowable period). Meanwhile the recipient has been placed on cardiopulmonary bypass in the transplant centre and cooled to below 20°C. The equivalent parts of the recipient's old heart are removed. The atria are sutured into place and then the pulmonary artery and aorta anastomosed and the recipient rewarmed. Postoperatively, artificial ventilation and inotropic support are usually required for about 24 hours.

Cardiopulmonary transplantation

The removal of the donor heart and lungs is carried out in the hospital in which the donor was being treated. Through a median sternotomy the lungs are freed from the pulmonary ligaments and then the circulation arrested by cold cardioplegia solution inserted into the aortic root (some surgeons prefer to cool through cardiopulmonary bypass). The aorta and trachea are transected and the right atrium separated from the venae cavae. The heart and lungs can then be removed in total and packed in ice for transfer to the transplant centre. Under cardiopulmonary bypass and cooling to below 20°C the recipient's heart and lungs are removed in the same way as for the donor organs (but usually removing the heart and lungs separately) and only three sutures are required, around the posterior right atrium, the trachea and the aorta. Immediate postoperative care is similar to that for cardiac transplantation although the donor lungs are usually slower to recover and a longer period of ventilation is usually required. Another complication is that the bronchi are not innervated (the trachea above the anastomosis is) so that spontaneous coughing does not occur unless secretions reach the trachea.

After either operation immunosuppressive therapy is started at once with prednisolone, azathioprine and cyclosporin, and this is usually continued for 3 months and then prednisolone and azathioprine gradually withdrawn. Serial endomyocardial biopsies are carried out for heart transplants every 2 weeks or more frequently if there are signs of rejection. To do this a sheath is inserted percutaneously into the internal jugular vein and a bioptome passed into the right ventricle and three or more specimens removed from the right side of the interventricular septum. In heart–lung transplants the lungs are likely to show evidence of rejection before the heart and therefore transbronchial biopsies are done instead.

The need for repeated biopsies is another reason why transplantation is technically more demanding in young children.

Patients usually spend about 3 weeks on average in hospital following heart transplantation and 4–5 weeks following heart–lung transplant. Particularly in the first year, repeated visits to the transplant centre are necessary for review and biopsy and patients, parents and their medical attendants are issued with guidelines from the transplant centre.

Chapter 6

Acyanotic lesions with left-to-right shunts

Patent ductus arteriosus

Definition

The ductus arteriosus, which *in utero* serves to divert blood from the lungs into the descending aorta, normally closes functionally within 10–15 hours of birth. Closure is brought about by constriction of specialized tissue, confined to the ductus, which is present from 25 weeks of intrauterine life and shows progressive maturation over the next 10–12 weeks (Gittenberger-de-Groot, 1979).

Incidence

In mature infants, persistent patency of the ductus probably results from a primary anatomical defect of this specialized tissue in the ductal wall (Gittenberger-de-Groot, 1977). Such patients account for about 7% of all congenital heart defects. Patency of the ductus in premature infants has increased as smaller babies survive (see page 77). Patency of the ductus arteriosus in association with other lesions such as pulmonary atresia is related to arterial hypoxaemia, and is dealt with under the respective primary lesion.

Natural history

The natural history is related to the size of the ductus and to the changes which occur in the pulmonary circulation after bith. If the ductus does not close during the first two weeks of life, spontaneous closure thereafter is rare, except in premature infants in whom spontaneous closure may occur up to 3 months after birth. Campbell (1968) calculated that, after infancy, only 0.6% of all ducts would close spontaneously every year. By the age of 60 years about 20% will have closed. In Cosh's series (1957) of 69 patients with patent ductus arteriosus, closure occured in 4 at the following ages – 15, 23, 23 and 29 years. The ductus closed in only 1 of the 48 adults reviewed by Mark and Young (1965). The general prognosis for patients with a small ductus is good but a number deteriorate in the third or fourth decades (Campbell, 1955). As with so many congenital heart lesions the most dangerous periods are infancy and then the third and fourth decades. By the age of 45 years about 42% of those untreated patients who survived infancy will have died (Campbell, 1968).

Prostaglandins have been demonstrated in high concentrations in the area of the ductus and can be shown to play a part in maintaining the normal patency prior to delivery (Olley and Coceani, 1979). This discovery has led to the possibility of pharmacological manipulation of the ductus (Olley *et al.*, 1979).

Clinical examination
Symptoms usually occur 3–7 days after birth, but when the respiratory distress syndrome is present these may be obscured. The respiratory rate rises and lower costal and intercostal recession becomes apparent. The liver enlarges and the pulse volume is usually increased. There is a short systolic murmur in the pulmonary area and often a short diastolic murmur in the mitral area, although this is less obvious than in the mature infant. Chest radiographs show generalized enlargement of the heart, and it may be possible to see increased size of pulmonary vessels.

Diagnosis
Since, in a premature infant, patent ductus is the most likely cause of symptoms, it is usually possible to make a presumptive diagnosis on clinical grounds. Cardiac catheterization in a very small baby is generally regarded as too traumatic and unnecessary.

Echocardiography shows enlargement of the left atrium and a value 1.5 times higher than the aortic dimension indicates a large ductus. If necessary Doppler studies can be done to demonstrate the left-to-right shunt through the ductus. Other intracardiac abnormalities can be excluded to make sure there is not a duct-dependant abnormality.

Echocardiography is also useful in monitoring the response to treatment with indomethacin by showing a reduction in size of the left atrium if the ductus is closing.

Treatment
Fluids should be restricted to 150 ml/kg/day and sufficient oxygen given (usually 30% is adequate) to prevent hypoxia which tends to keep the duct open. A $TcPo_2$ of 60–80 mmHg is satisfactory. The haematocrit should be maintained at 0.4–0.45, if necessary by small blood transfusions. Hypoglycaemia and hypocalcaemia must be corrected. Frusemide 1 mg/kg i.m. (once or twice daily) is given to control heart failure. If the heart failure is difficult to control and the baby cannot be weaned off the ventilator, the duct must be closed. There are two choices, medical treatment using indomethacin or surgical closure.

Most neonatalogists try indomethacin first, but contra-indications are: poor urinary output, hyperbilirubinaemia or a bleeding disorder (indomethacin causes alteration in platelet function (Kocsis *et al.*, 1973)). There is still argument about the time to give the drug, the route and the dose. Giving indomethacin as a prophylactic measure before heart failure develops has been tried and although the degree of shunting was less, that was offset by the presence of complications due to indomethacin.

When indomethacin is necessary, the following regime is recommended:
> 0.2 mg/kg body weight intravenously at 12-hourly intervals for a total of three doses.

The second or third dose should not be given if there are complications such as bleeding and further doses should be omitted if the duct has already closed. If the duct remains open after three doses, early surgical closure should be undertaken.

The results of surgery are now excellent, transfer in ventilator-incubators reduces transport risks and it is unwise to delay.

It has become recognized that early closure of the ductus not only saves lives but also leads to a reduction in morbidity. Cotton *et al.* (1978) reported 38 premature infants with patent ductus treated without surgical or pharmacological intervention. Of these, 11 died. Many of the survivors had persistent pulmonary complications attributable to prolonged artificial ventilation, and 5 had retrolental fibroplasia.

The reversed ductus

The term 'reversed ductus' refers to a patent ductus arteriosus associated with severe pulmonary hypertension in which there is a right-to-left shunt through the ductus. This is the Eisenmenger syndrome (Wood, 1958).

There seem to be two groups of cases. In one there is a high pulmonary vascular resistance from birth and, although initially there may be a left-to-right shunt, it is not of sufficient size to cause symptoms: any heart murmur is insignificant (see Figure 6.1) and heart disease usually remains undiagnosed for several years. In the second group there is initially a large left-to-right shunt in infancy and a high pulmonary vascular resistance develops as a secondary phenomenon. Although shunt reversal can occur in childhood, it is rare. If there is already reversal of flow when the child is first seen, it may be difficult to establish on historical grounds whether a significant left-to-right shunt was present in infancy. Cyanosis is usually not obvious and may be missed completely if the toes are not examined and their colour compared with the fingers. The right arm is usually still perfused with fully oxygenated blood coming through the ductus and the legs receive a greater quantity of desaturated blood. This means that when the reversal has been present for some time, there is clubbing of the toes, mild clubbing of the left hand but no clubbing of the right hand.

Left-sided obstructive lesions should always be looked for. If such a lesion is operable, the pulmonary pressure may then fall and the shunt through the ductus becomes left to right and be operable. If there are not such associated lesions, closure of a ductus with a right-to-left shunt is dangerous and not advised.

Other causes of continuous murmurs

Although the signs of a patent ductus arteriosus are usually characteristic and further investigation is not required, there are other lesions which give rise to continuous murmurs and may sometimes cause difficulty in diagnosis. The site of these murmurs is usually different from that of a patent ductus and they lack the characteristic 'systolic rattle' and the crescendo quality in systole so characteristic of a patent ductus.

Venous hum

The venous hum is caused by flow of blood in the large veins in the neck. It varies with the position of the neck, being loudest when the neck is extended. The hum can be abolished or minimized by firm pressure over the jugular veins or by turning the neck. It disappears when the patient lies flat.

Aortopulmonary window

Aortopulmonary window is a fistulous connection between the aorta and pulmonary artery close to their origins. It is usually associated with pulmonary

2. Muscular defects
Inlet defects in the inlet portion of the muscular septum.
Trabecular defects in the trabecular portion of the muscular septum, and these may be multiple (Figure 6.5).
Outlet defects are in the outlet portion of the muscular septum and may be difficult to distinguish from perimembranous outlet defects at echocardiography.

3. Doubly-committed subarterial defects
These are roofed by the conjoint aortic and pulmonary valve rings and the rest of the rim is formed by the muscular outlet septum. (These were previously called supracristal defects.)

Natural history

The natural history of this lesion has proved to be a fascinating one. Bloomfield's retrospective study in 1964 helped to clarify it and the study of this lesion illustrates more than any other that congenital heart disease is not a static condition, changes continuously take place as the child grows, but the most dramatic changes take place in infancy.

The prognosis depends on the size of the defect, its position in the ventricular septum and the physiological changes which take place as a result of blood flowing through the defect. Now that the position of the defect can be defined at echocardiography it would be helpful to know which defects are likely to close. More studies are required over a long period, starting in infancy, but the prospective studies of Sutherland and Godman (1986) give guidance as to which defects are more likely to close than others. Their results were as follows:

Position of defect

1. Perimembranous
Inlet   (64 infants). Only 2 closed but the remainder did tend to become smaller due to tricuspid valve tissue adhering to the margins of the defect and forming a pseudoaneurysm (Figure 6.6). The majority of this type will therefore improve clinically and become smaller as early as the first year of life, even though they do not tend to close completely in childhood. Only 3 cases required surgery in this group.
Outlet   (28 infants). None closed spontaneously and 11 infants required surgery. The 3 cases that improved did so because they had developed infundibular stenosis. There is no tendency for pseudoaneurysm to occur in this group (since they are not related to the tricuspid valve tissue), but a true aneurysm may form as the margins of the defect approximate to one another.
Confluent   (22 infants). Five of these closed spontaneously by pseudoaneurysmal formation but 12 required surgical closure because of their large size. The remaining 5 defects did develop pseudoaneurysms but remained large.

2. Muscular defects
Inlet   (7 infants). None of these was large and they tended to remain unchanged during the 3-year period of study.
Outlet   (13 infants). In 10 cases there was no change in size but 1 closed spontaneously, 1 developed infundibular stenosis and 1 required surgery.

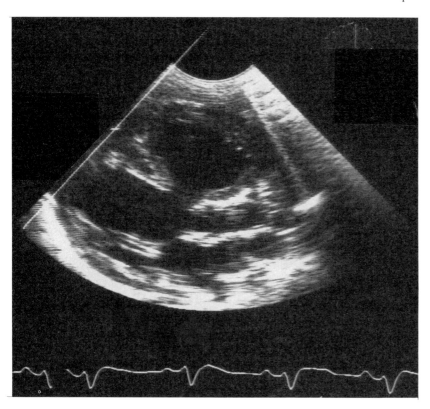

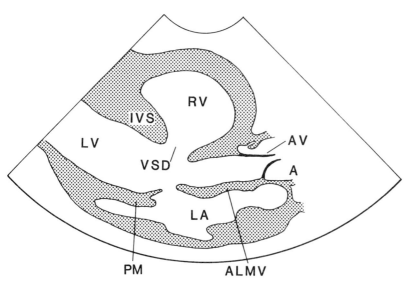

Figure 6.5 Cross-sectional echocardiogram of long-axis view showing large muscular ventricular septal defect. A, aorta; ALMV, anterior leaflet of mitral valve; AV, aortic valve; IVS, interventricular septum; LA, left atrium; LV left ventricle; PM, papillary muscle; RV, right ventricle, VSD, ventricular septal defect

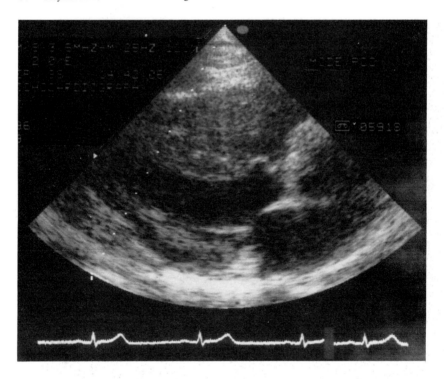

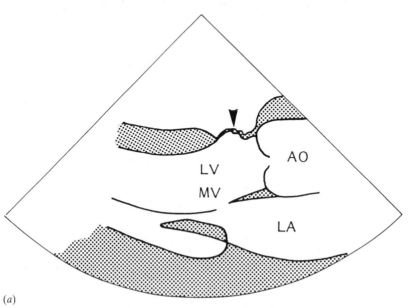

(a)

Figure 6.6 (a) Long-axis view of aneurysm of interventricular septum (arrowed) caused by adherence of tricuspid tissue to a ventricular septal defect. An, aneurysm; AO, aorta; LA, left atrium; LV, left ventricle; MV, mitral valve; PM, papillary muscle; RV, right ventricle; VS, ventricular septum

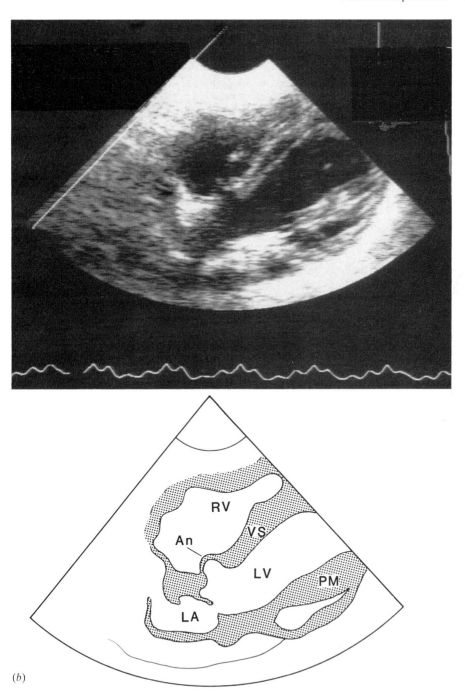

(b)

Figure 6.6 (b) Subcostal view showing ventricular septal defect closing by aneurysmal formation (for key see *Figure 6.6* (a))

Trabecular (19 infants with *large* defects). Ten of these large defects closed spontaneously, 4 required surgery because of intractable heart failure, 5 have become smaller.

(66 infants with *small* defects). Twenty-nine of these closed and the others diminished in size.

All these trabecular defects closed by muscle overgrowth on the right ventricular side.

3. Double-committed defects

Although none was seen in this series, these defects are invariably large and need closure in infancy. Prolapse of the aortic valve leaflet into the defect may reduce the size of the defect but result in important aortic regurgitation.

Physiological changes

Small defects

There are no significant haemodynamic changes within the heart or the pulmonary circulation. Pulmonary hypertension does not occur. Alpert *et al.* (1979) reported that of 50 patients with small defects followed from birth, 75% had closed by 10 years of age, the majority by 2 years.

Large defects

There is a high flow of blood from the left to the right ventricle and this results in equal pressures in the right and left ventricles. Assuming there is no obstruction to flow in the right ventricle, this high systemic pressure is transmited to the pulmonary artery. Several possible changes may occur as the child grows:

1. The defect becomes smaller, the left-to-right shunt diminishes, the pulmonary artery pressure falls and the patient follows a favourable course.
2. The defect goes on to close.
3. Infundibular stenosis develops which limits the left-to-right shunt. The patient improves and will do well in early life until the infundibular stenosis increases and surgery is required.
4. The defect remains large and as a result of the high flow of blood at high pressure into the pulmonary circulation, changes begin to occur in the medium-sized pulmonary arteries. The muscular coat thickens and there is proliferation of the intima. The lumen of these arteries narrows and causes a resistance to flow of blood into the lungs, i.e. an increase in pulmonary vascular resistance. At first this is beneficial because it limits the flow of blood into the lungs, but as the resistance to flow increases further a stage is reached when the changes in the pulmonary arteries become irreversible. If closure of the defect is not carried out before this irreversible state develops then the vascular resistance will go on rising until it is greater than the systemic resistance; a right-to-left shunt occurs, the patient becomes cyanosed and the Eisenmenger complex results. All the evidence available shows that the changes in the lungs are reversible if surgery is carried out before 12 months of age. In Down's syndrome, however, they may be irreversible at an even earlier age (see Chapter 21).

Clinical presentation

This varies with the size of the defect and pulmonary vascular changes, so for clarity the cases are divided into four groups.

Group 1. Small ventricular septal defects
The patients have no symptoms and grow and develop normally. The heart disease is discovered during routine examination. The murmur is not heard at birth but develops over the first few days. The heart is normal in size or very slightly enlarged, there is a pansystolic murmur and thrill maximal in the third and fourth interspaces at the left sternal edge. The second sound is normal. In *tiny* defects there may be no thrill and the systolic murmur is short as the defect closes as systolic contraction occurs and blood ceases to flow through it before the end of systole. Jordan (1985) showed on echocardiography that the majority of patients with early systolic murmurs had a pseudoaneurysm of the membranous septum due to adherence of tricuspid valve tissue. Pulsed Doppler studies did not show any evidence of a shunt but there was early systolic reflux through the tricuspid valve and this seems to be the cause of the early systolic murmur in the majority.

Radiology   shows slight or no cardiac enlargement and there may be slightly increased or normal pulmonary vascularity.

Electrocardiography   The electrocardiogram may be normal or show slight increase in left ventricular activity.

Investigation   Cross-sectional echocardiography may show the site of the defect. Very small defects, however, may not be visible but the flow through the defect may be picked up by Doppler studies. The gradient measured between the two ventricles will confirm the normal or near normal right ventricular pressures.
   Cardiac catheterization is unnecessary.

Treatment   No treatment is required in this group other than prophylaxis against bacterial endocarditis.

Group 2. Medium-sized ventricular septal defects
Medium-sized ventricular septal defects will often cause symptoms in infancy; the child is breathless on feeding, takes longer to feed and often does not finish his feeds. His weight gain is slower than normal. He is prone to chest infections, which take longer to resolve than in a normal child. Heart failure may develop in the first three months of life, often precipitated by a chest infection, but responds readily to treatment. Slow but steady progress is made and when spoon-feeding is introduced the infant feeds better, is less exhausted than by sucking a bottle and his weight gain improves. As he gains more weight the defect often becomes relatively smaller; he becomes less breathless and his general condition improves. Thereafter he makes reasonable progress although lagging behind normal. He may rest more than his friends. He is more disturbed by chest infections than a normal child but these distress him less as he becomes older and by the time school age is reached he is symptomatically little different from normal.
   On examination, in infancy, there may be slight breathlessness at rest. There is some cardiac enlargement with prominent activity of the left ventricle and some increase in the right ventricular activity. A well marked thrill is felt in the third and fourth left interspaces close to the sternum and there is a loud, harsh, impressive pansystolic murmur maximal in the same area and conducted all over the chest. A mid-diastolic murmur can be heard in the mitral area where it is fairly localized and gives a to-and-fro rhythm. The presence of this murmur indicates that there must

be a moderate or large left-to-right shunt through the defect, for, when a large amount of blood flows to the lungs, there is a large amount of blood returning to the left atrium and flowing through the normal mitral valve. This excessive flow through a normal valve causes the mitral diastolic murmur. It usually occurs when the amount of blood flowing to the lungs is more than twice that flowing in the systemic circulation.

The second sound may be normally split, but in cases where the pulmonary artery pressure is increased the splitting may be closer than normal and the second element increased in intensity.

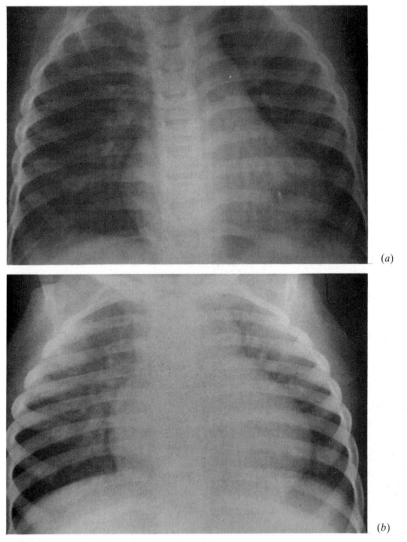

(a)

(b)

Figure 6.7 Radiology of ventricular septal defects. (a) Fairly small defect (pulmonary to systemic flow ratio 2:1 with normal pulmonary artery pressure). The left ventricle is enlarged and there is minimal plethora. (b) Moderate-sized defect (P:S about 4:1 and slight elevation in pulmonary artery pressure). The heart is enlarged and there is pulmonary plethora

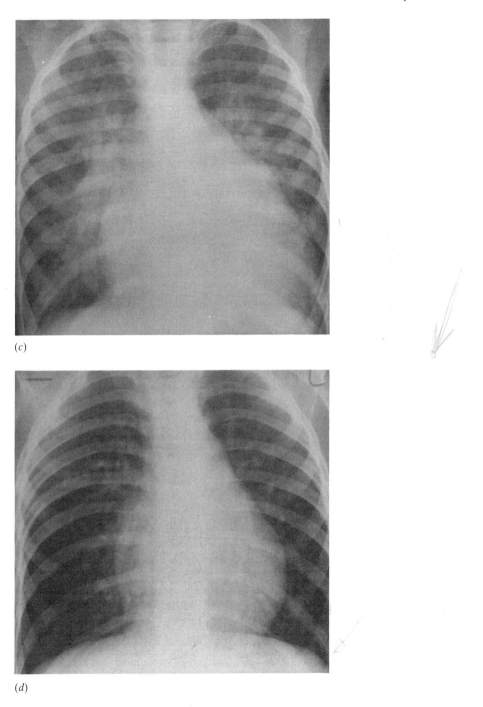

(c)

(d)

Figure 6.7 (c) Large defect with equal pulmonary artery and aortic pressures and P:S flow ratio 4:1. (d) Large defect and high pulmonary vascular resistance (P:S flow ratio 1.5:1). The heart is not enlarged overall, the main pulmonary artery is prominent but the peripheral vessels are pruned

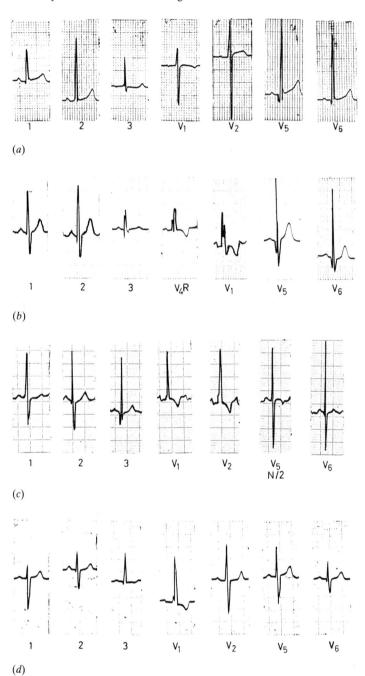

Figure 6.8 Electrocardiograms of patients with ventricular septal defects whose haemodynamic states correspond to those of Figure 6.7. (*a*) Mild left ventricular hypertrophy (10-year-old). (*b*) Left ventricular hypertrophy and mild right ventricular hypertrophy (3-year-old). (*c*) Biventricular hypertrophy (3-year-old). (*d*) Right ventricular hypertrophy with normal left ventricular activity (3-year-old)

Some patients with medium-sized defects have normal pulmonary artery pressures, but with others it is raised although not as high as systemic level.

Radiology Radiology shows moderate cardiac enlargement, a prominent pulmonary artery, moderately increased hilar vessels and an increased vascularity of the lungs (Figure 6.7b).

Electrocardiography The electrocardiogram shows an increase in right and left ventricular activity, the left greater than the right. Frequently the right ventricular hypertrophy appears as a right bundle branch block type pattern (Figure 6.8).

Investigation Echocardiography will demonstrate the position of the hole and the flow through it can be measured by Doppler studies. The gradient across the defect will give a guide to the right ventricular and pulmonary artery pressure. Additional lesions can be excluded. If the defect is in a position where it is likely to get smaller or to close and there is no worrying rise in pulmonary artery pressure then the patient can be followed-up clinically and by serial echocardiographic studies. Catheterization is unnecessary. If, however, the defect is in a position where it is unlikely to change in size and the estimated pulmonary artery pressure is near systemic, then catheter studies can be carried out to measure the pulmonary vascular resistance and help to make the best decision about management (Figure 6.9).

Treatment Heart failure, if present, must be treated (see Chapter 15) and prompt therapy must be given for respiratory infections or the child will deteriorate rapidly. Babies will often feed better from a spoon and begin to gain weight. If serial studies show that the hole is becoming smaller and the child improves symptomatically, surgery is not required. If the pulmonary artery pressure is near systemic, the infant

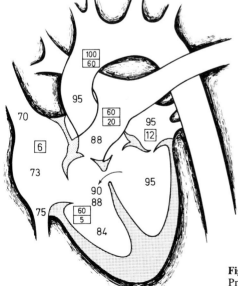

Figure 6.9 Ventricular septal defect of moderate size. Pressures in mmHg, within squares; percentage oxygen saturations, unsquared

must be carefully monitored, and if there is no evidence that the pressure is falling or the hole becoming smaller and the infant has symptoms, then surgery should be advised. The majority of infants in this age group have little in the way of symptoms by the time they are of school age and can be left alone. If patients still have impaired exercise tolerance, an enlarged heart and pulmonary plethora on the radiograph by the age of 4 years, then closure should be recommended before the child starts school.

Group 3. Large defects

Children with large defects are very ill early in life. Some of these have multiple defects in the septum. Symptoms occur in the second or third weeks of life (see page 235) and heart failure develops in the next few weeks, often precipitated by a chest infection. The first symptom is inability to feed adequately because of breathlessness and this gradually worsens. Despite poor feeding the baby may apparently gain weight, but this is due to fluid retention because of heart failure. Doctors and nurses must be aware of this and not reassure parents that all is well because the scale shows a satisfactory weight gain. Even after heart failure is treated the infants do not thrive and slow progress is often interrupted by deterioration due to repeated chest infections.

Infants show marked dyspnoea at rest (Figure 6.10). The heart is markedly enlarged with increased activity of both ventricles. A systolic thrill is palpable in the

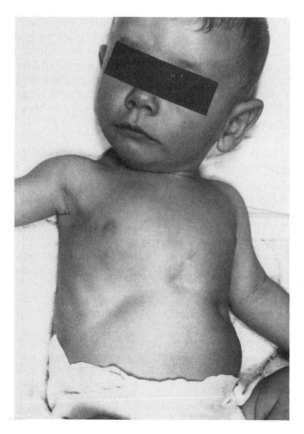

Figure 6.10 Infant aged 4 months with large ventricular septal defect. Note the incession of the lower chest. At the age of 5 years the patient was symptom-free and had only a very small defect, which did not require closure

third and fourth left intersapces where the systolic murmur is maximal. The thrill and murmur do not, however, occupy the whole of systole because there is some increase in pulmonary vascular resistance and the systolic pressures in the two ventricles equalize before the end of systole. In very large defects, the systolic murmur may be unimpressive and only an ejection systolic murmur is heard in the pulmonary area. The most impressive murmur is often the mid-diastolic murmur at the cardiac apex due to increased blood flow through the mitral valve. The second sound is loud and single.

Radiology shows marked cardiac enlargement with a very large pulmonary artery, large hilar vessels and increased peripheral vascularity (see Figure 6.7c).

Electrocardiography The electrocardiogram shows marked increase in both right and left ventricular activity and sometimes there are inverted T waves over the left ventricular leads.

Echocardiography This shows enlargement of the left atrium and both ventricles. The hole will be seen easily and there is no gradient between the two ventricles. Flow through the hole is demonstrated by Doppler echocardiography. Any additional lesions are looked for and complex abnormalities such as single ventricle, double outlet right ventricle and truncus arteriosus excluded.

Cardiac catheterization may not be required if the hole is in a position where it is likely to become smaller or to close and the patient can simply be followed by serial echocardiographic studies. If, however, the hole is in an unfavourable position for closure and serial studies show no improvement during the first year of life, then surgery is likely to be necessary and cardiac catheterization is done to measure the pulmonary vascular resistance. However, as echocardiography improves even further and yields more and accurate information, then cardiac catheterization will rarely be required in patients with ventricular septal defect.

Treatment It is in this group that surgery is most likely to be required. Patients with a high flow of blood entering the pulmonary circuit at systemic pressure are the ones who will develop pulmonary vascular disease. These patients must be monitored carefully in the first few months of life and if the hole is not becoming smaller and the pulmonary artery pressure falling, or infundibular stenosis developing, then closure of the defect should be carried out to prevent pulmonary vascular disease developing. Banding of the pulmonary artery to reduce the pulmonary artery pressure distal to the band is now reserved for infants with multiple ventricular septal defects where surgery is extremely difficult and carries an increased risk; when the child is bigger, further surgery will be required to close the defects and reconstruct the pulmonary artery. Some of the defects and occasionally all of them may have closed after banding.

Group 4. Large ventricular septal defects with high pulmonary vascular resistance
It used to be relatively common to see patients with large defects who had improved at the expense of developing pulmonary vascular changes and who had not been referred for surgery. (This is rare nowadays because patients are referred to special centres in infancy before irreversible changes occur.) When seen early in life this group have few if any symptoms, the heart is not enlarged or only slightly

so. The left ventricle is not over-working because any left-to-right shunt is small, the right ventricular activity is increased because of the systemic pressure within it. There are no thrills. The systolic murmur is ejection in type. The second sound is very loud and single and may be palpable. The resistance to flow of blood into the lungs continues to increase until the pulmonary vascular resistance is greater than the systemic resistance, the flow through the defect is reversed and the patient becomes cyanosed, presenting the picture of the Eisenmenger complex (see page 259).

Radiology   Radiology shows only a slight increase in heart size or a normal size. The pulmonary artery is prominent, the hilar vessels are large but there is poor vascularity in the periphery of the lungs, an appearance often described as 'pruning' (from its resemblance to a pruned tree with spindly new growth) (see Figure 6.7).

Electrocardiography   The electrocardiogram shows right ventricular hypertrophy and there is often a qR pattern in V_4R and V_1. The left ventricular activity is normal (see Figure 6.8).

Echocardiography   This demonstrates the defect, shows that there is no gradient across it and the pulmonary flow is consistent with pulmonary hypertension. No, or very little, flow is detectable through the defect despite its large size.

Cardiac catheterization   is unnecessary in patients who are cyanosed and indeed should be avoided because it carries an increased risk. In others who are not yet cyanosed, catheterization will simply confirm the high pulmonary vascular resistance which the clinical findings suggest.

Treatment   The pulmonary vascular resistance in this group is inevitably more than half the systemic resistance and closure of the defect is not advised. The only treatment possible for such patients is a heart–lung transplant later in life when they have developed the Eisenmenger syndrome and symptoms justify the risks.

It must be emphasized that dividing the lesion into groups for the purpose of description is somewhat artificial. Patients will move from one group to another as they grow. Some will move from Group 2 to Group 1 as they improve and the defect becomes smaller and eventually closes. On the other hand, patients in Group 3 could move to Group 4 if surgery is not carried out in time to prevent pulmonary vascular disease developing. Other patients will develop infundibular stenosis and become indistinguishable from those with tetralogy of Fallot.

Ventricular septal defect with aortic regurgitation

In these patients the defect lies below the aortic valve and is most commonly a perimembranous defect but may also be doubly committed subarterial. It is usually the right coronary cusp which prolapses but occasionally it is the non-coronary cusp. Aortic regurgitation is uncommon in infancy but develops in the early years of life and gradually increases. Some also develop infundibular stenosis. Patients with ventricular septal defect should always be carefully examined for the presence of an early diastolic murmur of aortic regurgitation. The defect may apparently become smaller because of the aortic cusp prolapsing into it. The pansystolic murmur plus early diastolic murmur may mimic a patent ductus arteriosus murmur. As the aortic incompetence increases the heart enlarges, left ventricular activity is more prominent and the pulses become collapsing. Echocardiography demonstrates the site of the ventricular septal defect and the prolapse of the right coronary cusp but prolapse of the non-coronary cusp is more difficult to determine. Doppler studies show the regurgitation in about a third of cases (Craig *et al.*, 1985).

Treatment

If the degree of aortic incompetence is increasing, closure of the ventricular septal defect should be carried out in the hope of halting its progress (Somerville, Brandao and Ross, 1970). Plication of the aortic cusp is carried out if required. If the aortic regurgitation is severe, aortic valve replacement may be necessary to relieve the patient's symptoms.

Left ventricle to right atrial communication (Gerbode defect)

In the Gerbode defect there is a fault in the part of the septum between the left ventricle and the right atrium, at the base of the tricuspid valve, which is frequently cleft. The precise anatomical abnormality is variable but in every case as the left ventricle contracts, a jet of blood streams into the right atrium.

Clinically a patient presents as with a ventricular septal defect but the electrocardiogram frequently shows an rSr' complex in V_4R and V_1 and peaked P waves indicate right atrial hypertrophy. The radiograph shows a prominent right atrium with left ventricular enlargement.

Echocardiography will demonstrate the defect and a high velocity jet will be detected in the right atrium on Doppler studies.

Atrial septal defects

It is best to classify these as:

1. *Simple* atrial septal defects in which the defect lies in the septum around the region of the fossa ovalis (known as ostium secundum defect) or lies near the mouth of the superior vena cava (known as sinus venosus defect). The latter is usually accompanied by an anomalous pulmonary vein.
2. *Complex* atrial septal defects which form part of endocardial cushion defects, now known as atrioventricular defects (previously atrioventricular canal). This complex variety will be discussed under atrioventricular defects.

Ostium secundum defects

Incidence
Eight per cent of congenital heart defects are simple atrial septal defects and most are of the ostium secundum type.

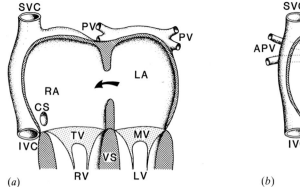
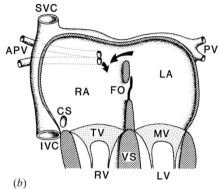

Figure 6.11 Atrial septal defects. (*a*) Ostium secundum defect (arrowed) (*b*) Sinus venosus defect (arrowed). APV, anomalous pulmonary vein; CS, coronary sinus; FO, fossa ovale; IVC, inferior vena cava; LA, left atrium; LV, left ventricle; MV, mitral valve; PV, pulmonary vein; RA, right atrium; RV, right ventricle; SVC, superior vena cava; TV, tricuspid valve; VS, ventricular septum

Definition
There is an opening between the two atria in the region of the fossa ovalis (Figure 6.11(a)). There may be more than one opening. The amount of blood shunting through the defect depends more on the filling resistances of the two ventricles than on the size of the defect. In the early months of life, the right and left ventricles have walls of equal thickness and, since the filling characteristics of the two ventricles are similar, very little blood flows through the defect. As the pulmonary vascular resistance falls, so does the right ventricular pressure, and the right ventricular muscle becomes thinner. The right ventricle becomes more distensible and offers less resistance to filling than the left ventricle and so blood flows from the left to the right atrium to enter the right ventricle.

Atrial septal defects are often associated with partial anomalous drainage of pulmonary veins which enter the superior vena cava or the right atrium directly. The haemodynamic effect of this anomalous drainage is the same as that of atrial septal defect and it is not possible to determine clinically whether there is anomalous drainage as well as an atrial septal defect. Occasionally, partial anomalous pulmonary venous drainage occurs without an atrial septal defect.

A special type of atrial septal defect occurs near the entrance of the superior vena cava and is associated with one or more pulmonary veins from the right lung draining into the superior vena cava. This is called a sinus venosus defect (Figure 6.11(b)).

Natural history
It is very uncommon for an atrial septal defect alone ever to give rise to symptoms in infancy, when the resistance to filling in the two ventricles is the same. Only in very large shunts are symptoms present in childhood and more usually a heart murmur is found during a routine examination. Most patients do well in childhood and rarely develop symptoms before the third decade. They may then develop pulmonary hypertension, heart failure or atrial arrhythmias. Pregnancy often aggravates the condition and causes heart failure.

Pulmonary hypertension is rare before the third decade, but when it becomes severe the right ventricle hypertrophies and is less compliant, the flow through the defect becomes from right to left and cyanosis occurs. The reason why pulmonary hypertension does not occur in childhood is probably related to the fact that the left atrial pressure never rises significantly and so the pulmonary venous pressure is normal (unlike with ventricular septal defects and patent ductus arteriosus). The pulmonary hypertension in atrial septal defects is secondary to increased pulmonary flow.

Clinical presentation
Only when there is a very large flow of blood through the atrial septal defect do the patients have symptoms. They are excessively tired and breathless on exertion and may suffer from frequent chest infections. Most children are free of symptoms.

The patients are usually normal in size but some are tall and thin with long fingers and toes. When the shunt is large they may be below average weight. The patient is pink, the pulses are normal or of small volume and usually do not show any respiratory variation in rate. The heart is only slightly enlarged or normal in size but there is palpable pulsation of the right ventricle. There is no thrill but an ejection systolic murmur is heard which is loudest in the second left interspace. This murmur is due to excessive flow through the normal pulmonary valve. When the amount of blood flowing to the lungs is more than twice that flowing to the systemic circulation, an additional, diastolic murmur can be heard in the tricuspid area due to increased flow of blood through the tricuspid valve. This murmur increases with inspiration and fades with expiration. Flow through the defect causes no murmur as the defect is large and there is no pressure gradient and therefore no turbulence. The two components of the second sound are more widely split than normally and the splitting no longer varies with respiration and is described as being 'fixed'.

Occasionally the patient may have a tinge of cyanosis due to some inferior vena-caval blood being deflected to the left atrium by a large eustachian valve on the inferior vena cava, so that desaturated blood enters the systemic circulation.

Radiology
The degree of cardiac enlargement varies with the size of the shunt, the right atrium is prominent and the pulmonary artery and its branches are enlarged and there is increased vascularity in the periphery of the lungs (Figure 6.12). In the lateral view the right ventricle bulges forward under the sternum. The aorta is small and the superior vena cava shadow is not usually visible.

Electrocardiography
The electrocardiogram shows right axis deviation and right ventricular hypertrophy. Leads V_4R and V_1 show an rsR' complex and this is present in 95% of all ostium secundum atrial septal defects (Figure 6.13) – its *absence* makes the diagnosis of ostium secundum suspect. It must be stressed, however, that this rsR' complex occurs in other lesions and its *presence* does not mean that the lesion is an atrial septal defect. The P–R interval may be prolonged but the P waves are usually normal. The rhythm is usually regular; atrial fibrillation is rare in childhood but occurs in adults.

Investigation
The diagnosis can be made with certainty clinically in most cases. Echocardiography will demonstrate the defect (Figure 6.14) and Doppler studies can evaluate the

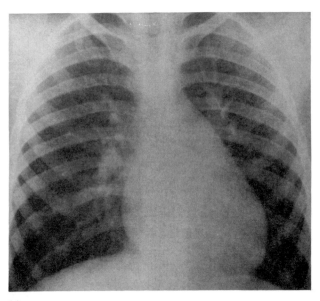

(a)

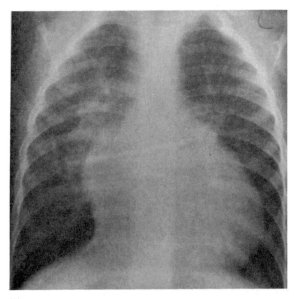

(b)

Figure 6.12 Chest radiographs of patients with atrial septal defects. (a) Ostium secundum defect, pulmonary flow four times systemic. The right ventricle is enlarged, the main pulmonary artery is prominent and there is moderate pulmonary plethora. (b) Ostium primum defect. The heart is larger and the pulmonary vessels more prominent

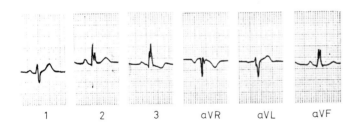

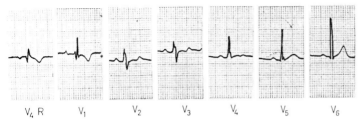

(a)

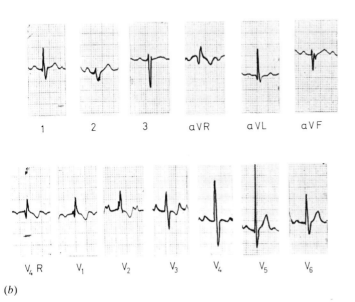

(b)

Figure 6.13 Electrocardiograms in atrial septal defect. (*a*) Ostium secundum defect. Right bundle branch block pattern and right axis deviation (+110 degrees). (*b*) Ostium primum. Right bundle branch block pattern and left axis deviation (−60 degrees) with P–R interval of 0.20 s which is above the normal limit for the age (3 years) of the patient

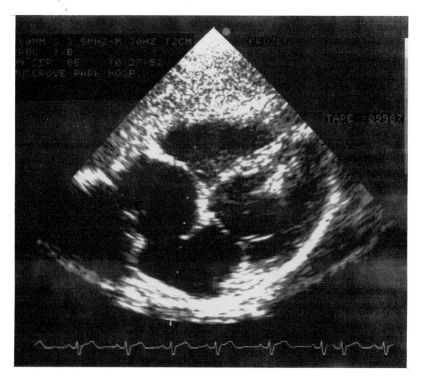

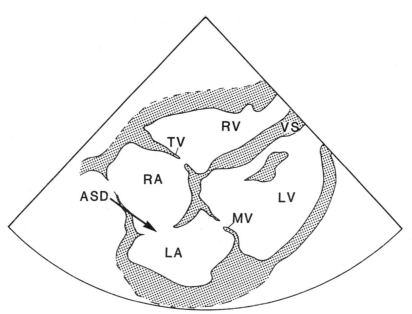

Figure 6.14 Cross-sectional echocardiogram, four-chamber subcostal view, showing ostium secundum atrial septal defect (arrowed). ASD, atrial septal defect; LA, left atrium; LV, left ventricle; MV, mitral valve; RA, right atrium; RV, right ventricle; TV, tricuspid valve; VS, ventricular septum

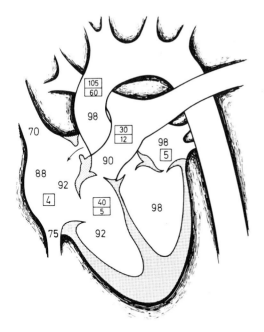

Figure 6.15 Ostium secundum defect. Pressures in mmHg, within squares; percentage oxygen saturations, unsquared

degree of left-to-right shunting by assessing the increase in tricuspid and pulmonary blood flow. Cardiac catheterization is performed nowadays only if an additional lesion is suspected but even so echocardiography will give much information about additional lesions prior to catheterization. A right heart catheterization shows a rise in oxygen saturation in the right atrial samples (Figure 6.15) and the defect is usually crossed by the catheter.

Diagnosis
Difficulty is sometimes experienced in distinguishing the systolic murmur of a small atrial septal defect from a functional murmur. The second heart sound is the best guide, for if it shows clear variation with respiration, a defect large enough to warrant surgical closure can definitely be excluded.

With large defects the main problem is to exclude a more complicated lesion. Total anomalous pulmonary venous connection produces similar signs, and the degree of cyanosis may be mild enough to escape detection clinically. It is also important to exclude obstruction to the the left side of the heart, or left ventricular disease, both of which increase the amount of left-to-right shunting. Certainly, if cardiac failure occurs in childhood a more complex lesion should be suspected.

Treatment
Ostium secundum defects are closed using cardiopulmonary bypass. The hole may be sutured directly or by using a patch to cover it. Operation is advised in childhood when the shunt is more than 2:1. It is usually done at about 4 or 5 years old, but earlier if symptoms demand it. The mortality rate is less than 0.5%.

Atrioventricular defects

Definition

In the partial and mildest form (called ostium primum defect) there is a defect in the lowest part of the atrial septum and there is always a cleft in the anterior leaflet of the mitral valve (Figure 6.16(a)). In the most severe form (complete atrioventricular defect) (previously called atrioventricular canal) there is a defect in the lower part of the atrial septum and the upper part of the ventricular septum. The mitral and tricuspid valves are no longer separate and leaflets common to both orifices bridge the defect (Figure 6.16(b)). There is an intermediate type in which the ventricular component is small and may become closed off by valve tissue.

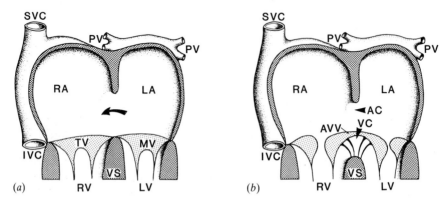

Figure 6.16 Atrioventricular defects, as viewed anteriorly. (*a*) Ostium primum (arrowed). (*b*) Common atrioventricular canal. AC, atrial component (ostium primum); AVV, bridging atrioventricular valve; IVC, inferior vena cava; LA, left atrium; LV, left ventricle; MV, mitral valve; PV, pulmonary veins; RA, right atrium; RV, right ventricle; SVC, superior vena cava; TV, tricuspid valve; VC, ventricular component; VS, ventricular septum

Ostium primum defect

The haemodynamic changes are similar to those of ostium secundum defects but there is mitral incompetence in addition. The degree of mitral incompetence is determined by the size of the cleft in the mitral valve; it may range from a trivial to a severe degree. The presence of mitral regurgitation increases the left-to-right shunt through the defect. If there is a cleft in the tricuspid valve there is also tricuspid regurgitation.

Natural history

The overall prognosis in patients with ostium primum defects is much worse than in those with ostium secundum defects. Patients fail to thrive and require treatment at an earlier age than those with ostium secundum defects. This is due to the effect of the associated mitral regurgitation.

Clinical presentation

If there is no significant mitral incompetence the situation is the same as with an ostium secundum defect and there are no symptoms. There is more disability, however, when mitral regurgitation is significant and half the patients have excessive dyspnoea, are easily tired and have frequent chest infections.

The patient presents as with an atrial septal defect with mitral incompetence. There is no cyanosis and the pulse is small or normal in volume. Children are often below normal size and may show a sulcus around the chest and a bulging precordium. The heart is usually enlarged and there is increased left, as well as right, ventricular activity. The murmurs are as described in the secundum defects with the additional apical pansystolic murmur of mitral incompetence. The apical murmur is not always very obvious, however, even when there is significant mitral regurgitation.

Radiology
As in secundum defects, the right ventricle is enlarged and the pulmonary artery is prominent. There is an increased vascularity of the hilar and peripheral pulmonary vessels. The left atrium and left ventricle are also enlarged when there is a significant degree of mitral incompetence (see Figure 6.12). Overall, cardiomegaly is much commoner than in ostium secundum defects.

Electrocardiography
The electrocardiogram is very characteristic and helpful in making the diagnosis (see Figure 6.13). There is left axis deviation and evidence of hypertrophy of both ventricles. The rsR′ pattern in leads V_4R and V_1 found in secundum defects, is often present, but there is usually a greater degree of right ventricular hypertrophy. The P waves may be tall due to right atrial hypertrophy but when there is considerable mitral regurgitation they are bifid due to left atrial enlargement. Splintered S waves are common in leads 2, 3 and aVF. The P–R interval is frequently prolonged.

Echocardiography
As in ostium secundum defects there is evidence of overloading of the right side of the heart but there is also increased volume overloading of the left ventricle when significant mitral regurgitation is present. The defect is best seen in the four-chamber subcostal view and careful scanning will show the cleft in the left atrioventricular valve, directed towards the ventricular septum. Doppler studies can assess the degree of left-to-right shunting and can give some indication of the degree of mitral regurgitation (Figure 6.17(a)).

Cardiac catheterization
This is not necessary now in most patients but if the degree of mitral regurgitation is in doubt, left ventricular angiography will help to assess it (Figure 6.18).

Treatment
Operation is required in patients with obvious symptoms or with progressive cardiac enlargement on radiography. Since these patients deteriorate more rapidly than those with ostium secundum defects, surgery is usually advised at an earlier age, at 2–3 years. The results of operation are good and the mitral valve can usually be repaired satisfactorily, leaving trivial or no incompetence. Occasionally, however, the shortness of chordae tendineae and a wide cleft makes repair impossible and mitral valve replacement is necessary. The proximity of the atrioventricular bundle to the defect resulted in a high incidence of postoperative heart block in early series, but this has not proved as common in recent years.

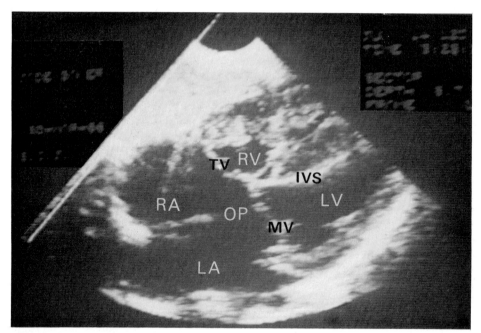

Figure 6.17 Cross-sectional echocardiogram, apical four-chamber view showing ostium primum defect (OP). IVS, interventricular septum; LA, left atrium; LV, left ventricle; MV, mitral valve; RA, right atrium; RV, right ventricle; TV, tricuspid valve

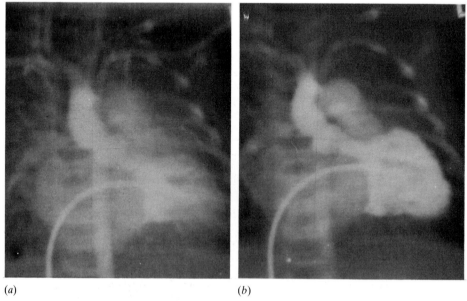

(a)   (b)

Figure 6.18 Left ventricular angiogram of a 3-week-old infant with an atrioventricular defect. (a) Systole. The medial wall of the left ventricle is irregular due to the abnormal mitral valve. (b) Diastole. The mitral valve balloons abnormally far into the outflow region of the ventricle producing a 'goose-neck' deformity

Complete atrioventricular defect

Natural history
The prognosis is poor. Infants usually have repeated episodes of chest infection and cardiac failure and there is a high death rate. Of those who survive infancy, improvement may occur because of the development of pulmonary vascular disease. About one-third of patients with atrioventricular defects have Down's syndrome and atrioventricular defect is one of the commonest lesions in the 40% of Down's syndrome infants who have congenital heart disease.

Clinical presentation
Symptoms occur in the first few weeks of life. The infants feed poorly, are slow to gain weight and are excessively breathless. Cyanosis usually occurs, but may be slight. Congestive heart failure commonly occurs in the first few months. Examination reveals a breathless, slightly cyanosed infant with a markedly enlarged heart. The pulses are normal or of small volume. There is usually evidence of pulmonary hypertension with a loud single second sound and a heaving right ventricle. There is an ejection systolic murmur over the pulmonary area and very often a tricuspid diastolic murmur due to excessive flow of blood through the tricuspid valve. There may be a pansystolic murmur at the apex due to mitral incompetence.

Radiology
There is marked cardiac enlargement with pulmonary plethora and often interstitial oedema. The left atrium is usually enlarged but may be difficult to identify in the presence of generalized cardiac enlargement.

Electrocardiography
The electrocardiogram shows left axis deviation with combined right and left ventricular hypertrophy. Deep and splintered S waves are seen in leads 2, 3 and aVF. The P–R interval is usually prolonged.

Echocardiography
This produces superb anatomical detail of the abnormality and is superior to the pictures obtained at angiocardiography. In the four-chamber subcostal view, the atrioventricular valves are seen and careful scanning along the crest of the septum will be required to demonstrate whether there are separate right and left valves or a common atrioventricular valve (Figure 6.19).

Cardiac catheterization
This is not necessary for diagnosis but is required to assess the pulmonary vascular resistance when surgery is being considered. In complete atrioventricular defects the pulmonary vascular resistance can rise with alarming rapidity, especially in Down's syndrome, and even at the age of 6 months the pulmonary vascular resistance may be 50% of the systemic resistance.

Treatment
Medical treatment is first required to control heart failure. This is often unsuccessful, especially when there is severe mitral regurgitation.
    Total correction is possible but still carries a high mortality in infants. Most

surgeons are unwilling to operate if the pulmonary vascular resistance is more than 50% of the systemic resistance. At operation the atrial and ventricular components of the defect are patched and the mitral and tricuspid valves repaired – or occasionally replaced.

The special problems of Down's syndrome are discussed in Chapter 21.

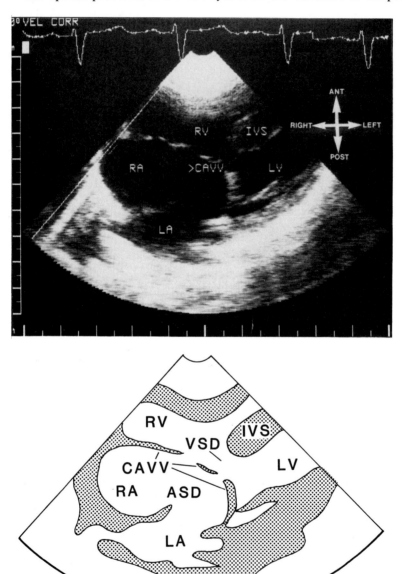

Figure 6.19 Cross-sectional echocardiogram, subcostal four-chamber view showing complete atrioventricular defect. ASD, atrial component of defect; CAVV, common atrioventricular valve; IVS, interventricular septum; LA, left atrium; LV, left ventricle; RA, right atrium; RV, right ventricle; VSD, ventricular component of defect

Bibliography and references

Patent ductus arteriosus

Campbell, M. (1955) Patent ductus arteriosus. Some notes on prognosis and on pulmonary hypertension. *British Heart Journal*, **17**, 511–533

Campbell, M. (1968) Natural history of persistent ductus arteriosus. *British Heart Journal*, **30**, 4–13

Cosh, J. A. (1957) Patent ductus arteriosus: a follow-up study of 73 cases. *British Heart Journal*, **19**, 13–22

Cotton, R. B., Stahlman, M. D., Bender, H. W., *et al.* (1978) Randomized trial of early closure of symptomatic patent ductus arteriosus in small premature infants. *Journal of Paediatrics*, **93**, 647–651

Cotton, R. B., Stahlman, M. D., Catterton, W. Z., *et al.* (1978) Medical management of small preterm infants with symptomatic patent ductus arteriosus. *Journal of Paediatrics*, **93**, 467–473

Gibson, G. A. (1900) Clinical lectures in circulatory affections. 1. Persistence of the arterial duct and its diagnosis. *Edinburgh Medical Journal*, N.S.8, 1

Gittenberger-de-Groot, A.C. (1977) Persistent ductus arteriosus: most probably a primary congenital malformation. *British Heart Journal*, **39**, 610–618

Gittenberger-de-Groot, A.C. (1979) Patent ductus arteriosus in the newborn: histological observations. In *Paediatric Cardiology*, Vol. 2 (eds M. J. Godman and R. M. Marquis), Churchill Livingstone, London

Hallidie-Smith, K.A. and Girling D. J. (1971) Persistent ductus arteriosus in ill and premature babies. *Archives of Disease in Childhood*, **46**, 177–181

Keys, A. and Shapiro, M. J. (1943) Patency of the ductus arteriosus in adults. *American Heart Journal*, **25**, 158–186

Kocsis J., Hernandovich J., Silva M. J., *et al.* (1973) Duration of inhibition of platelet prostaglandin formation and aggregation by ingested aspirin or indomethacin. *Prostaglandins*, **3**, 141–144

Mark, H. and Young, D. (1965) Congenital heart disease in the adult. *American Journal of Cardiology*, **15**, 293–302

Olley, P. M. and Coceani, F. (1979) Mechanism of closure of the ductus arteriosus. In *Paediatric Cardiology*, Vol. 2 (eds M. J. Godman and R. M. Marquis), Churchill Livingstone, London, pp. 15–31

Olley, P. M., Rowe, R. D., Freedom R. M., *et al.* (1979) Pharmacological manipulation of the ductus arteriosus. In *Paediatric Cardiology*, Vol. 2 (eds M. J. Godman and R. M. Marquis), Churchill Livingstone, London, pp. 32–44

Rudolph, A. M. (1977) In *Paediatric Cardology* 47 (eds R. H. Anderson and E. A. Shinebourne, Churchill Livingstone, London, pp. 409–412

Rudolph, A. M., Mayer F. E., Nadas, A. S. *et al.* (1958) Patent ductus arteriosus. A clinical and hemodynamic study of 23 patients in the first year of life. *Pediatrics, Springfield*, **33**, 892

Wood, P. H. (1958) The Eisenmenger syndrome. *British Medical Journal*, **2**, (i) 701; (ii) 755–762

Ventricular septal defect

Alpert, B. S., Cook, D. H., Varghese, P. J. *et al.* (1979) Spontaneous closure of small ventricular septal defects: ten year follow-up. *Pediatrics, Springfield*, **63**, 204–206

Bloomfield, D. K. (1964) The natural history of ventricular septal defect in patients surviving infancy. *Circulation*, **29**, 914–955

Jordan, S. C. (1985) Two-dimensional and pulsed Doppler investigations of children with early systolic murmurs. *British Heart Journal*, **54**, 618

Sutherland, G. R. and Godman, M. J. (1986) The natural history of ventricular septal defects. A long-term prospective cross-sectional echocardiographic study. Chapter 16 in *Clinical Echocardiography* (eds A. S. Hunter and R. J. C. Hall), Castle House Publications, Tunbridge Wells

Ventricular septal defect with aortic regurgitation

Craig, B., Smallhorn, J., Burrows, P., *et al.* (1985) Two-dimensional echocardiographic features of aortic valve prolapse associated with ventricular septal defect. *Abstracts of Second World Congress of Paediatric Cardiology*, Springer-Verlag, Berlin, p. 48

Somerville, J., Brandao, A. and Ross, D. N. (1970) Aortic regurgitation and ventricular septal defect. Surgical management and clinical features. *Circulation*, **41**, 317–330

Chapter 7

Acyanotic lesions with left heart obstruction

Aortic valve stenosis

Incidence

Aortic stenosis accounts for about 5% of all congenital heart disease presenting in infancy and childhood. In the Bristol series 5.7% of cases had aortic stenosis as their main or only lesion, but it occurred in association with other lesions, particularly coarctation, in almost another 6%. Isolated aortic stenosis is about 4 times as common in boys as in girls. It is significantly more common in Turner's syndrome, although less so than coarctation. According to Campbell, bicuspid aortic valves which are not stenotic in childhood occur much more frequently, with an incidence close to 3.5 per 1000 of the population generally, again more common in men, so that if these are included the total incidence is about 4 per 1000, or slightly greater than that of ventricular septal defect.

Pathology and definition

By definition there must be sufficient narrowing of the aortic valve orifice in systole to cause obstruction to flow from left ventricle to aorta. The anatomy is variable (Figure 7.1) but the majority have only two cusps with partial fusion of one or both commissures. This applies more to the mild or moderate forms. Severe stenosis is more often seen in unicuspid or non-cusped valves. About 10% have clinically detectable regurgitation although this may not be noted in the first few years.

Natural history

Campbell's study in 1968 showed a 1.2% mortality per annum over the first two decades of life, but this series contained rather few patients presenting symptomatically in the neonatal period. In the Bristol series 1.1% had died by the end of the first year, 0.7% without surgical intervention and 0.4% with surgery. However, three-quarters of all deaths occurred in patients with other recognizable abnormalities: 10 had some degree of left ventricular hypoplasia (left ventricular diameter less than half predicted normal for size), 2 had dilated left ventricles with endocardial fibroelastosis, and 3 had severe mitral valve abnormalities. The overall mortality for surgery for aortic stenosis under 1 year was 41%, but all but 2 of these deaths occurred in patients with other lesions. Campbell showed that the annual mortality in the 3rd, 4th, 5th and 6th decades was 3.0, 3.5, 6.0 and 8.5%

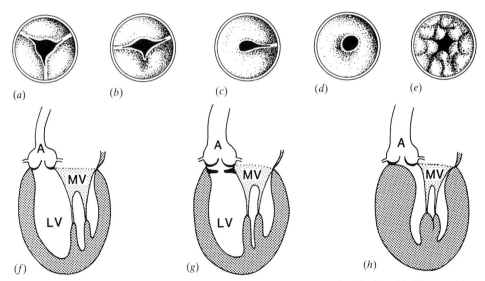

Figure 7.1 Types of aortic obstruction. (*a*) to (*e*) are types of valvar stenosis: (*a*) tricuspid; (*b*) bicuspid; (*c*) unicuspid; (*d*) non-cusped; (*e*) myxomatous; (*f*) Supravalvar stenosis; (*g*) discrete subaortic stenosis; (*h*) hypertrophic obstructive cardiomyopathy. A, aorta; LV, left ventricle; MV, mitral valve

respectively so that 60% of patients had died by the age of 40 years. This was, of course, before the days when aortic valve replacement was available.

Most of the patients who died have had symptoms, and sudden death is rare. Infective endocarditis occurs commonly in adults but is rare under the age of 10, at any rate in countries where prophylactic measures against infective endocarditis are undertaken routinely. Only 2 cases out of a total of 245 in Bristol had this complication.

The most important long-term factor producing deterioration is the development of calcification in the valve cusps, a process which may start in adolescence but rarely becomes important before the fifth decade in men and later in women.

Clinical presentation

Severe aortic stenosis may be seen in infancy, when it causes heart failure or sudden death (Scott and Feldman, 1964). In older children the heart murmur is discovered at a routine examination and few have any symptoms. When symptoms do occur they are breathlessness, substernal pain on effort and syncope or dizziness on effort.

The patient is acyanotic and the pulse is usully normal in character except in severe stenosis when the characteristic small volume pulse is felt. Severe stenosis can, however, exist with a normal pulse. There is forceful pulsation of the left ventricle and in moderate and severe stenosis there may be a presystolic impulse at the cardiac apex, due to forceful atrial contraction filling the ventricle. In children, a systolic thrill may not be felt at the base of the heart but is obvious in the suprasternal notch and over the carotid vessels. If a thrill is not palpable the obstruction is usually mild. The systolic murmur is ejection in type and is best heard in the aortic area, but is also loud at the cardiac apex. It is well conducted up into the neck over the carotid arteries. When the aortic valve is mobile the murmur is preceded by an ejection click, usually best heard at the apex during expiration. The more severe the stenosis, the closer the ejection click becomes to the first sound, because the rapid rise of pressure in the left ventricle opens the aortic valve soon after the mitral valve has closed. The second heart sound is normal in mild stenosis but in severe stenosis it may be single due to prolonged left ventricular systole and the aortic element occurring late. In very severe stenosis the aortic closure sound may occur after the pulmonary closure and this results in paradoxical splitting with respiration.

Radiology

The overall heart size is usually normal but there may be rounding of the apex due to thickening of the left ventricle. The ascending aorta commonly shows poststenotic dilatation. In very severe obstruction the left ventricle may enlarge and there may be a prominent left atrium.

Electrocardiography

When the electrocardiogram shows evidence of left ventricular hypertrophy and strain the aortic stenosis is severe. On the other hand, severe aortic stenosis may exist in the presence of a normal electrocardiogram. The presence of symptoms or clinical evidence of severe aortic stenosis is more reliable than the electrocardiogram.

In severe stenosis the P waves in lead 2 are broad and bifid. In moderate stenosis the QRS axis in the standard leads is normal but there is increased voltage of the R wave in all standard leads and the precordial leads V_5 and V_6 which are over the left ventricle. In severe stenosis the electrical axis is directed more posteriorly and there are deep S waves in the anterior chest leads V_2 and V_3. As the disease increases in severity the T waves in V_5 and V_6 become flattened and then inverted, and the QRS duration may be increased (see Figure 4.8).

Echocardiography

Using suitable techniques it is now possible to obtain detailed information on valve structure and function and this is now the most important investigation in aortic stenosis. Serial measurements enable changes to be documented and surgical intervention carried out at the optimum time.

Cross-sectional studies of the valve show thickening and restricted opening of cusps (Figure 7.2(a)) and show the number of cusps. M-mode had been used to demonstrate the eccentric closure of the bicuspid valve (Figure 7.2(b)) but is less accurate. The degree of left ventricular hypertrophy can be accurately assessed and left ventricular function studies made by M-mode.

Doppler studies allow estimation of the aortic valve gradient (see Chapter 4 for details of technique and calculations), but for all but small gradients continuous-wave mode is required. This is usually done from the suprasternal notch and the maximum velocity of the jet allows the gradient to be calculated. However, it is often not possible to make allowance for the angle between the jet (which may not

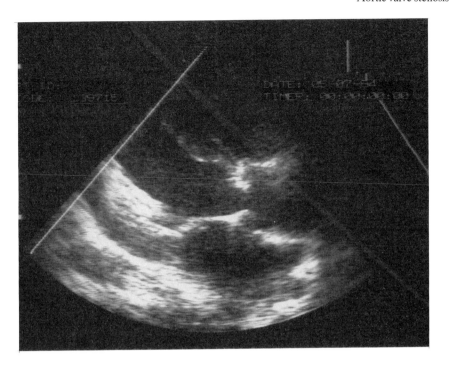

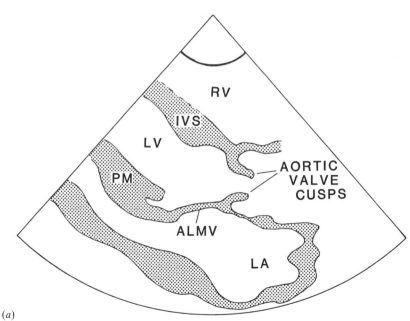

(a)

Figure 7.2 (a) Cross-sectional echocardiogram, long axis view, showing thickened aortic valve cusps with restricted opening in left ventricular systole from case of aortic valve stenosis. ALMV, anterior leaflet of mitral valve; IVS, interventricular septum; LA, left atrium; LV, left ventricle; PM, papillary muscle; RV, right ventricle.

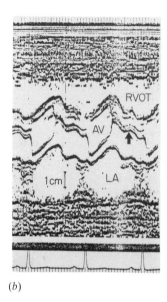

(b)

Figure 7.2 (b) M-mode echocardiogram showing eccentric closure but normal opening of bicuspid aortic valve

be parallel to the aortic wall) and the direction of the ultrasound beam. For this reason it is useful to make estimations from apical and subcostal positions and also from the right parasternal position. The maximum velocity is used to calculate the gradient (Figure 7.3). Partly because the patient is unsedated (and may be active) and partly because this technique measures the maximum instantaneous gradient rather than the peak-to-peak gradient as in catheter studies, the calculated gradients are somewhat higher than those at catheterization. Aortic regurgitation can be detected, particularly by using pulsed-wave Doppler to focus on the area just below the aortic valve. Flow patterns in the aortic arch allow some quantification of regurgitation by comparing the sizes of the forward and retrograde flow.

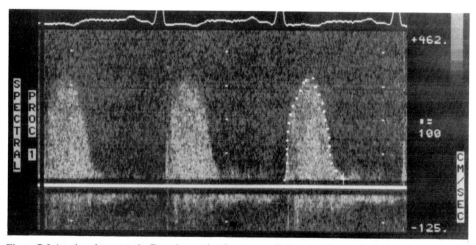

Figure 7.3 Aortic valve stenosis. Doppler tracing from ascending aorta. The maximum gradient is calculated from the maximum velocity 3.23 m/sec^2×4, i.e. 41.7 mmHg

Cardiac catheterization

Cardiac catheterization is now seldom used to investigate aortic stenosis, since more information can be obtained by echocardiography. If there is a discrepancy between the echo and clinical findings it may be useful to measure the gradient by catheter (Figure 7.4). The valve is usually approached retrogradely via the femoral artery, but it is sometimes difficult to pass the catheter back across the stenotic valve into the left ventricle. In neonates and some infants it may be possible to enter the left atrium and left ventricle through the foramen ovale, but this closes rather earlier if there is left-sided obstruction. From the age of 1 year onwards the atrial septum can be punctured using the Brockenbrough catheter and needle and

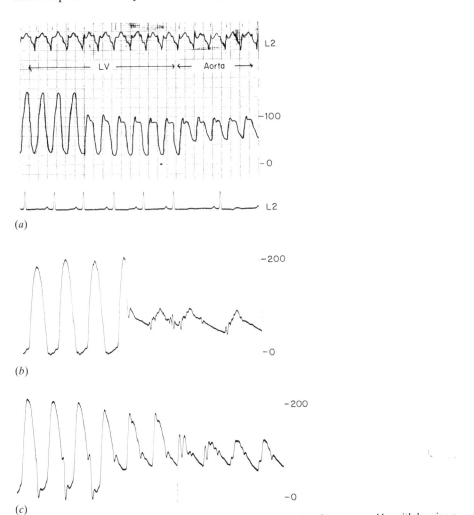

Figure 7.4 Pressure gradients in different types of aortic obstruction demonstrated by withdrawing a catheter from the left ventricle into the aorta. (*a*) Hypertrophic obstructive cardiomyopathy in a 3-month-old infant. The gradient is within the ventricle and the aortic pressure shows a rapid upstroke. (*b*) Aortic valve stenosis in a 10-year-old boy. (*c*) Supra-aortic stenosis in a 4-year-old girl who had facies of infantile hypercalcaemia and also multiple pulmonary artery stenosis

the catheter then passed into the left ventricle. Ideally the cardiac output should also be measured since a relatively small increase or decrease in cardiac output has a disproportionately large effect on the gradient. In severe aortic stenosis the gradient at rest will be between 60 and 100 mmHg.

Treatment

Mild stenosis

Children with mild aortic stenosis do not require treatment or restrictions in physical activity. Mild stenosis implies clinically a murmur without a thrill, normal volume pulses and a normal cardiac output. On the echocardiogram there will be normal thickness of left ventricular walls for the age and the Doppler gradient will be under 20 mmHg. The electrocardiogram will be normal, but this does not in itself imply mild stenosis.

Moderate stenosis

This is diagnosed when the pulse is normal but there is a thrill in the aortic area or suprasternal notch and the electrocardiogram shows at most some increase in left ventricular voltages. The echocardiogram shows up to 30% increase in left ventricular wall thickness and the estimated Doppler gradient is up to 50 mmHg. Such children should not be allowed to undertake competitive athletics, games or swimming but can do games which do not involve all-out effort or endurance training. The disadvantages of overactivity in this group is more the development of a very hypertrophied ('muscle-bound') ventricle which may predispose to arrhythmias, which may occasionally result in sudden death.

Severe stenosis

This may present as sudden cardiovascular collapse in the neonatal period, heart failure in infancy or as a symptomatic or apparently asymptomatic child with small volume pulses, conspicuous left ventricular hypertrophy and a long murmur with or without a thrill. The electrocardiogram will generally show clear evidence of left ventricular hypertrophy and may show flattening or inversion of T waves over the left ventricle. The echocardiogram shows usually a very hypertrophied left ventricle but sometimes shows dilatation and impaired contractility. These patients are candidates for surgical treatment. Medical treatment has virtually no place in the treatment of aortic stenosis except temporarily in infants presenting with heart failure.

Surgical treatment

Surgical treatment of aortic stenosis in childhood is unsatisfactory for two reasons. If a conservative operation is carried out it will usually only be possible to convert severe stenosis into moderate stenosis with mild regurgitation or, if the surgeon is too aggressive, mild stenosis with moderate or severe regurgitation. However, valve replacement is impossible in infants and unsatisfactory in older children since the valve, whether tissue or prosthetic, will not grow with the child. In addition, tissue valves have a limited life span (degeneration occurs more rapidly than in adults) and prosthetic valves require anticoagulants which, although they can be controlled successfully, do impose restrictions on active children. It is for these reasons that only severe stenosis is treated surgically. Aortic valvotomy is carried out under cardiopulmonary bypass and limited incision of the fused commissures is performed.

If at all possible further operation is postponed until adult life, but in some children there is continued deterioration due either to failure adequately to relieve the stenosis or to the production of severe aortic regurgitation.

If valve replacement is required during the growing period the best results are usually obtained with homograft replacement, including, if necessary, excision of the aortic root and enlargement of the left ventricular outflow. This is a specialized operation and best left to surgeons who have had special experience in the technique. An alternative procedure is to transfer the patient's own pulmonary valve to the aortic position and replace the pulmonary valve (where some deterioration in function is better tolerated) with a homograft.

As an alternative to surgical valvotomy, balloon dilatation of the aortic valve has been tried. There appears to be a greater risk of causing severe damage to the valve and the overall risk is probably greater than for aortic valvotomy (less than 1% over the age of 1 year), but it is likely that with greater experience the results can be improved.

In moderate, unoperated aortic stenosis or operated severe stenosis there is clearly a need for close supervision at all times including regular reassessment by echocardiography. The clinical state of the child will vary and the paediatrician and paediatric cardiologist must be prepared to react promptly to changes which call for intervention. Failure to do so will result in impairment of left ventricular function, which may be permanent, or sudden deterioration, or death.

Stringent dental hygiene and adequate antibiotic cover for dental or other operations is clearly essential. Infective endocarditis, although uncommon, is particularly dangerous in aortic stenosis. If the infection is not promptly diagnosed and adequately treated the valve cusps may tear or perforate leading to severe aortic regurgitation. Any paediatrician or paediatric cardiologist treating infective endocarditis on the aortic valve should always be in touch with the nearest paediatric cardiac centre to allow prompt transfer should there be evidence of aortic regurgitation developing. Urgent surgery to replace the valve may be required.

Aortic regurgitation

Incidence

Aortic regurgitation occurs both as a congenital lesion and as a result of acute rheumatic fever. Occasionally it is produced by acute bacterial endocarditis on a previously normal valve, and subacute bacterial endocarditis can convert a slightly stenotic bicuspid aortic valve into a freely regurgitant one. At present congenital aortic regurgitation is rather more common than the acquired forms in childhood. Several of our patients have had a family history of a similar abnormality. In the congenital form the lesion is only about one-tenth as common as aortic stenosis.

Definition

Severe regurgitation occurs as a result of rolling up and rigidity of the cusps or from weakness and prolapse of one or more cusps. It also occurs in association with aneurysms of the sinuses of Valsalva, and with high ventricular septal defects which extend into the fibrous ring of the aortic valve and weaken it. Marfan's syndrome is associated with dilatation of the aorta and aortic regurgitation due to prolapse of valve cusps.

Clinical presentation

Severe aortic regurgitation may present with heart failure in infancy or with breathlessness in older children. Most patients, however, are asymptomatic and are referred because a murmur has been heard on routine examination. The pulses are of large volume or collapsing if the regurgitation is severe, capillary pulsation is visible in the fingers and the muscles of arms and legs are felt to pulsate. The blood pressure shows a high systolic and a low diastolic pressure. The left ventricle is palpably enlarged and hyperdynamic. As well as the characteristic early diastolic murmur heard at the aortic area and left sternal border, there is usually also a systolic murmur due to the high stroke output. Occasionally a short, mid-diastolic (Austin Flint) murmur is heard at the apex. This has been shown by echocardiography to be due to fluttering of the anterior cusp of the mitral valve due to the combined effects of the regurgitant jet on one side and the normal flow through the mitral valve on the other. In addition, the rapid rise in pressure in the left ventricle in diastole may close the mitral valve prematurely so that flow is restricted to the early part of diastole, and has therefore to be more rapid than normal.

In mild aortic regurgitation the only abnormality is the soft, early diastolic murmur usually best heard in the 3rd left intercostal space.

Radiology

In moderate or severe regurgitation the left ventricle is enlarged. Owing to the large stroke volume there is a considerable difference in the size of the heart in different parts of the cardiac cycle. Single films are therefore unreliable, but screening the heart gives a better idea of its size.

Electrocardiography

The electrocardiogram shows left ventricular hypertrophy of a degree commensurate with the degree of regurgitation.

Echocardiography

Cross-sectional echocardiography usually enables the cause of the aortic regurgitation to be determined without difficulty. There may be thickening and failure of closure of the cusps, lengthening of the free edges causing prolapse or a high ventricular septal defect or sinus of Valsalva aneurysm allowing prolapse. In Marfan's syndrome the dilatation of the aortic root with anatomically normal cusps stretched but unable to close the orifice is seen. On the M-mode, fluttering of the anterior cusp of the mitral valve with early closure is the classic sign. The left ventricular size and calculated stroke volume give a good indication of the severity of the regurgitation and serial studies allow any deterioration in left ventricular size or function to be detected. Actual detection of regurgitation is best done using pulsed-wave Doppler, looking from the apical window. The sampling spot is located just below the aortic valve and anterior to the mitral valve (so as to avoid confusion with normal mitral valve flow). It is only possible to give a rough idea of the severity, based on how far back to the apex of the left ventricle the regurgitant jet can be detected. Doppler sampling in the aortic arch allows the volume of the normal, anterograde and regurgitant, retrograde flow to be compared and a better estimate of the severity made. Echocardiography also allows the detection of associated defects such as a high ventricular septal defect and also the occasional lesion such as an aorto–left ventricular tunnel which mimics valvar regurgitation.

Cardiac catheterization

This is seldom needed for diagnostic reasons but may be used if there is doubt about other associated lesions. The definitive examination is the aortogram, which gives a semi-quantitative indication of the severity and helps to show the basic pathology in the valve.

Treatment

Infants may present with heart failure and require diuretics and digoxin. Surgical treatment should generally be avoided in childhood, but in some patients with prolapsing cusps it may be possible to stop or minimize the regurgitation by repairing the valve. The operation consists of shortening the commissures and buttressing them through the aortic wall onto Teflon pledgets. Where there is an associated high ventricular septal defect it is usually possible to close the defect with a patch and support the cusp attachment by buttress sutures. If the regurgitation is part of a dysplastic valve or due to previous surgery or infective endocarditis, repair is seldom possible and valve replacement is the only surgery possible (see under Aortic valve stenosis).

Supravalvar aortic stenosis

There is a diffuse or localized narrowing immediately above the aortic sinuses and coronary arteries. Most commonly the condition occurs as part of Williams' syndrome (see page 332) but may occur sporadically or as a Mendelian dominant in families. Many patients have peripheral pulmonary artery stenosis in addition to supra-aortic stenosis. From the outside the aorta looks almost normal, but the wall is extremely thick, being composed of fibrous tissue and the lumen narrowed, often to about a third of the normal diameter. There is usually severe, concentric hypertrophy of the left ventricle, often out of proportion to the actual gradient. Fibrosis in the myocardium is common and has been attributed to myocardial ischaemia, which is accentuated by the fact that the stenosis may impair retrograde flow into the coronary arteries in diastole. The aortic narrowing may extend into the arch and, rarely, into the descending aorta. Stenosis of the origins of the arteries arising from the arch is also common.

The clinical presentation is similar to aortic stenosis but the murmur is not as well heard at the left sternal border and the thrill is often best felt over the carotids. The usual clue, however, is the characteristic facies of Williams' syndrome.

The electrocardiogram usually shows left ventricular hypertrophy often with inversion of T waves over the left ventricle. Cross-sectional echocardiography demonstrates the typical narrowing, best seen in the long-axis parasternal and the suprasternal views. When the stenosis is localized to the immediate supra-aortic region it is possible to measure the gradient with continuous-wave Doppler, but this may not be possible if the stenosis extends into the aortic arch. Cardiac catheterization is now seldom used, but will demonstrate the gradient (see Figure 7.4) and angiography confirms the degree of stenosis.

Operation is advised if there is a gradient of 60 mmHg or over, or if the left ventricle looks severely thickened on the echocardiogram. The narrow area is enlarged with a gusset of Dacron to relieve the stenosis as far as possible. This, of course, requires cardiopulmonary bypass. The operation sounds very straightforward, but arrhythmias, poor cardiac output and cardiac arrest are common in the postoperative period, related to the myocardial abnormalities, and most surgeons are cautious about the results of this operation.

Subaortic stenosis

Incidence

Discrete subaortic stenosis is about one-tenth as common as congenital aortic valve stenosis and accounts for about 0.5% of all congenital heart disease.

Definition and pathology

There is a fibrous diaphragm just below the aortic valve. It is attached both to the anterior cusp of the mitral valve and to the interventricular septum. It may also be directly attached to the underside of the aortic valve. Often the diaphragm has a spiral course so that it is attached to the septum and the mitral valve at different levels. It has only recently become clear that the whole subaortic region is abnormal and that there is a covering of fibrous tissue, continuous with the actual diaphragm, around the subaortic region. In addition, the actual subaortic region is frequently narrowed, adding a tunnel type of stenosis to the more obvious diaphragm. The main atrioventricular conducting tissue lies just below this fibrous tissue. About a third of patients with subaortic stenosis also have some degree of valvar stenosis, although this is usually mild. The condition is also seen in association with other left-sided abnormalities, particularly coarctation.

Clinical presentation

When the stenosis is severe, symptoms similar to those of aortic stenosis – breathlessness, chest pain and effort syncope – occur, but it is rare for the stenosis to be severe enough to cause heart failure or collapse in the neonatal period. As in aortic valve stenosis, the murmur is often discovered at routine examination. As with any stenotic murmur it is present from birth. The murmur is usually best heard at the mid left sternal border and in the neonatal period is often mistaken for the murmur of a small ventricular septal defect (which is not normally heard immediately after birth, however). Later, when its radiation to the aortic area becomes more obvious, it simulates aortic valve stenosis, but the absence of a click should arouse the suspicion that the obstruction is subvalvar. A soft, early diastolic murmur is heard in about half of older children and adults with subvalvar stenosis. This is probably due to localized thickening and retraction of one of the aortic cusps due to the jet from the subaortic stenosis.

Radiology

The chest radiograph shows some rounding of the apex consistent with left ventricular hypertrophy, but, unlike valvar stenosis, there is no post-stenotic dilatation of the ascending aorta.

Electrocardiography

The electrocardiogram is the same as in aortic stenosis, showing left ventricular hypertrophy roughly in line with the degree of stenosis.

Echocardiography

The distinction between valvar and subvalvar stenosis can be made by echocardiography with little difficulty. The diaphragm is easily seen on cross-sectional, long-axis views (Figure 7.5) and the associated tunnel narrowing of the left ventricular outflow can be shown. It is usually possible to show the extent of attachment of the diaphragm to the aortic and mitral valve cusps. The M-mode tracings from the aortic valve show a characteristic pattern in which one of the cusps shows abrupt closure early in systole (Figure 7.5). This is due to the fact that the jet is usually eccentric and directed towards only one or two cusps, so that the other one is allowed to close. The aortic cusps also show vibration due to the jet. Left ventricular hypertrophy is assessed in the usual way and also left ventricular function. A careful search for other lesions, particularly of the aortic and mitral valves should be made. An assessment of the gradient can be made in the same way as for aortic valve stenosis using the continuous-flow Doppler probe.

Cardiac catheterization

This is seldom required, as the lesion can actually be better shown by echocardiography, but may be necessary if there is a discrepancy between clinical and echo assessment of severity, or if other lesions are present. The left ventricle is best catheterized retrogradely via the femoral approach and a withdrawal tracing indicates both the position and the severity of the gradient. Angiography may be used to show the diaphragm but, due to the obliquity and occasional spiral course may not show it very clearly.

Treatment

Since the diaphragm can be excised without interfering with the mitral and aortic valves, surgical treatment should be advised in all but the very mild cases. Apart from the risks of symptoms from the obstruction itself, the damage to the aortic valve from the jet tends to increase if the condition is left untreated. It used to be recommended that only enough of the diaphragm be excised to provide adequate relief of the stenosis, but it is now known that much better results are obtained if the whole of the fibrous subaortic region is dissected away from the septum, the aortic valve and the mitral valve. This gives a much larger outflow to the left ventricle and prevents to a large extent the subsequent development of a diffuse tunnel stenosis. The only area where the original lining of the left ventricular outflow is left is in the region of the atrioventricular bundle, to avoid as far as possible the production of complete heart block. Occasionally when the obstruction is mainly of the tunnel type, or after a previous inadequate operation, it may be necessary to insert a gusset between the mitral valve and the septum (on the opposite side to the conducting tissue) to provide adequate enlargement.

Occasionally the mitral valve is abnormal, either with redundant tissue or with abnormal attachment to the septum, so that efforts to free the left ventricular outflow are followed by mitral regurgitation. These cases, and those where the mitral valve is congenitally stenotic, should, if possible, be left until the child is old enough to allow mitral valve replacement with a low profile valve such as the

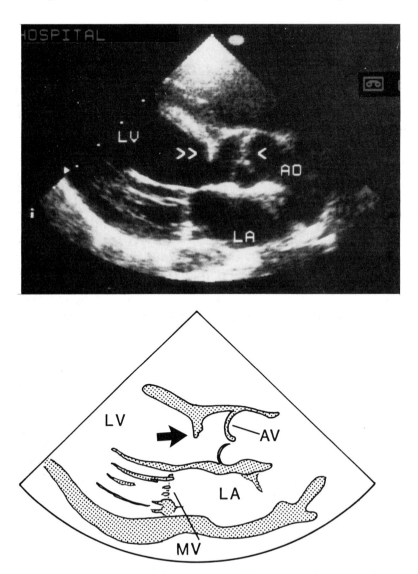

Figure 7.5 Parasternal long-axis view. Subaortic stenosis (arrowed). AV, aortic valve; LA, left atrium; LV, left ventricle; MV, mitral valve

Bjork–Shiley. Since the anterior mitral valve leaflet, which forms the posterior part of the left ventricular outlet, is removed, this automatically relieves the subaortic stenosis and only the protruding part of the diaphragm needs to be removed.

Subaortic stenosis seems to be particularly prone to infective endocarditis, which actually occurs on the aortic valve cusps, causing regurgitation, so that scrupulous prophylactic measures are called for.

Coarctation of aorta

Incidence

This was 6% in the Bristol series.

Definition

The term 'coarctation' is used to describe a constriction in the region of the aorta where the ductus joins it. There is often a discrete shelf of tissue in the aorta at the site of constriction and the aorta proximal to the constriction may show hypoplasia of varying degrees.

Developmental anatomy and pathophysiology

Coarctation is probably caused by spread of the specialized ductal tissue into the adjacent aorta, forming a sling round the aorta (Ho and Anderson, 1979). In *severe* coarctation which presents in the neonatal period, there is usually some degree of isthmic hypoplasia and the ductus is initially patent (Figure 7.6). Blood flow continues as in the fetus from the pulmonary artery through the ductus to the descending aorta. The presence of a coarctation is not evident until the ductus closes. When this happens blood can only enter the descending aorta through the tight coarctation. There is a markedly reduced flow of blood to the kidneys, liver and gastrointestinal tract. Left ventricular failure develops, there is poor urinary output and the baby becomes acidotic, hypoglycaemic and hypocalcaemic.

Associated lesions

Over half the patients with coarctation have other lesions. Ventricular septal defect, mitral valve abnormalities and aortic stenosis are the commonest in the infant group.

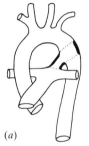 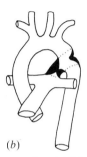 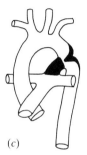 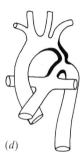

(a)   (b)   (c)   (d)

Figure 7.6 Development of coarctation. (*a*) Prior to birth. (*b*) Immediately following closure of the arterial duct. (*c*) Obliteration of the aortic end of the duct leads to further obstruction. (*d*) Tubular hypoplasia of the isthmus. The contractile tissue, normally confined to the duct, is shown in solid black

Few patients with severe coarctation survive the neonatal period without treatment. Mild coarctation, however, causes no symptoms in early life but Campbell (1970) estimated that 50% of these die by the age of 32 years and 75% by 46 years if no treatment is given.

Coarctation in the newborn

Clinical presentation of severe coarctation

An infant who has been apparently well for the first few days of life suddenly becomes acutely ill. Symptoms occur at some time between the second and tenth days of life but occasionally are delayed if the ductus remains open longer. Symptoms are dramatic. The baby ceases to take feeds and becomes breathless, grey and collapsed with a poor peripheral circulation. The liver enlarges, there is oliguria or anuria and the infant presents a picture of cardiac and renal failure. The brachial pulses are palpable initially and the femoral pulses weak or absent but as the baby's condition deteriorates, all the pulses are poor. Occasionally the ductus may open up temporarily and the pulses in the legs improve again; the clinical picture may vary from hour to hour but there is a gradual downhill course. Heart murmurs are absent or unimpressive. Blood pressure in the arms is higher than in the legs but in collapsed infants the pressure in the arms is not raised above normal. The pulses should be felt in both arms because occasionally the site of the coarctation is *above* the left subclavian artery, the left arm pulses are poor and the blood pressure in the left arm is the same as that in the legs.

Radiography

Chest radiograph shows generalized cardiac enlargement and pulmonary venous congestion.

Electrocardiography

In the newborn there is usually marked right ventricular hypertrophy on the electrocardiogram.

Fetal echocardiography

Allen *et al.* (1988) have shown that the diagnosis of coarctation of the aorta can be made in prenatal life. The finding of increased dilatation of the right ventricle and pulmonary artery compared with the normal, raises the possibility of coarctation; study of the aortic arch shows hypoplasia and Doppler studies demonstrate a diminution of aortic blood flow. These combined findings give a high degree of accuracy as early as 18 weeks of gestational age.

To be able to predict the diagnosis in coarctation is extremely valuable; the echocardiogram can be repeated after birth to confirm the diagnosis and the baby safely referred for sugery before he has become acutely ill.

Echocardiography

This has proved to be a most valuable investigation in confirming the clinical diagnosis of coarctation in newborn infants. The baby lies on his back with padding under the shoulders so that the head and neck extend backwards. The probe is inserted in the suprasternal notch and the echo beam is directed downwards diagonally along the line of the ascending aorta, the arch and the descending aorta. If the coarctation is not seen in that view, the 'ductus view' as described by Smallhorn and Macartney (1984) should be used. The transducer is moved to the left and more into a transverse plane down the left pulmonary artery to the descending aorta. Echocardiography will not only demonstrate the coarctation but also the size of the aorta above the coarctation and the position of the subclavian artery. In most cases a clear anatomical picture is obtained; catheterization is unnecessary and indeed should be avoided if at all possible. It is only done nowadays if echocardiography is unsatisfactory or there is doubt about the aortic arch being interrupted or there are important associated lesions seen on echocardiography.

Treatment

Urgent resuscitation is essential. *Coarctation of the aorta is one of the most important emergencies in babies.* Dramatic improvement results from giving prostaglandins intravenously to open up the ductus and ensure a flow of blood to the lower part of the body. The babies are also severely acidotic, hypoglycaemic and hypocalcaemic and in heart failure. As soon as the prostaglandins are given (in a dose of 0.05 µg/kg/min for the first hour, reducing to 0.02 µg/kg/min), diuretics are begun and the hypocalcaemia, hypoglycaemia and acidosis are corrected. Dopamine in a medium-dose range of 2–10 µg/kg/min intravenously gives immediate inotropic support to the failing myocardium and by dilating peripheral vascular beds reduces some of the after-load on the heart and improves renal function.

A marked improvement occurs in 24 hours and the baby is then referred for surgery when his condition is relatively good. The operation of choice is the subclavian flap operation (Figure 7.7). The aorta is incised longitudinally across the coarctation, the incision is extended up into the left subclavian artery which is then ligated and divided. The coarctation and any shelf-like tissue within the aortic lumen are removed and the subclavian flap is brought down as a gusset. This not only enlarges the size of the aortic lumen but also leaves an elongated rather than a circumferential scar so that there is less tendency for a stricture to redevelop with the growth of the child. Some surgeons believe, however, that ductal tissue may be incorporated into the anastomosis in the newborn infant and cause constriction and they prefer an end-to-end anastomosis for that reason. Re-coarctation occurs in some patients whichever operation is done.

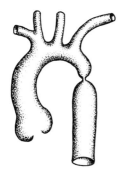 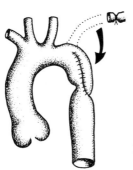

Figure 7.7 Subclavian flap operation for coarctation

It must be emphasized that the use of echocardiography and prostaglandins has revolutionized the management of coarctation in the newborn. The infant is no longer subjected to cardiac catheterization and angiography which caused deterioration in his condition, and the use of prostaglandins allows effective treatment of heart failure and biochemical upset, so that the infant goes for surgery in a much better state than previously. Operative mortality has fallen dramatically.

Balloon dilatation of coarctation

This is not yet in use for naturally occurring coarctation in the newborn but if re-coarctation occurs as the child grows, balloon dilatation can first be tried before further surgery (Figure 7.8). Reduction of the gradient across the coarctation is usually but not always achieved (Lababidi, Daskalopoulos and Stoeckle, 1984).

Certainly, follow-up of postoperative patients by echocardiography is now invaluable and the gradient across the coarctation can be measured by Doppler echocardiography. If the gradient increases and hypertension is developing in the upper limbs, balloon dilatation is advised. If this procedure is unsatisfactory then further surgery is recommended.

Coarctation in newborns associated with ventricular septal defect

If the ventricular septal defect is small, the amount of blood flowing through it is small and the treatment is the same as isolated coarctation.

If the defect is large, the best results are achieved by banding the pulmonary artery at the same time as operating on the coarctation (de Leval, 1986).

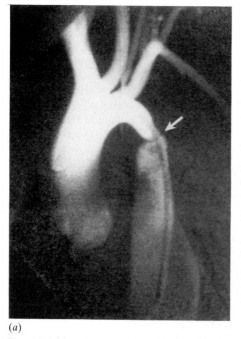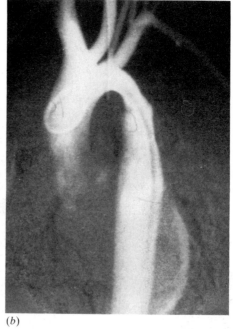

(a)   (b)

Figure 7.8 (*a*) Aortogram before dilatation (angioplasty) shows site of coarctation (arrowed). Radio-opaque dye is diluted below the coarctation. (*b*) Aortogram after angioplasty shows marked improvement at site of narrowing and good concentration of dye in the descending aorta

Coarctation in older children

Clinical presentation

In patients who do not have symptoms in infancy, the diagnosis is usually made at a routine medical examination. The classic sign which establishes the diagnosis of coarctation is that the femoral pulses are absent or weak in the presence of normal or increased brachial pulses. Delayed but easily palpable femoral pulses occur only when there is an *extensive* collateral circulation between the aorta proximal and distal to the coarctation. This is uncommon in early childhood but is seen after the age of 10 years. The blood pressure in the arms is higher than normal. It is important to feel the brachial pulses in both arms because occasionally the coarctation occurs above the origin of the left subclavian artery and the left arm pulses are reduced. The systolic pressure in the legs is lower than that in the arms and there is a reduced pulse pressure. From about the age of 6 years, it is possible to feel collateral vessels in the intercostal spaces down the medial borders of the scapulae. Short systolic murmurs can be heard in the same area. The left ventricular activity is increased but there are no significant precordial murmurs to be heard.

Examination may reveal the presence of associated lesions such as bicuspid aortic valve, mitral valve lesions and ventricular septal defect.

Radiology

The heart may appear normal, but left ventricular enlargement is frequently seen. In severe cases the left atrium is prominent. In an overpenetrated posteroanterior film the aorta assumes a figure 3 shape, the first bulge being the aorta above the coarctation and the second bulge the poststenotic dilatation. The barium-filled oesophagus is similarly indented to give a reverse-3 pattern. In older children and adults notching of the ribs by the collateral vessels is evident. This is rarely seen before 6 years of age (Figure 7.9).

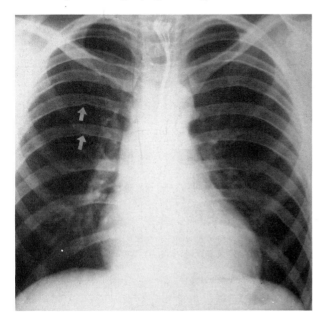

Figure 7.9 Chest radiograph of a patient with coarctation of the aorta, showing left ventricular enlargement and notching of the ribs (arrowed)

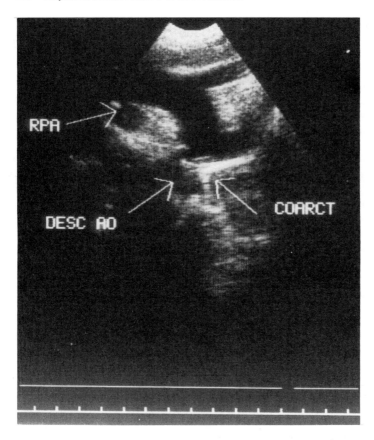

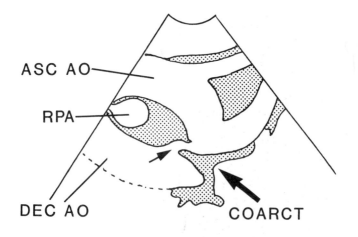

(a)

Figure 7.10 (a) Suprasternal view shows coarctation of aorta (COARCT). ASC AO, ascending aorta; DEC AO, descending aorta; RPA, right pulmonary artery

Electrocardiography

The electrocardiogram may be normal or show left ventricular hypertrophy, depending on the severity of the lesion. Severe left ventricular hypertrophy with inverted T waves over V_5 and V_6 is rare in childhood and its presence usually means that there is an additional lesion such as aortic stenosis. A right bundle branch block pattern is sometimes seen.

Echocardiography

This will demonstrate the presence of other lesions and the gradient across the coarctation can be measured by Doppler studies. The site of the coarctation is defined (Figure 7.10(a)) and as long as there is clinical evidence of a collateral circulation, surgery is advised without further investigation by cardiac catheterization.

Treatment

Operation is carried out nowadays as soon as the diagnosis is made except in *very* mild cases where there is very little hypertension and no collateral circulation. Follow-up studies have shown that if a patient is left with systemic hypertension for some years, then it will not return to normal even after successful surgery (Nanton and Olley, 1976). Now that the subclavian flap operation is available or a Gore-Tex graft may be inserted, there is no reason to delay surgery. Some patients may require further treatment for re-coarctation but this may be resolved by balloon dilatation. If it is not, then it is better to have a second operation and for the patient to become normotensive than to leave him with a high blood pressure.

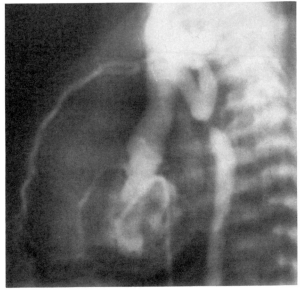

(b)

Figure 7.10 (*b*) Left lateral view of angiogram of coarctation. The catheter has been passed through the foramen ovale and lies in the left ventricle where radio-opaque dye was injected

The mortality of operation is less than 1%. Reactive hypertension may occur within 36 hours of operation but it usually responds quickly to treatment with hypotensive drugs for a few days. Now that patients are diagnosed earlier and operated on without delay, it is very rare to see the so-called 'postcoarctectomy syndrome' in which patients had severe hypertension postoperatively accompanied by abdominal pain, nausea and vomiting. In such patients the hypertension is difficult to control and the abdominal distension and discomfort persist for 3 or 4 weeks but eventually subside. Laparotomy is best avoided unless perforation of the gut is suspected. Bacterial endarteritis remains a risk after surgery and prophylaxis should always be given against it.

Residual hypertension sometimes occurs in the adolescent, particularly if he has been operated on in late childhood. It is also found in patients who have a residual gradient across the coarctation site. Treatment with hypotensive drugs such as atenolol 50–100 mg daily orally is effective.

The blood pressure should be checked routinely at out-patients after repair of coarctation. If hypertension is found re-coarctation must be looked for and if present treated surgically. Hypertension without re-coarctation may persist after operation for coarctation at any age but is less frequent when operation is done early in life. Persistent hypertension should be treated with beta-blockers.

Exercise testing will show systolic hypertension in some patients after operation with or without re-coarctation. If re-coarctation is present it should be relieved. If there is no re-coarctation, drugs will not relieve exercise-induced hypertension in most cases (Martinez *et al.*, 1988).

Aortic ring

In the course of development of the great arteries, the only primitive aortic arch which remains complete is the fourth left arch, which forms the definitive aortic arch. Occasionally, only the right fourth arch remains, this occurring particularly in association with Fallot's tetralogy. Functionally it is of no significance. Very rarely, both left and right fourth arches persist and a vascular ring then encircles the trachea and oesophagus, leading to stridor and difficulty in swallowing in early infancy. There are no abnormal signs in the cardiovascular system, but good radiographs of the chest show compression of the trachea and a barium swallow shows compression of the oesophagus. These findings can be confirmed by oesophagoscopy and laryngoscopy. Angiography is required to show which of the arches is the larger (Figure 7.11), and the opposite arch is divided at thoracotomy.

Anomalous right subclavian or innominate arteries

Atrophy of the proximal rather than the distal portion of the right fourth aortic arch results in a right subclavian artery (less commonly an innominate artery) which arises from the descending aorta and passes behind the oesophagus or between the oesophagus and trachea. Stridor may occur during childhood, and in later life mild dysphagia may occur. Occasionally, a continuous murmur is produced. Otherwise there are no abnormal signs. A barium swallow shows an oblique impression across the oesophagus.

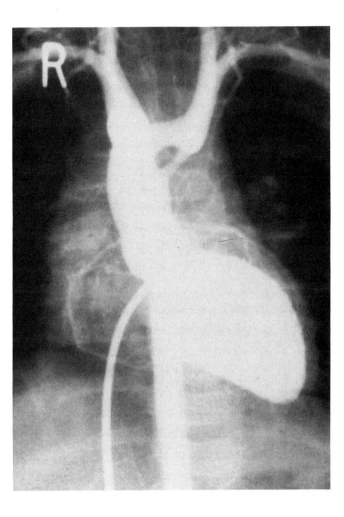

Figure 7.11 Double aortic arch. In this patient the left arch is, unusually, much smaller than the right

Aortic atresia

Complete atresia of the aortic valve is dealt with in the chapter on heart disease in the newborn (page 239).

Mitral stenosis

Isolated congenital mitral stenosis is a very rare lesion although it occurs occasionally in association with aortic atresia and coarctation. The valve cusps are poorly formed and often myxomatous. Breathlessness or pulmonary oedema occurs at any time from the neonatal period onwards. Occasionally, the presentation is that of pulmonary hypertension. The murmur so characteristic in adolescents and adults is frequently not heard in the neonatal period, but in older children it enables the condition to be diagnosed clinically. Otherwise, radiological evidence of pulmonary oedema, and left atrial enlargement, is a helpful guide to the diagnosis which can be confirmed at cardiac catheterization by demonstrating a gradient during diastole between the left atrial (or pulmonary wedge) and left ventricular pressures. Owing to the poor cusp development valvotomy is seldom satisfactory but may, in a young child, produce relief until the child is large enough for prosthetic valve replacement.

Mitral atresia

Complete obstruction of the mitral valve is one cause of the 'hypoplastic left heart syndrome' and is dealt with in Chapter 14 (page 239).

Mitral regurgitation

Formerly mitral regurgitation was regarded as being invariably due to rheumatic fever, but the diminution in the disease together with the early investigation of infants with heart disease, has shown up a small number of patients with isolated congenital mitral regurgitation. In addition, mitral regurgitation is well recognized in endocardial cushion defects, L-(corrected)transposition, endocardial fibroelastosis, hypertrophic obstructive cardiomyopathy and in association with coronary artery or myocardial disease causing left ventricular dilatation. In reviewing isolated mitral regurgitation, Berghius and co-workers (1964) found cleft anterior mitral valve cusps, shortened or absent chordae tendineae, accessory orifices, redundant posterior cusps and deficient posterior cusps.

Natural history

Severe lesions can cause death in infancy. Minor defects are compatible with a normal life-span.

Clinical presentation

Apart from those patients who have heart failure in infancy the lesion is usually discovered at routine examination. Left ventricular enlargement is palpable in moderate or severe disease. In all but the most trivial lesions (when the murmur may be late systolic) there is a loud apical pansystolic murmur. With a large regurgitant flow there is also a short diastolic murmur due to rapid filling of the left ventricle. Signs of pulmonary arterial hypertension may be present.

Radiology

The left atrium and left ventricle are enlarged in moderate and severe regurgitation and the pulmonary veins are congested. If the left atrial pressure is very high, signs of pulmonary oedema (either a diffuse hilar haze or Kerley lines) may be seen. When the lesion is complicated by reactive pulmonary hypertension the main pulmonary artery is prominent.

Electrocardiography

The electrocardiogram shows left atrial and left ventricular hypertrophy.

Echocardiography

The nature and degree of the abnormalities are well shown on echocardiography. Mitral valve prolapse, either from elongated chordae tendineae or absence of chordal attachment of part of the anterior cusp are best seen in the long-axis parasternal view. Clefts in the anterior cusp are well shown in the short-axis view, as is the large single papillary muscle found in parachute mitral valve. Accessory mitral valve orifice is also best seen in short axis. If the left ventricle is dilated and poorly contracting with a mitral valve which looks anatomically normal but stretched over the mitral valve ring without closing in systole, the diagnosis is primary myocardial disease with secondary mitral regurgitation. Estimation of left ventricular stroke volume from M-mode or cross-sectional studies gives some idea of the degree of regurgitation.

To detect mitral regurgitation, the Doppler probe sampling site is positioned initially in the middle of the left atrium, using the apical four-chamber view. The sample is then moved towards the valve centre and then from side to side until the high velocity signal is detected. Colour-flow Doppler is undoubtedly the most sensitive technique and the extent of the regurgitant jet is well shown. Without this, it is possible to get some idea of the severity by seeing how extensively the regurgitant jet can be picked up in the left atrium. Forward flow through the mitral valve in diastole is increased and, by comparing this with tricuspid flow some indication of the regurgitant fraction can be obtained.

Cardiac catheterization

In general, cardiac catheterization and angiography add little to the information obtained by cardiac ultrasound. The left atrial or wedge pressure is usually normal in mild or moderate regurgitation at rest and may be little elevated in severe regurgitation. Pulmonary hypertension may accompany severe forms, but always regresses following successful operation, so that its detection does not influence treatment. Left ventricular angiography gives a semi-quantitative indication of the degree of regurgitation but is less good at indicating the cause than echocardiography.

Treatment

Minor abnormalities require no treatment or restriction. Antibiotic prophylaxis is required for any mitral abnormality. The treatment of major abnormalities is discussed on page 132.

Mitral valve prolapse

In children as well as adults mitral valve prolapse has been increasingly reported over the past decade, although it appears to be uncommon under the age of 10 years, except in association with Marfan's syndrome. Becker and de Wit (1979) have drawn attention to the variable length of chordae tendineae and cusps and it is probable that those diagnosed as 'floppy valves' are one end of a spectrum.

The classic signs are a loud midsystolic click (or series of clicks) and a late systolic murmur. Occasionally the murmur is pansystolic. The signs in mild cases may vary

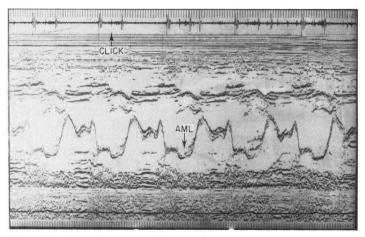

Figure 7.12 Echocardiogram and phonocardiogram of patient with midsystolic click due to mitral valve prolapse. There is an abrupt backward movement of the anterior mitral leaflet (arrowed) in midsystole corresponding to the click recorded on the phonocardiogram

from day to day and according to posture – often being loudest when the child is standing. Occasionally the murmur is very loud when the child stands up and a loud honk is heard. The condition is usually diagnosed without difficulty clinically, but can be elegantly shown by either M-mode or two-dimensional echocardiography (Figure 7.12). Apart from the risk of bacterial endocarditis the condition is benign and requires no treatment or restriction other than penicillin cover for dental extractions.

The question of when mitral valve prolapse becomes mitral regurgitation is usually settled by regarding children with either a midsystolic clock or a late systolic murmur as having mitral valve prolapse and those with a pansystolic murmur as having mitral regurgitation, even if the cause is a floppy or prolapsing valve. The distinction is empirical but useful as those with mitral valve prolapse show no evidence of progression whereas those with pansystolic murmurs will include some with haemodynamically significant lesions and also show a tendency to progress. In addition, a click or late systolic murmur always means prolapse, while a pansystolic murmur may indicate regurgitation due to other mitral pathology.

Treatment of major mitral valve abnormalities

Cross-sectional echocardiography has enabled better diagnosis of the underlying abnormalities and enables those valves which can be repaired to be distinguished from those which will need replacement. The latter are best treated conservatively if at all possible, since mitral valve replacement in children is unsatisfactory (see below). Valves with clefts in the anterior cusp or redundant tissue can be treated by repairing the cleft or plicating the redundant cusp tissue. Where there is a deficiency of the posterior cusp and in some patients with anterior cusp deficiency it is possible to advance the posterior cusp by inserting a patch of pericardium to lengthen the cusp. When the annulus is dilated (provided that myocardial function is normal or only slightly impaired) the annulus can be reduced in size by annuloplasty, that is taking two tucks in the annulus and left atrial wall in the region of the two commissures. Some improvement in parachute mitral valves can be produced by incising the single papillary muscle longitudinally and fenestrating the valve cusps to effectively lengthen the chordae tendineae. This usually improves the mitral obstruction but may make regurgitation worse. Supravalve rings can usually be excised without damage to the mitral valve, but there may be hypoplasia or thickening of the valve itself which makes operation less than curative.

Mitral valve replacement is practicable in children from about 5 years onwards and in some younger children with dominant regurgitation where the valve ring is generally larger than normal. Tissue valves have proved very disappointing, despite their apparent advantage of not requiring anticoagulants, in that degeneration of the cusps proceeds at a much faster rate than in adults so that stenosis and retraction of cusp tissue may make reoperation necessary as early as a year after insertion. The only valves which have proved useful are the tilting disc type such as the Bjork–Shiley. Permanent anticoagulants are required, but have not proved significantly more difficult to control than in adults. The anticipated life of such valves is in the region of 30 years, but when valve replacement has been necessary in the first 5 years of life, replacement with a larger size is usually necessary in adolescence. Echocardiography, particularly measurement of the gradient by Doppler and checking for regurgitation, is part of the follow-up of such patients.

Cor triatriatum

An unusual defect, cor triatriatum consists of a diaphragm, usually with a small hole in it, across the left atrium, separating the pulmonary veins from the mitral valve orifice. The condition is thought to arise either from failure of incorporation of the common pulmonary vein into the left atrium, or from an incorrect positioning of the septum primum. Physiologically the condition simulates mitral stenosis.

Patients usually present in the first two years of life either with cough and breathlessness due to pulmonary oedema or with signs of pulmonary hypertension. There are no murmurs. Radiology shows right ventricular enlargement and pulmonary venous congestion or oedema. Unlike the picture in mitral stenosis the left atrial appendage is not prominent. The electrocardiogram shows right ventricular hypertrophy and, a helpful pointer, left atrial hypertrophy.

Echocardiography is usually successful in making the diagnosis, but it should be noted that the high pressure in the proximal left atrial chamber pushes the diaphragm against the mitral valve, so that it does not occupy the position across the centre of the left atrium shown in anatomical and surgical papers, but it is usually possible to see it extending beyond the mitral valve annulus, thus distinguishing it from a supravalve diaphragm. The other important distinction is that the atrial appendage is on the low-pressure side and therefore small in cor triatriatum.

Cardiac catheterization reveals pulmonary artery hypertension with raised pulmonary artery and pulmonary wedge pressures. Contrast medium injected into the pulmonary artery outlines the left atrium and shows the septum after circulation through the lungs.

The septum can be excised using cardiopulmonary bypass and the heart is then anatomically and physiologically normal. The pulmonary hypertension regresses.

Bibliography and references

Aortic valve stenosis

Campbell, M. (1968) The natural history of congenital aortic stenosis. *British Heart Journal,* **30,** 514
Blackwood, R. A., Bloom, K. R. and Williams, C. M. (1978) Aortic stenosis in children. Experience with echocardiographic prediction of severity. *Circulation,* **57,** 263
Glew, R. H., Varghese, P. J., Krovetz, J., *et al.* (1969) Sudden death in congenital aortic stenosis. A review of eight cases with an evaluation of premonitory clinical features. *American Heart Journal,* **78,** 615
Gundry, S. R. and Behrendt, D. M. (1986) Prognostic factors in valvotomy for critical aortic stenosis in infancy. *Journal of Thoracic and Cardiovascular Surgery,* **92,** 747–754
Hossack, K. F., Neutze, J. M., Lowe, J. B., *et al.* (1980) Congenital valvar aortic stenosis. Natural history and assessment for operation. *British Heart Journal* **43,** 561
Johnson, A. M. (1971) Aortic stenosis, sudden death and the left ventricular baroreceptors. *British Heart Journal,* **33,** 1
Mulder, D. G., Katz, R. D., Moss, A. J., *et al.* (1968) The surgical treatment of congenital aortic stenosis. *Journal of Thoracic and Cardiovascular Surgery,* **55,** 786
Phillips, R. R., Gerlis, L. M., Wilson, N., *et al.* (1987) Aortic valve damage caused by operative balloon dilatation of critical aortic stenosis. *British Heart Journal,* **57,** 168–70
Roberts, W. C. (1970) The congenitally bicuspid aortic valve. *American Journal of Cardiology,* **26,** 72
Scott, L. P. and Feldman, B. H. (1964) Aortic stenosis in infancy. *Pediatrics, Springfield,* **33,** 931
Shackleton, J., Edwards, F. R., Bickford, B. J., *et al.* (1972) Long-term follow up of congenital aortic stenosis after surgery. *British Heart Journal,* **34,** 47
Somerville, J. and Ross, D. N. (1977) Atypical aortic valve stenosis – a diffuse congenital cardiovascular disease – recognition and surgical treatment. *British Heart Journal,* **39,** 930

Subaortic stenosis

Krueger, S. K., French, J. W., Forker, A. D., *et al.* (1979) Echocardiography in discrete subaortic stenosis. *Circulation,* **59,** 506
Somerville, J., Stone, S. and Ross, D. (1980) Fate of patients with fixed subaortic stenosis after surgical removal. *British Heart Journal,* **43,** 629

Coarctation of aorta

Allen, L. D., Chita, S. K., Anderson, R. H., *et al.* (1988) Coarctation of the aorta in prenatal life: an echocardiographic, anatomical, and functional study. *British Heart Journal,* **59,** 356–360
Campbell, M. (1970) Natural history of coartation of the aorta. *British Heart Journal,* **32,** 633–640
Ho, S. Y. and Anderson, R. H. (1979) Coarctation of the aorta. In *Paediatric Cardiology* Vol. 2 (Heart Disease in the Newborn) (eds M. J. Godman and R. M. Marquis), Churchill Livingstone, London, p. 173
Lababidi, Z. A., Daskalopoulos, D. A. and Stoeckle, H. Jnr (1984) Transluminal balloon coarctation angioplasty: experience with 27 patients. *American Journal of Cardiology,* **54,** 1288–1291
de Leval, M. R. (1986) Editorial, 'Surgical management of the neonate with congenital heart disease'. *British Heart Journal,* **55,** 1–3
Martinez, J., Vergara, F., Amaral, F., *et al.* (1988) Systemic hypertension after operation for coarctation of the aorta. Abstract. Association of European Paediatric Cardiologists, Lisbon
Nanton, M. A. and Olley, P. M. (1976) Hypertension after coarctectomy in children. In *The Child with Congenital Heart Disease After Surgery* (eds Langford Kidd and Richard Rowe), Futura Press, London, p. 143
Smallhorn, J. F. and Macartney, F. J. (1984) Suprasternal cross-sectional echocardiography in the assessment of congenital heart disease. In *Echocardiography* (eds A. S. Hunter and R. J. C. Hall), Churchill Livingstone, Edinburgh, pp. 289–302

Mitral regurgitation

Berghuis, K. H., Kirklin, J. W., Edward, J. E. *et al.* (1964) The surgical anatomy of congenital mitral insufficiency. *Journal of Thoracic and Cardiovascular Surgery,* **47,** 799

Cor triatriatum

Ahn, C., Hosier, D. M. and Sirak, H. D. (1968) Cor triatriatum. A case report and review of other operative cases. *Journal of Thoracic and Cardiovascular Surgery,* **56,** 177

Chapter 8

Acyanotic lesions with right heart abnormalities

Pulmonary valve stenosis

Incidence

Isolated pulmonary valve stenosis accounts for 8% of all cases of congenital heart disease.

Definition

The pulmonary valve cannot open normally. The valve cusps are not well formed and the valve is dome-shaped with a central or near central orifice (Figure 8.1(b)). It is thickened and at times almost cartilaginous in consistency. The size of the orifice varies in diameter from 1 mm to two-thirds of that of the valve ring. The right ventricle thickens in relation to the severity of the stenosis and in severe stenosis the cavity of the right ventricle is reduced by the hypertrophied muscle which can cause secondary obstruction to blood flow. The pressure gradient between the right ventricle and pulmonary artery varies from 10–20 mmHg in very mild stenosis, to 100 or even 200 mmHg in severe stenosis. The gradient increases with activity when the cardiac output increases.

Natural history

Severe stenosis may cause death in infancy from right heart failure. Longitudinal studies have helped to clarify what happens with growth. The gradient across the valve varies with the size of the orifice and the amount of blood flowing through it. In mild stenosis, the orifice increases in size with growth and although the blood flow also increases, the increase is relatively less. Since the gradient is related to the fourth power of the diameter of the orifice, a small increase in orifice size can cause a significant reduction in the gradient. If there is severe stenosis there is relatively little increase in orifice size with growth and the increase in pulmonary flow makes the gradient larger. In summary, mild stenosis improves with growth, severe stenosis becomes worse. Although pulmonary stenosis does not cause symptoms in childhood except when it is severe, the right ventricular muscle thickens progressively and the infundibulum becomes narrowed and itself forms further obstruction.

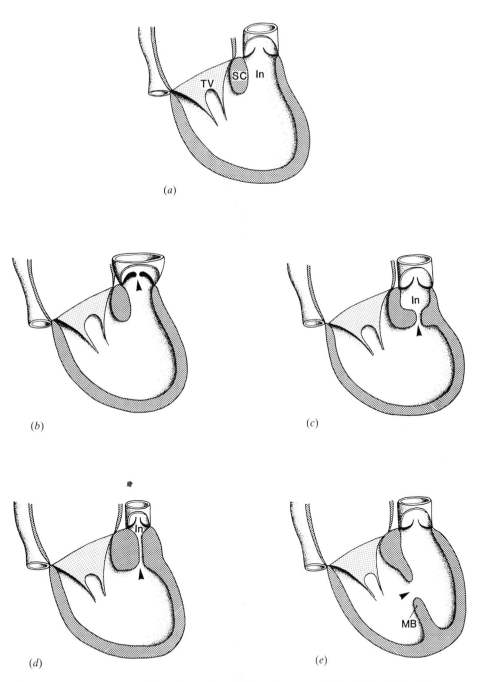

Figure 8.1 Types of right ventricular obstruction. (*a*) Normal anatomy of the right ventricle. (*b*) Pulmonary valve stenosis. (*c*) Localized infundibular stenosis. (*d*) Generalized muscular thickening of the infundibulum. (*e*) Double-chambered right ventricle (obstruction by anomalous muscle bundle). The obstruction sites are arrowed. In, infundibulum; MB, Anomalous muscle bundle; SC, supraventricular crest; TV, tricuspid valve

Clinical presentation

The heart murmur is usually an incidental finding and the child has no symptoms even though the stenosis is severe. When the cardiac output becomes low, however, breathlessness, fatigue, ischaemic chest pain and syncope follow and relief of the stenosis becomes urgent or sudden death may occur, probably due to arrhythmias. Palpitations due to extrasystoles may occur.

The physical appearance is often helpful in making the diagnosis. The child is well nourished, chubby and healthy looking with a moon face and rather a high colour. The lips and tongue, however, are quite pink. The extremities are often cold with peripheral vasconstriction. The peripheral pulses are normal in mild to moderate stenosis but are reduced when there is severe obstruction. In moderate stenosis the A wave in the jugular pulse is accentuated but in severe stenosis it may be 5 cm or more in height and may be palpable. Presystolic pulsation of the liver may also then be felt. There is increased heaving over the right ventricle and this increases with the severity of the stenosis. The left ventricle at the apex may be difficult to feel or is 'tapping' in quality. A systolic thrill in the second left interspace is palpable except in the mildest and most severe forms.

Auscultation is valuable in assessing the severity of the stenosis. The first heart sound is normal and is followed by an ejection click which occurs when the dome-shaped stenotic valve is fully open. The valve must be mobile for an ejection click to occur so it is not heard when the valve is dysplastic and immobile. The click is best heard in the second left interspace and is loudest in expiration. As the stenosis becomes more severe the right ventricular pressure rises more rapidly and the valve opens earlier so that the click occurs earlier. In very severe stenosis the click may disappear completely. The systolic murmur is a rough, loud ejection murmur and is well conducted to the lung apex and particularly over the left lung because the jet through the stenotic valve is carried into the left pulmonary artery which originates as a continuation of the main pulmonary artery. In infants with pinpoint pulmonary stenosis, the stenotic murmur may be very soft. In mild stenosis, right ventricular systole is only slightly prolonged so the murmur is symmetrical and ends before the aortic component of the second sound. In moderate stenosis the murmur ends after the aortic component and in severe stenosis the aortic component may be obliterated by the murmur which is longer because of the prolongation of the emptying of the right ventricle (Figure 8.2).

The second sound also gives clues to the severity of the stenosis. The more severe the stenosis, the longer the duration of the right ventricular ejection; pulmonary valve closure is therefore delayed and the split between the aortic and pulmonary components of the second sound widens. In severe stenosis the split is fixed and in the most severe stenosis the pulmonary component may be inaudible.

Noonan's syndrome (see Chapter 21)

Children with this syndrome have the phenotype of a Turner's syndrome but the chromosomes are normal. One often sees children who have a characteristic facies with widely separated and downward sloping eyes, often with a flattened nasal bridge, and have none of the other features of Noonan's syndrome, but who, like those with Noonan's syndrome, have pulmonary stenosis in which the valve is thick and dysplastic and associated with a small valve ring. Such cases are much more difficult to operate on than the classic thin dome-shaped valves and it is being increasingly recognized that many of these children have cardiomyopathy as well.

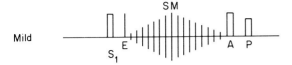

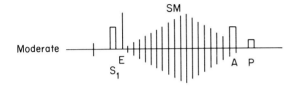

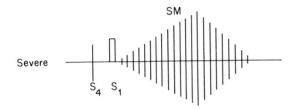

Figure 8.2 The systolic murmur in pulmonary valve stenosis. S_1, first heart sound; A_2, aortic component of second sound; E, ejection click; P_2, pulmonary component of second sound; SM, systolic murmur; S_4, fourth heart sound. *Note*: The ejection click is heard nearer to the first heart sound as the severity of the stenosis increases; in very severe stenosis it disappears

Radiology

The most striking finding is dilatation of the pulmonary artery with a heart of normal size and no increase in the vascularity of the lungs (Figure 8.3). There is no direct correlation between the size of the pulmonary artery and the degree of pulmonary stenosis – it is sometimes obvious in mild stenosis and small in severe stenosis. It is due to the jet of blood coming through the narrowed pulmonary valve and impinging on the wall of the pulmonary artery. There is prominence of the right atrium in moderate and severe cases and in this group the peripheral vascularity in the lungs is diminished. The small size of these vessels is thought to be due to lack of pulsatile flow in them because all the output from the right ventricle must in fact enter the lungs and there is no diminution in the amount of blood reaching them. Enlargement of the heart usually occurs only when the patient is developing symptoms and the heart is beginning to fail(Figure 8.3).

Electrocardiography

The degree of right ventricular hypertrophy is a good guide to the severity of the stenosis. Typical tracings of mild, moderate and severe stenosis are shown in Figure 4.9 (p. 32). In moderate and severe stenosis there is evidence of right atrial hypertrophy (peaked P waves in lead 2).

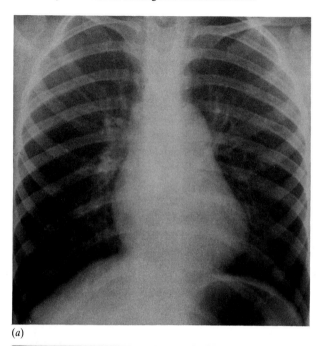

(a)

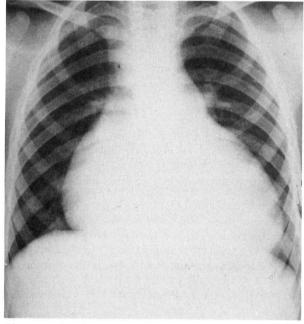

(b)

Figure 8.3 Pulmonary stenosis; chest radiographs. (a) Usual picture in moderate or severe stenosis. The main pulmonary artery is prominent (poststenotic dilatation) but there is no generalized cardiac enlargement. (b) Uncommon picture in a 7-year-old girl with severe pulmonary stenosis who presented with effort syncope and a right ventricular pressure over 200 mmHg at rest. The right atrium and right ventricle are dilated and the lungs are oligaemic

Investigation

Although the clinical findings, electrocardiogram and radiograph can reliably make the diagnosis and tell us whether the stenosis is mild, moderate or severe, nowadays it is usual to carry out echocardiography with Doppler studies. This is not only helpful at the initial examination but will demonstrate changes with the passage of time as the child grows. If the gradient across the valve at rest is less than 30 mmHg, no further investigation or treatment is required and the child should be reviewed in 2–3 years. If the gradient is between 30 and 50 mmHg then the child should be reviewed in a year and if the gradient is increasing treatment may be required. If the gradient is more than 50–60 mmHg then cardiac catheterization with a view to pulmonary valvuloplasty is recommended.

Differential diagnosis

Mild pulmonary stenosis may be confused with a *small* atrial septal defect, but the differentiation of these lesions is not important since neither of them requires treatment. In significant pulmonary stenosis there is a thrill palpable and in atrial septal defect of significant size a tricuspid diastolic flow murmur is heard.

Treatment

The attitude towards treatment of pulmonary stenosis has changed since pulmonary valvuloplasty using a balloon catheter has become possible. Previously an open valvotomy using cardiopulmonary bypass was necessary and was not advised until the gradient was 70 mmHg or more at rest. The situation is now different; we have sufficient knowledge of the natural history of pulmonary stenosis to predict that if a young child has a gradient of 50–60 mmHg at rest, then this will increase with growth and treatment will be required at some time. It seems logical then to relieve the stenosis in such cases as early as possible if we can be sure it will be successful. All the evidence so far shows that a 60–75% reduction in valve gradient is achieved by balloon valvuloplasty and stenosis does not recur. It has been found that balloons which are 20–30% larger than the diameter of the valve are safe and produce a greater reduction in valve gradient than the smaller balloons (Kan *et al.*, 1984; Lock, Keane and Fellows, 1986; Radtke *et al.*, 1986) The exception to this form of treatment is severe stenosis in the newborn infant (see Chapter 14).

Technique
Initial measurement of pressure is carried out to confirm the gradient and right ventricular angiography is done to allow estimation of the size of the pulmonary annulus (Figure 8.4).

An end-hole catheter is used to position a guidewire with a flexible tip in the left pulmonary artery and is then withdrawn. The balloon catheter is introduced percutaneously over the guidewire and is passed across the pulmonary valve. Dilute contrast medium is injected by hand into the balloon and as it inflates 'waisting' of the balloon confirms the correct position (Figure 8.5). As more dye is introduced the waisting disappears and the balloon assumes its full cylindrical shape. The right ventricular pressure rises when the valve is obstructed by the balloon and then the systemic pressure falls. When the balloon is deflated, however, the systemic

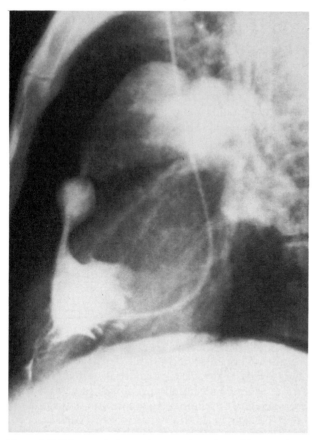

Figure 8.4 Right ventricular angiogram of a patient with pulmonary valvar stenosis (left lateral view). The right ventricle is hypertrophied, especially in the infundibular part, the pulmonary valve is thickened and domed and there is a jet of contrast medium through the centre. The main pulmonary artery shows poststenotic dilatation

pressure rises again and assuming the valvuloplasty has been successful, the right ventricular pressure becomes low. The gradient across the valve is measured after the procedure. In severe cases of pulmonary stenosis there may be some secondary infundibular stenosis due to muscular thickening and a gradient will remain immediately after valvuloplasty, but assuming this has been successful this infundibular gradient will disappear some months later. In most patients the gradient will be reduced by more than two-thirds (Lababidi and Wu, 1983; Kan *et al.*, 1984). Pulmonary regurgitation occurs only rarely after valvuloplasty and does not cause any problems in the low-pressure pulmonary system. Long-term follow-up is not yet available but in the short term there seems to be no evidence of re-stenosis. The electrocardiogram shows that the right ventricular hypertrophy disappears and Doppler echocardiography confirms the abolition of the gradient.

Pulmonary valvuloplasty is now the treatment of choice in isolated pulmonary valve stenosis. The procedure is cheaper, simpler and the child has no scars.

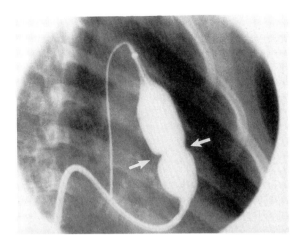

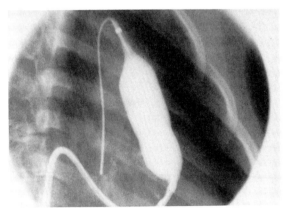

Figure 8.5 Balloon valvuloplasty. Upper frame shows 'waisting' of balloon (arrowed) by narrowed pulmonary valve. Lower frame shows disappearance of 'waisting' after valvuloplasty

Dysplastic pulmonary valve and Noonan's syndrome

In this type of pulmonary stenosis the valve is thick and dysplastic and associated with a small valve ring. Valvuloplasty does not help this type of valve as there is no commissural fusion to tear in the majority of cases (Musewe *et al.*, 1987). Surgical treatment is also difficult and a patch annuloplasty is usually necessary, sometimes with actual excision of the valve. Children with dysplastic valves usually have the features of Noonan's syndrome (see Chapter 21).

Pulmonary infundibular stenosis

Definition

The cavity of the right ventricle is separated into inflow and outflow portions by a band of muscle, the crista supraventricularis. The outflow portion of the ventricle, between the crista supraventricularis and the pulmonary valve, is called the infundibulum, and stenosis of any portion of this chamber is known as infundibular stenosis.

In tetralogy of Fallot infundibular stenosis is common and is associated with ventricular septal defect, but isolated infundibular stenosis associated with an intact ventricular septum is rare, occurring only about one-tenth as commonly as pulmonary valve stenosis. The stenosis may be fibrous, muscular or a combination of both. Two types are described, according to the size of the chamber between the stenosis and the pulmonary valve. A large infundibular chamber is usually associated with a fibrous stricture and a small chamber with muscular narrowing (see Figure 8.1(c)).

Presentation

When there is no interatrial communication there are usually no symptoms. When an atrial septal defect or patent foramen ovale is present, cyanosis may occur due to the right-to-left interatrial shunt. In severe obstruction there may be an accentuated 'a' wave in the venous pulse. The cardiac impulse is usually normal but a loud systolic murmur is heard, maximal in the third or fourth left intercostal space, usually with a thrill. There is no ejection click and the pulmonary element of the second heart sound is usually faint or inaudible.

Investigation

Radiographs of the chest in the frontal view are usually unremarkable unless there is a right-to-left shunt, in which case the lung fields are oligaemic. In the lateral view the right ventricle may be seen to be prominent. The electrocardiogram usually shows right ventricular hypertrophy.

Diagnosis

Although the lower site of the murmur and the absence of an ejection click are useful in distinguishing the condition from pulmonary valvar stenosis, cardiac catheterization is usually required to establish the diagnosis. On withdrawal of the catheter from the pulmonary artery, the pulmonary artery and infundibular systolic pressures are normal but a gradient is shown on further withdrawal into the body of the right ventricle (Figure 8.6). The angiogram demonstrates the obstruction.

Treatment

Operation is usually advised if the pressure in the right ventricle proximal to the obstruction is 80 mmHg or more at rest. Cardiopulmonary bypass or profound hypothermia is required and the obstruction is excised through a right ventriculotomy.

Double-chambered right ventricle

Occasionally, obstruction due to muscle bands is found below the level of the infundibulum. The effect is to divide the right ventricle into two roughly equal chambers (see Figure 8.1(e)). The physical signs are the same as for infundibular stenosis, but the electrocardiogram frequently does not show right ventricular hypertrophy, owing to the relatively small size of the proximal, high pressure chamber.

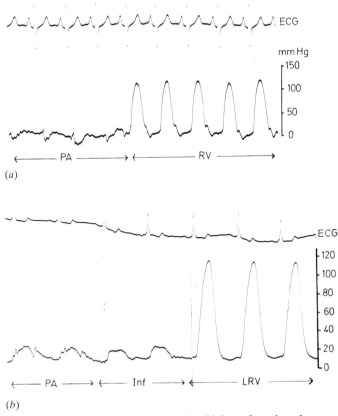

(a)

(b)

Figure 8.6 Pressure traces as the catheter is withdrawn from the pulmonary artery to the body of the right ventricle. (a) Pulmonary valvar stenosis. PA, pulmonary artery; RV, right ventricle. (b) Infundibular stenosis. Inf, infundibulum; LRV, low right ventricle. The systolic pressure in the infundibulum is the same as in the pulmonary artery, the diastolic pressure the same as in the body of the right ventricle

Right ventricular involvement in hypertrophic obstructive cardiomyopathy

In patients with hypertrophic obstructive cardiomyopathy the interventricular septum may bulge into the right ventricle, producing obstruction. A gradient of up to 50 mmHg may be found at cardiac catheterization.

Pulmonary regurgitation

Isolated pulmonary regurgitation is extremely rare. A few of the patients are shown to have complete absence of the pulmonary valve. The condition may complicate disease of connective tissue, such as Marfan's syndrome. (Functional pulmonary regurgitation occurs in severe pulmonary hypertension and a mild degree is common after repair of Fallot's tetralogy.)

Presentation

The condition is asymptomatic in children although tiredness and right heart failure have been reported in patients in late middle-age. A murmur is heard on routine examination or a routine chest radiograph draws attention to the condition. Usually the only sign is a soft diastolic murmur or systolic and distolic murmurs heard in the pulmonary area, but absence of the pulmonary component of the second sound may be noted. The electrocardiogram in children is normal but in adults may show a right bundle branch block pattern. The chest radiograph in older children shows dilatation of the main pulmonary artery, which becomes more marked with increasing age.

Treatment

The condition is benign and no restrictions are required except for prophylaxis against bacterial endocarditis.

Absence of the pulmonary valve

This rare abnormality is associated with a ventricular septal defect. The valve is represented by small nodules of tissue like primitive valve tissue and is grossly incompetent. There is infundibular stenosis. The right and left pulmonary arteries are markedly dilated and there is associated tracheobronchial dysplasia.

Symptoms occur immediately after birth. There is pulmonary incompetence and the heart dilates, often resulting in heart failure. The baby may be cyanosed due to some right-to-left shunting through the ventricular septal defect, but as the pulmonary vascular resistance falls the shunting becomes left to right and the baby is pink. The finding of systolic and diastolic thrills at the left sternal edge is pathognomonic of an absent pulmonary valve and there are systolic and early diastolic murmurs giving a to-and-fro rhythm. Respiratory infections occur because of the tracheobronchial dysplasia and pressure on the bronchi by the large dilated arteries. Such infections occur repeatedly during the first year and require frequent hospitalization as the infants become critically ill.

Radiography

There is marked enlargement of the heart with huge dilated pulmonary arteries.

Electrocardiography

There is right ventricular hypertrophy and if there is a large left-to-right shunt, left ventricular activity is also increased.

Treatment

Conservative treatment is best, although occasionally obstructive emphysema occurs and requires surgery. Attempts have been made to reduce the size of the pulmonary arteries to prevent pressure on the bronchi. Alternatively, the pulmonary artery may be ligated above the valve ring (thus creating pulmonary atresia), a Blalock–Taussig shunt having previously been carried out. The risk of any operation is high in this lesion and markedly so in infants under 1 year of age.

Pulmonary artery stenosis

Obstruction to the flow of blood on the right side of the heart may occur from stenosis of the main pulmonary artery above the valve or from multiple stenoses of peripheral branches.

Peripheral pulmonary stenoses may be caused by maternal rubella. It also occurs in tetralogy of Fallot and in association with the Williams' syndrome (see Chapter 21). Dilatation of the stenoses with balloon catheters has shown encouraging results (Ring, Bass and Marvin, 1985).

Tricuspid stenosis

This is a very rare lesion in childhood. If it is severe, its presentation resembles that of tricuspid atresia, but if mild it causes no symptoms.

Ebstein's anomaly

Although about one-fifth of patients with Ebstein's anomaly are acyanotic, the majority present with a right-to-left shunt at atrial level and are cyanosed. The lesion is discussed in detail in Chapter 9.

Bibliography and references

Acyanotic lesions with right heart abnormalities

Kan, J. S., White, R. I., Mitchell, S. E., *et al.* (1984) Percutaneous transluminal balloon valvuloplasty for pulmonary valve stenosis. *Circulation*, **69**, 554–560

Lababidi, Z. and Wu, J-R. (1983) Percutaneous balloon aortic valvuloplasty. *American Journal of Cardiology*, **52**, 560–562

Lock, J. E., Keane, J. F. and Fellows, K. E. (1986) The use of catheter intervention procedure for congenital heart disease. *Journal of the American College of Cardiology*, **7**, 1420–1423

Musewe, N. N., Robertson, M. A., Benson, L. N., *et al.* (1987) The dysplastic pulmonary valve: echocardiographic features and results of balloon dilatation. *British Heart Journal*, **57**, 364–370

Radtke, W., Keane, J. F., Fellows, K. E., *et al.* (1986) Percutaneous balloon valvotomy of congenital pulmonary stenosis using over-sized balloons. *Journal of the American College of Cardiology*, **8**, 909–915

Ring, J. C., Bass, J. L. and Marvin, W. (1985) Management of congenital stenosis of a branch pulmonary artery with balloon dilatation angioplasty. Report of 52 procedures. *Journal of Thoracic and Cardiovascular Surgery*, **90**, 35–44

Chapter 9

Cyanotic lesions with diminished pulmonary blood flow

Tetralogy of Fallot

Incidence

This accounted for 5% in the Bristol series and *after the first year of life* it is the commonest cyanotic heart lesion.

Definition

Of the four abnormalities which make up the tetralogy of Fallot, the two important ones are pulmonary stenosis and ventricular septal defect (Figure 9.1). The ventricular septal defect is large, about the size of the aortic orifice, and it lies beneath the aortic valve more anteriorly than usual. Stenosis is present in the infundibulum and at the pulmonary valve. The other two components of the 'tetralogy' are hypertrophy of the right ventricle and over-riding of the aorta across the ventricular septal defect.

There is a spectrum of severity of this lesion and the factor which determines the severity is the degree of infundibular and pulmonary valve stenosis. When that narrowing is severe more of the desaturated blood from the right ventricle enters the aorta through the ventricular septal defect. When the stenosis is mild, most of the right ventricular blood enters the pulmonary artery and it is only during exercise that a significant amount of right ventricular blood enters the aorta.

Immediately after birth in some infants the degree of pulmonary stenosis may be so mild that there is a left-to-right shunt through the ventricular septal defect. As the child grows, the degree of infundibular narrowing increases, the left-to-right shunt ceases and gradually a right-to-left shunt occurs.

The right ventricular hypertrophy and over-riding aorta are not important in understanding the haemodynamics of the lesion. The size of the right-to-left-shunt is determined by the pulmonary valve and infundibular stenosis and not by the amount of over-ride of the aorta. The right ventricular hypertrophy is secondary to the increased pressure in the right ventricle. This pressure is always systemic pressure because the right ventricle is in contact with the aorta through the large high ventricular septal defect.

A small number of patients are seen in whom there is severe narrowing of the outflow tract from the right ventricle and who also have aortopulmonary collateral vessels supplying the lungs. Such cases more closely resemble pulmonary atresia with ventricular septal defect, but usually have central pulmonary arteries present, albeit small.

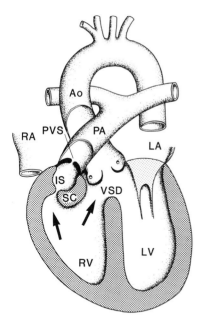

Figure 9.1 Anatomy of Fallot's tetralogy. The aorta (Ao) over-rides the ventricular septal defect (VSD) and both valvar (PVS) and infundibular (IS) pulmonary stenoses are illustrated. LA, left atrium; LV, left ventricle; PA, pulmonary artery; RA, right atrium; RV, right ventricle; SC, supraventricular crest

Natural history

The natural history was not documented before surgical help became possible and will never now be accurately known. In Abbott's series (1936) the average age at death was 12 years. There is a high death rate in severe cases in the first year of life and this falls after 2 years of age but most children gradually deteriorate in the first 3 or 4 years of life. The study of Bertranon *et al.* (1978) shows that without treatment only half the children born with this lesion survive their third birthday. There is then a progressive deterioration around puberty and death usually occurs in the second decade.

Patients who have little or no right-to-left shunt may remain virtually asymptomatic well into middle age, but even in those patients polycythaemia tends to develop and thromboembolism may occur.

Clinical presentation

The majority of infants are pink at birth and gradually become cyanosed as they grow. Initially some infants present with signs of a ventricular septal defect with a left-to-right shunt and minimal pulmonary stenosis; gradually, after a variable period, the pulmonary stenosis increases and the resistance to flow of blood into the lungs becomes greater than the systemic resistance and a right-to-left shunt occurs and the patient becomes cyanosed.

Some infants, usually around 4–6 months of age, present with 'cyanotic attacks'. These attacks most commonly occur in the mornings after breakfast and after the infant has had a good night's sleep. The infant becomes irritable and cries as though in pain, becomes increasingly cyanosed and breathless and then loses consciousness. The attack is due to spasm of the infundibulum which prevents right

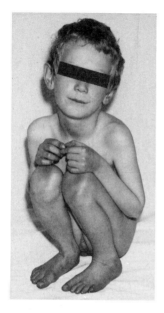

Figure 9.2 Squatting demonstrated by a patient with Fallot's tetralogy

ventricular blood reaching the lungs and it therefore flows into the aorta. As the child loses consciousness the infundibulum relaxes and recovery gradually occurs. Nevertheless some infants may die during an attack or suffer from the effects of cerebral anoxia. Interestingly, some of the worst cyanotic attacks occur in babies who appear to be pink between the attacks and the serious significance of the attacks is often ignored. The mother may be the only person who observes them. Although the heart murmur due to blood flowing through the narrowed infundibulum disappears when the infundibular spasm occurs, it recurs when the child recovers. *All children, therefore, who have a history of such attacks should be examined for the presence of a heart murmur and if a murmur is present, they must be referred to a cardiac unit without delay.*

Some children do not have attacks but gradually become more cyanosed with limitation of activity. This often becomes evident when the child begins to walk and after bouts of exercise the child may be observed to squat. He sits with his knees up to his chest and, as he does so, becomes gradually less cyanosed and less breathless, and then resumes activity again (Figure 9.2). *Squatting* is a very important finding because its occurrence makes tetralogy of Fallot the most likely diagnosis. Squatting in any other lesion is exceptionally rare.

The way in which squatting benefits the patient has been imperfectly understood. It is best first to consider what happens when a patient with tetralogy of Fallot exercises. During the period of exercise a large oxygen debt is built up, the muscle vascular beds are dilated and there is an increase in the extraction of oxygen locally so that the amount of oxygen in the systemic venous blood is reduced more than usual. In tetralogy of Fallot such a reduction of oxygen in the venous blood causes a further fall of oxygen content in the arterial blood, because some of the venous return to the right heart is shunted directly into the aorta. Furthermore, the vasodilatation in the muscles lowers the systemic vascular resistance, and thus lowers the systemic blood pressure which favours an increase in the amount of blood flowing from the right ventricle into the aorta. The patient therefore becomes intensely blue.

Squatting helps to counteract the effects of exercise in two ways.

1. The arterial blood flow to the legs is reduced during squatting and this helps to maintain the systemic resistance so that more blood enters the lungs.
2. The venous return from the legs is slowed and therefore the oxygen debt after exercise can be paid off over a longer period and this corrects the sudden fall in arterial oxygen saturation.

Gunteroth and co-workers (1968) have shown that there is a diminished flow of blood in the inferior vena cava in the squatting position and this is accompanied by a rise in systemic arterial pressure and a rise in arterial oxygen saturation.

In some children the progress of the disease is slow and they continue to live reasonable, though slightly restricted, lives until they reach puberty. It is worth mentioning that heart failure in tetralogy of Fallot is extremely rare in childhood. Its presence makes the diagnosis doubtful or raises the possibility of bacterial endocarditis complicating the disease.

The degree of cyanosis and clubbing of fingers and toes varies with the severity of the disease. The conjunctivae are often injected. A prominent 'a' wave may be seen in the neck. There is usually a systolic thrill in the second, third and fourth left interspaces close to the left of the sternum and a systolic murmur of the ejection type is heard in the same area. The murmur is caused by infundibular stenosis and not by blood flowing through the ventricular septal defect – it must be remembered that the peak systolic pressure is the same in both ventricles.

Blood count

The red cell count and haematocrit level are elevated. This usually correlates well with the severity of the arterial desaturation and the severity of the pulmonary stenosis. An exception occurs when the infant is iron deficient. The haemoglobin may then be normal or low although there is nearly always some polycythaemia and a normal or raised packed cell volume.

Radiology

The heart is not enlarged. The aortic arch can usually be identified lying on either the left or the right side of the trachea (Figure 9.3). It is on the right side in 25% of patients. The size of the ascending aorta can often be assessed. The small apex of the heart suggests right ventricular enlargement. Marked concavity in the upper left cardiac border suggests a small pulmonary artery; a convex shadow in that region suggests that the pulmonary artery is of good size. The vascularity of the lungs is reduced to a degree depending on the severity of the pulmonary stenosis.

Electrocardiography

In the newborn infant, the electrocardiogram may differ little from normal, although the T wave may be positive in V_1 in infants with tetralogy of Fallot. As the infant with the severe form of the disease becomes older, severe right ventricular hypertrophy is seen. The R wave in V_4R and V_1 is tall and there is an S wave in V_5 and V_6. The P wave in lead 2 is often peaked in appearance, indicating right atrial

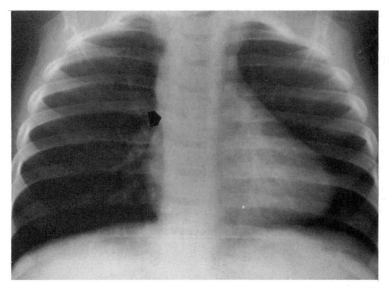

Figure 9.3 Chest radiograph in Fallot's tetralogy. The arrow points to the right-sided aorta

hypertrophy. A Q wave in V_4R or V_1 is unusual in tetralogy of Fallot and suggests the possibility of corrected transposition of the great vessels with pulmonary stenosis, or severe pulmonary stenosis and atrial septal defect.

Echocardiography

In cross-sectional echocardiography the ventricular septal defect is seen just below the aortic valve and the aorta can be seen to over-ride the ventricular septum to varying degrees (Figure 9.4(a)). The narrowed outflow tract to the lungs can be seen (Figure 9.4(b)) and Doppler echocardiography can estimate the gradient across the outflow tract. Stenoses of the main pulmonary arteries should be looked for and assessed. The size of the right pulmonary artery can be checked using the suprasternal view.

Cardiac catheterization

If echocardiography shows the anatomy to be straightforward cardiac catheterization is not necessary, but if there are additional abnormalities such as stenosed pulmonary artery branches then angiography will give the surgeon a clearer picture of the abnormal anatomy (Figure 9.5). Nevertheless, as echocardiography produces better pictures, invasive investigation will become unnecessary.

Complications

Cerebral thrombosis
Cerebral thrombosis is most common in severely cyanosed infants and young children and may cause hemiplegia. Such children may have high haematocrit values and should always be kept well hydrated so that the viscosity of their blood is

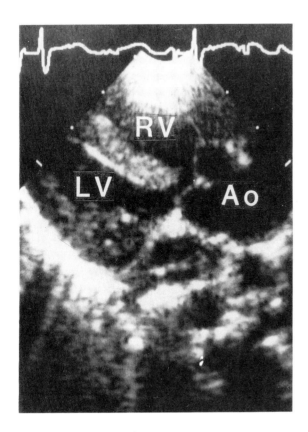

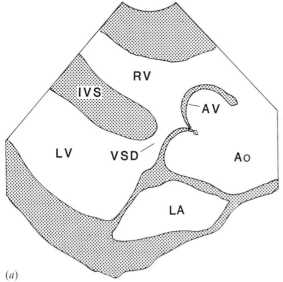

(a)

Figure 9.4 (a) Cross-sectional echocardiogram, long-axis view, showing over-riding of the aorta in tetralogy of Fallot. Ao, aorta; AV, aortic valve; IVS, interventricular septum; LA, left atrium; LV, left ventricle; RV, right ventricle; VSD, ventricular septal defect.

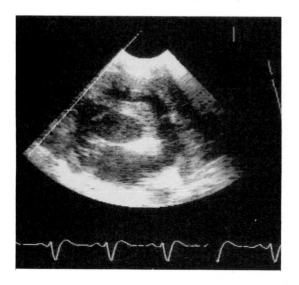

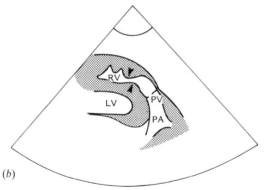

(b)

Figure 9.4 (b) Echocardiogram of tetralogy of Fallot. This is a systolic frame showing infundibular narrowing (arrowed) LV, left ventricle; PA, pulmonary artery; PV, pulmonary vein; RV, right ventricle

not further increased by dehydration. Martelle and Linde (1961), however, have found a closer relationship between the presence of relative anaemia and hemiplegia, than between high haematocrit levels and hemiplegia.

Cerebral abscess
A diagnosis of cerebral abscess should always be considered in a child with tetralogy of Fallot who presents with headaches, fever and a change of personality followed by vomiting, convulsions and localizing cerebral signs. A hemiplegia may occur insidiously. Cerebral abscess is hardly ever associated with bacterial endocarditis. It is possible that there is some localized cerebral damage following thrombosis and that infection subsequently occurs when there is a systemic bacteraemia. Early diagnosis with prompt treatment nowadays carries a good prognosis in this condition. It must be stressed that a shunt operation does not alter the incidence of cerebral abscess and is another reason why complete correction is a

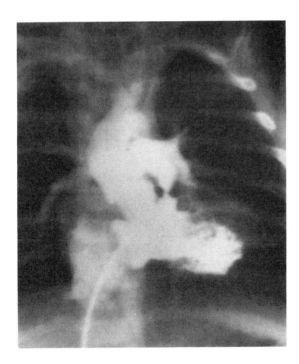

Figure 9.5 Right ventricular angiogram of a 6-month-old infant with Fallot's tetralogy. The infundibular stenosis is well shown, the pulmonary arteries are small and most of the contrast has passed backwards through the ventricular septal defect and entered the aorta

preferable operation if the child's size permits it. Taussig *et al.* (1971), in their long follow-up study of patients who had shunt operations, found an incidence of 5.5%.

Bacterial endocarditis
Bacterial endocarditis should be suspected in patients with unexplained fever. The associated anaemia in bacterial endocarditis may not be appreciated in tetralogy of Fallot because the haematocrit value is usually very much higher than normal, so a normal blood count in a patient with tetralogy of Fallot indicates some degree of anaemia. The follow-up of Taussig *et al.* (1971) showed an incidence of bacterial endocarditis of 14.3% and a mortality rate of 21.4%.

Haemorrhagic tendency
Any operation in patients with tetralogy of Fallot may be associated with excessive bleeding. This is probably associated with the lowered platelet count and is best controlled by transfusing with fresh whole blood. Sudden blood loss in a child with tetralogy of Fallot may aggravate the hypoxia to a dangerous degree.

Treatment

Restriction of exercise is unnecessary since such patients restrict themselves. It should be ensured that infants and young children have adequate supplies of iron so that they do not become relatively anaemic. If a child with tetralogy of Fallot is found to have a *relatively* low haemoglobin the response to iron therapy may be dramatic and cause marked improvement in symptoms. There should be scrupulous care of the teeth and prophylactic penicillin should be given to cover dental extraction. Dehydration should be prevented during intercurrent illnesses. Loss of blood from any cause may require transfusion to prevent hypotension occurring.

Cyanotic attacks are thought to be due to infundibular spasm. Infants are helped by being placed in the knee–elbow position (a similar position to squatting) and 100% oxygen given by mask. If the attack continues propranolol 0.1 mg/kg i.v. as a bolus is of value. Morphine 0.2 mg/kg will help to terminate an attack. Acidosis develops during an attack and this should be corrected by giving intravenous sodium bicarbonate. An alternative method of terminating an attack is to give a drug which increases the peripheral vascular resistance such as metaraminol (0.2 mg/kg i.m. or i.v.). Digoxin should not be used in patients with cyanotic attacks and it is never indicated in tetralogy of Fallot; it increases the contraction of the heart muscle and may further narrow the outflow tract from the right ventricle.

Cyanotic attacks are an indication for surgical treatment but if for any reason this has to be delayed, then propranolol should be continued orally in a dose of 1.0 mg/kg, 6- or 8-hourly. The long-term results of propranolol are not as good as a successful shunt operation.

Surgical treatment

All patients require surgery at some time but the choice of operation and the time it is carried out varies with the clinical severity of the lesion, the type of anatomy demonstrated at investigation and the size of the child. It must be emphasized again that there is a wide spectrum of severity in patients with tetralogy of Fallot.

If the infundibular stenosis is localized and the pulmonary valve ring and pulmonary arteries are of a good size and free of stenoses, then total correction can be carried out any time that the child's symptoms justify it. The sooner such cases are operated on the better, because the child can grow up leading a normal life and the secondary effects of the lesion on the heart muscle regress. Also it avoids complications due to palliation such as kinking and narrowing of the pulmonary arteries. The operation is carried out using cardiopulmonary bypass. The infundibular muscle is resected and a pulmonary valvotomy carried out. The ventricular septal defect is closed with a patch.

At the other end of the spectrum are patients who have long and tortuous infundibular stenosis, a small pulmonary valve ring and small pulmonary arteries which have stenoses at their origins. The risks of early correction in such patients are high and palliative surgery is necessary. The palliative operation of choice is:

A shunt operation in which the subclavian artery is anastomosed to the right or left pulmonary artery so that the flow of blood to the lungs is increased (Blalock–Taussig operation) (see Chapter 5). If the subclavian artery is small a Gore-Tex graft can be inserted between the subclavian artery and the pulmonary artery. Moulton *et al.* (1985), in comparing the classic Blalock–Taussig shunt and modified Gore-Tex shunts in 45 patients, found that the modified shunts were best reserved for the newborn and patients with severe hypoplasia of the pulmonary or subclavian arteries and ensured a satisfactory shunt with immediate improvement. The classic Blalock–Taussig shunt should be used in other cases; it gives excellent long-term palliation and avoids the risks associated with the use of a prosthesis.

Following palliative surgery, definitive surgery is necessary at a time depending on the child's symptoms and size. Such patients usually require an onlay patch to enlarge the outflow tract. This patch may be confined to the infundibulum or extend across the valve ring into the pulmonary artery. The ventricular septal defect is closed with a patch.

Following definitive surgery almost all patients have a residual systolic murmur and a diastolic murmur due to pulmonary regurgitation – particularly those in whom a patch has been inserted across the pulmonary valve. There is usually a dramatic improvement in exercise tolerance and postoperative studies (Finnegan *et al.*, 1976) show near normal values.

As in most operations nowadays, the aim is to make the heart as normal as possible as soon as possible so that the heart muscle is not overloaded for a long time and can return to normal function after surgery as the child grows.

Late complications and results of definitive surgery

Ventricular ectopic beats may occur and should be treated with phenytoin or propranolol. If complete heart block occurs a pacemaker is necessary. Pulmonary incompetence is common but has little harmful effect. The work of Hegerty, Anderson and Deanfield (1987) suggests that progressive damage to the right ventricular muscle by fibrous tissue occurs with increasing age *before* surgery and there may be a lower incidence of ventricular ectopic beats when operations are performed early in life.

Fuster *et al.* (1980) report excellent late results in 87% of hospital survivors. Of those that died, 4% had a residual ventricular septal defect; 2% died from a cardiac cause and 2% from a non-cardiac cause. Three per cent died suddenly.

Tetralogy of Fallot with bronchopulmonary collateral arteries

Occasionally one sees patients with the anatomy of a tetralogy of Fallot with severe narrowing of the right ventricular outflow tract, who also have arteries coming from the aorta which either enter the lung directly at the hilum or enter the main pulmonary artery. It is as though the child was born with tetralogy of Fallot and naturally occurring shunts. The arteries usually have stenoses on them as they enter the lung or the central pulmonary arteries. These central pulmonary arteries are connected with the entire pulmonary vascular bed and palliative surgery using a shunt will help the pulmonary arteries to grow so that definitive surgery will be possible in the future (Ramsay, Macartney and Haworth, 1985).

Pulmonary atresia with ventricular septal defect

Incidence

This was 1% in the Bristol series.

Definition

In this deformity the ventricular septal defect lies in the same position as in tetralogy of Fallot – or even more anteriorly, but there is complete obstruction to flow of blood from the right ventricle to the pulmonary artery. All the right ventricular blood enters the aorta. The site of atresia varies. There may be atresia of the valve only and the central pulmonary artery and its branches are well formed (Figure 9.6(a)). More often there is complete obstruction of the infundibulum with small pulmonary arteries. Blood may enter the pulmonary arteries either by a patent ductus arteriosus or by major aortopulmonary collateral arteries or both.

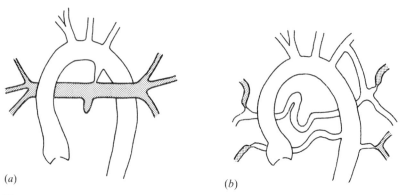

Figure 9.6 Blood supply to the lungs in pulmonary atresia with ventricular septal defect; ▨ = low resistance vascular bed. (*a*) The central pulmonary arteries are present and supply to the lungs is through the patent ductus arteriosus only. (*b*) The central pulmonary arteries are absent and supply to the lungs is through major aorto-pulmonary collateral arteries which arise from the aorta and have stenoses on them as they enter the lungs

These collateral arteries are large and tortuous and arise from the aortic arch or the upper part of the descending aorta. They usually have stenoses on them as they enter the lungs. The central pulmonary arteries are often small and seagull shaped but may be absent, in which case the aortopulmonary collateral arteries enter the lungs at the hilum (Figure 9.6(b)). Usually the amount of blood reaching the lungs is decreased but occasionally the patent ductus may be large and there are large aortopulmonary collateral vessels resulting in increased pulmonary blood flow.

Natural history

Patients who are dependent on a patent ductus for pulmonary blood flow die if the duct closes. Some patients who have a good pulmonary blood flow from collateral arteries lead a restricted life well into the third decade.

Clinical presentation

Cyanosis occurs earlier than in tetralogy of Fallot, usually in the newborn period. There are no cyanotic attacks subsequently and the patients never squat. There is no systolic murmur in the pulmonary area but if the ductus is patent a continuous murmur is heard in the pulmonary area. When there are collateral arteries, continuous murmurs are heard over the lungs anteriorly or posteriorly. Heart failure occurs in the rare cases with excessive pulmonary blood flow; such patients may be diagnosed as having a patent ductus but the widespread continuous murmurs, often well heard at the back, the slight cyanosis and right ventricular hypertrophy on the electrocardiogram, contradict this.

Radiology

Radiological appearances are similar to tetralogy of Fallot but there is marked pulmonary oligaemia and a longer left cardiac border.

Electrocardiography

The electrocardiogram resembles that seen in tetralogy of Fallot, with right axis deviation and right atrial and right ventricular hypertrophy.

Echocardiography

The large ventricular septal defect and over-riding aorta are clearly seen on cross-sectional echo. There is no pulmonary valve visible and no flow of blood from the right ventricle to the lungs on Doppler studies. The ductus may be seen and Doppler echocardiography shows blood flow through it into the pulmonary artery. In some patients no main pulmonary artery can be seen.

Cardiac catheterization

Investigation in this lesion is difficult and time-consuming. The nature of perfusion of the lungs is even more complex than used to be thought. A collateral artery may be the sole supply of blood to a particular region of lung, but at other times there are duplicate sources of pulmonary blood supply. Selective injections of collateral arteries are necessary to demonstrate this duplicate supply which Fäller *et al.* (1981) found in 65% of cases. It is also important to find out whether there are stenoses on these collateral vessels and to measure the pressure in them. It is essential to show whether central pulmonary arteries are present; they appear late in an angiocardiographic sequence when they fill retrogradely from collateral arteries. Injection into pulmonary veins will fill these low pressure central pulmonary arteries retrogradely and demonstrate their size (Singh, Astley and Rigby, 1980).

Treatment

The decision about treatment is related to the pulmonary blood supply and this is usually both complex and variable.

In the rare case in the newborn infant when the atresia is at the pulmonary valve only and the patient is dependent on flow through the ductus to supply the lungs, prostaglandins are given to keep the duct open until surgery can be arranged (see Chapter 2). A pulmonary valvotomy is done initially and closure of the ventricular septal defect deferred until later.

In the majority of cases, however, the pulmonary valve is absent and the outflow tract of the right ventricle ends blindly without any potential connection to the main pulmonary artery. Blood flows to the lungs through major aortopulmonary collateral arteries with or without a patent ductus. The central pulmonary arteries are often small and in some cases do not connect with enough lung segments to make a shunt operation beneficial. In others a shunt operation helps the child initially but further shunt operations may be required as the child grows. It is hoped that shunt operations will make the central pulmonary arteries grow but this does not always happen and the results are disappointing.

The aim subsequently is to carry out some definitive surgery but this is often difficult, or impossible. The factors which affect the possibility of correction are:

1. The presence and size of central pulmonary arteries;
2. The stenosis in central and intrapulmonary arteries (the stenoses may be distal to any suitable point for anastomosis);

3. The presence of pulmonary vascular obstructive disease;
4. The amount of lung parenchyma actually connected to the central pulmonary arteries.

If all the intrapulmonary arteries are connected to unobstructed confluent central pulmonary arteries (Figure 9.6(a)) a single pressure head supplies all the parenchyma of both lungs, i.e. there is a unifocal pulmonary blood supply, but this is infrequent. Usually the intrapulmonary arteries are supplied by major aortopulmonary collateral arteries directly or by way of the main pulmonary arteries, i.e. there is a multifocal pulmonary blood supply (Figure 9.6(b)) (Macartney, Scott and Deverall, 1974).

When there is a unifocal blood supply with pulmonary arteries of a good size, a conduit can be inserted from the right ventricle to the central pulmonary artery and the ventricular septal defect closed. When there is a multifocal blood supply a single stage repair is not possible. Attempts have been made to try to achieve unifocalization of the pulmonary blood supply with a view to definitive repair by anastomosing major aortopulmonary collateral arteries to central pulmonary arteries without sacrificing segmental perfusion (Sullivan et al., 1988). Although this resulted in improvement of symptoms and a rise in systemic oxygen saturation, there was an appreciable mortality (4 of 26 patients died). Furthermore, the central pulmonary arteries did not increase in size sufficiently to permit complete repair.

If there are no central pulmonary arteries the situation is even worse from the surgical point or view. Ingenious operations have been devised to try to connect the major aortopulmonary vessels together and make a unifocal blood supply. This means several operations and sometimes the patient is not improved.

It must be remembered that many patients have mild symptoms and live reasonable lives and some surgical procedures may make them worse – or no better. Older children will often have developed pulmonary vascular obstructive disease which then rules out any surgical help other than a heart–lung transplant.

Pulmonary atresia with intact ventricular septum

Incidence

Pulmonary atresia with intact ventricular septum comprises less than 1% of all cardiac malformations.

Definition

The right ventricular cavity is always small and often minute. Bull et al. (1982) proposed a revised classification of the right ventricular morphology. There are three components: inlet, trabecular and outlet portions. (The inlet portion incorporates the tricuspid valve and its apparatus; the trabecular portion is beyond the papillary muscles of the tricuspid valve towards the apex; the outlet portion leads up to the pulmonary valve.) In pulmonary atresia with intact ventricular septum, the trabecular portion is frequently almost obliterated by myocardial hypertrophy leaving a two-portion right ventricle. When the right ventricular hypertrophy is more severe, the outlet portion is obliterated also, leaving a tiny cavity consisting of an inlet portion only. Zuberbuhler et al. (1979) showed that the outflow tract obstruction is rarely at the pulmonary valve only. The tricuspid valve

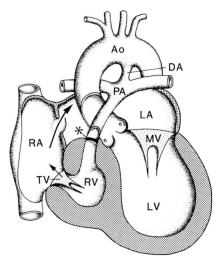

Figure 9.7 Pulmonary atresia with intact ventricular septum and hypoplastic right ventricle. Ao, aorta; DA, ductus arteriosus; LA, left atrium; LV, left ventricle; MV, mitral valve; PA, pulmonary artery; RA, right atrium; RV, right ventricle; TV, tricuspid valve. The atretic pulmonary valve is marked with an asterisk

is hypoplastic because of the hypoplastic ventricle and it is often thickened and dysplastic, or may have an Ebstein-like malformation. Unlike pulmonary atresia with a ventricular septal defect, there is always a central pulmonary artery supplied by a patent ductus arteriosus (Figure 9.7).

Natural history

Death usually occurs in the first few months of life if no treatment is available (Moller and co-workers, 1970).

Clinical presentation

Cyanosis is present on the first or second day of life. The baby becomes breathless and liver enlargement occurs. There are usually no heart murmurs, though occasionally the murmur of tricuspid incompetence occurs. Flow of blood to the lungs is entirely dependent on the ductus remaining patent and if it closes the patient dies.

Radiology

The chest radiograph shows some cardiomegaly after the first day or two of life. The right atrium is prominent. The pulmonary vascular markings are usually diminished unless the ductus is widely patent.

Electrocardiography

The electrocardiogram shows peaked, tall P waves indicating right atrial enlargement. There is a normal QRS axis. In the cases with hypoplastic right ventricle the anterior precordial leads (V_1 and V_2) show less right ventricular activity than is usually seen in infancy (or there may be left ventricular hypertrophy) and this pattern, in a severely cyanosed infant with oligaemic lung fields, is highly suggestive of pulmonary atresia with intact ventricular septum.

Echocardiography

The right ventricular morphology can be assessed by cross-sectional echocardiography, particularly in determining whether there is an outlet portion of the ventricle. Doppler echocardiography will exclude any flow of blood from the right ventricle into the pulmonary artery, confirming the atretic valve. The atrial septum is seen to bulge to the left. The ductus can be seen and the size of the pulmonary artery and its main branches assessed.

In the majority of cases echocardiography gives enough information in the newborn for a decision to be made regarding surgery.

Cardiac catheterization

This is carried out in the first instance only in patients who need an atrial septostomy (see below). At the same time angiography will show whether there are any right ventricular myocardial sinusoids which communicate with the coronary circulation. These sinusoids indicate a poor prognosis (see below). Cardiac catheterization is also performed if necessary before deciding about definitive repair of the lesion.

Treatment

All these infants are dependent for survival on the ductus remaining patent. Initially treatment is with intravenous prostaglandins (see Chapter 2) to ensure that the ductus remains patent to supply the lungs with blood. Surgical treatment is essential in all these infants and the type of surgery advised depends on the anatomy.

If there is an outflow portion of the right ventricle, a transpulmonary valvotomy should be performed in order to decompress the right ventricle in the hope that the massive hypertrophy will regress. In rare cass in which the right ventricle is of good size, this will suffice, but in the majority a shunt operation is also required to ensure an adequate blood flow to the lungs. Recently Hamilton et al. (1987) have described 6 infants in whom a balloon catheter was used to carry out the valvotomy. The catheter was introduced through a right ventricular stab incision and susbequently prostaglandin infusion was continued postoperatively until the blood gases were satisfactory. In 2 of the 6 patients the prostaglandins could not be withdrawn and shunt operations were required. In this group of patients with an outflow portion in the right ventricle, it is probably unwise to carry out an atrial septostomy because a high right atrial pressure will encourage forward flow through the poorly functioning right ventricle.

If there is no outflow portion in the right ventricle, atrial septostomy should be performed (so that there is no restriction of flow through the atrial septum) and this is followed by a shunt operation.

Further surgery will then be required at some later date depending on the child's progress. De Leval et al. (1985) have analysed their cases and discuss possible procedures:

1. A definitive repair is an operation in which the outflow tract obstruction can be relieved and the atrial septal defect and shunt closed.
2. A definitive palliation is an operation in which the outflow tract can be resected but it is still necessary to keep the shunt and atrial septal defect open because

there is doubt as to whether the right ventricle can function well enough to maintain the pulmonary circulation.
3. A complete separation of the systemic and pulmonary circulations is established using the Fontan procedure.

De Leval *et al.* (1985) concluded that if the right ventricle has all three parts present and the tricuspid valve diameter is above the lower 99% confidence limit of the normal mean, then a complete definitive repair can be carried out provided there is no major tricuspid incompetence. If there is no trabecular portion of the ventricle, but the crtieria for a Fontan operation are fulfilled (Chapter 11), then it is still possible to do a complete repair. This is not possible in the neonatal period when the pulmonary resistance is high.

The Fontan operation is reserved for patients who have only an inlet portion of the right ventricle with a small tricuspid valve. An atrial to pulmonary artery connection gives the best results.

Myocardial sinusoids

A peculiarity of pulmonary atresia with intact ventricular septum is the presence, in about one-third of all patients, of sinusoids leading from the right ventricle and connecting with the coronary arteries. These presumably develop *in utero* due to the excessive pressure in the right ventricle. They present a considerable obstacle to treatment because lowering the right ventricular pressure by valvotomy or reconstruction of the outflow tract may encourage coronary artery 'steal' and result in myocardial ischaemia. It is probably best to abandon any idea of relief of outflow tract obstruction and hope to do a Fontan operation later.

In the past the results of treatment of this lesion have been poor. It is hoped that the use of prostaglandins and a more aggressive approach surgically will result in improvement. Nevertheless, in some patients where the outflow tract has been adequately reconstructed and the tricuspid valve on echocardiography is of adequate size and competent, the results are still poor. The reasons for this are not clear. Poor right ventricular function is one cause but it may be that the thickened septal wall of the right ventricle bulges into the left ventricle and interferes with left ventricular function (Sideris and Olley, 1982). If this is so then pulmonary valvotomy should be recommended early in life to relieve the right ventricular hypertension.

Pulmonary valve stenosis with right-to-left shunt at atrial level

Incidence

The incidence of pulmonary valve stenosis is 8% and a few of these patients have critical stenosis resulting in a right-to-left shunt at atrial level.

Definition

The degree of stenosis at the pulmonary valve is severe, resulting in a very high right ventricular pressure. This causes a high right atrial pressure and the foramen ovale is forced open so that a right-to-left shunt at atrial level develops. Occasionally an atrial septal defect is present. It is of interest that some infants and children can withstand very high pressures in the right ventricle without any right-to-left shunt developing.

Natural history

The stenosis is usually so severe in these children that, if it is not relieved, heart failure and death occur in infancy or early childhood.

Clinical presentation

In the newborn period the patients usually feed well and gain weight and are often moon-faced healthy-looking babies. Slight cyanosis then develops and the baby is regarded as having a healthy colour. The cyanosis gradually increases, the baby becomes dyspnoeic and feeding is difficult. A heaving right ventricle is visible and palpable along the left sternal edge. A soft systolic murmur is heard in the pulmonary area but a thrill is usually absent because the stenosis is so severe. Heart failure develops and then a loud systolic murmur is heard over the tricuspid area due to tricuspid incompetence. The cardiac output falls and the baby quickly becomes critically ill.

Echocardiography

This is an invaluable investigation when the babies have become critically ill. The narrowed immobile valve and thick right ventricle are seen. Doppler echo will demonstrate a right-to-left shunt at atrial level and there is bowing of the septum to the left. It may not be possible to measure the gradient across the pulmonary valve. Sick infants can be referred directly for surgery without the risk of further deterioration at angiocardiography.

Cardiac catheterization

This is now unnecessary for diagnostic purposes but attempts may be made to dilate the valve with a balloon catheter. In the newborn period this is difficult and time-consuming and does not always give a good result (Ettedgui *et al.*, 1988). It may be successful in children presenting later in life although it is difficult to pass the catheter through the severely narrowed valve. If the infant is sick, surgery is probably safer.

Treatment

This is urgent if the baby is blue and dyspnoeic or has heart failure. Medical treatment is of no avail and operation using cardiopulmonary bypass and transarterial pulmonary valvotomy is the operation of choice, although some surgeons have achieved good results with inflow occlusion and transarterial pulmonary valvotomy.

Ebstein's anomaly

Incidence

Ebstein's anomaly is rare and affects less than 1% of children with congenital heart disease. Recently a sudden increase in the number of cases was shown to be associated with the drug lithium being taken by the mother.

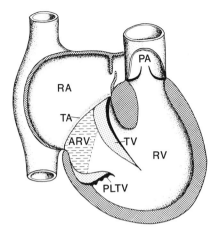

Figure 9.8 Ebstein's anomaly of the tricuspid valve. The posterior leaflet of the tricuspid valve (PLTV) originates within the ventricular cavity, so there is a portion of the right ventricle cavity (ARV) which is 'atrialized' as far as pressure is concerned; this region is shown hatched. PA, pulmonary artery; RA, right atrium; RV, right ventricle; TA, tricuspid annulus; TV, tricuspid valve

Definition

The posterior and septal leaflets of the tricuspid valve are not attached to the annulus fibrosus but to the endocardium of the right ventricle below the annulus (Figure 9.8). The anterior leaflet usually arises normally. The leaflets are often thickened and inserted into chordae tendineae which are attached directly to the wall rather than to the papillary muscles, and the valve assumes a conical shape. It is narrowed and incompetent. The part of the heart above the valve has atrial and ventricular portions, although both are functionally atrium, and it is divided into these two parts by the annulus fibrosus. The ventricle distal to the valve is small and the atrial and ventricular muscle is unusually thin. The infundibulum is thick and muscular. There is usually a patent foramen ovale or atrial septal defect. The right ventricle is unable to eject the normal blood volume and the flow of blood to the lungs is reduced. The right atrium and ventricle proximal to the valve are dilated and a right-to-left shunt may occur between the two atria.

The degree of the abnormality varies and there is a whole spectrum of these malformations ranging from mild to severe forms.

Natural history

The effects of the condition are manifest most strikingly soon after birth, when the high pulmonary vascular resistance produces an obstruction to forward flow which the right ventricle is unable to overcome with an incompetent tricuspid valve. If the first few days of life are survived the prognosis in childhood is good except for the few who have severe cyanosis or attacks of paroxysmal tachycardia.

Symptoms

Breathlessness, mild cyanosis and congestive heart failure occur in infancy in the more severe forms, but in the milder forms symptoms develop later with mild cyanosis and excessive dyspnoea becoming apparent after exercise.

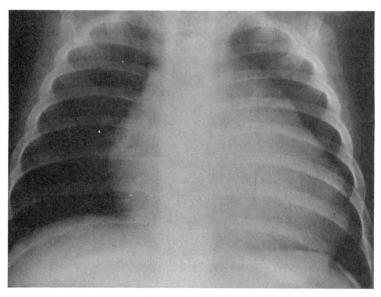

Figure 9.9 Ebstein's anomaly. Chest radiograph showing right atrial and right ventricular enlargement and pulmonary oligaemia in a 9-month-old infant with a right-to-left shunt through an atrial septal defect

Signs

Although a few patients are acyanotic, the majority show mild cyanosis associated with mild clubbing. The pulse has a small volume and the venous pulse may show prominent 'a' or 'v' waves, but is often normal. The heart action is quiet and the apex beat diffuse and difficult to locate. A systolic murmur at the left sternal edge occurs when there is significant tricuspid regurgitation. Three or four heart sounds can be heard, giving rise to a triple or quadruple rhythm. A characteristic scratchy diastolic murmur is usually present, best heard at the lower left sternal edge.

Radiology

Radiology is characteristic in the overt case, there being marked cardiac enlargement with a large right atrium and oligaemia of the lung fields (Figure 9.9). In milder forms, prominence of the right atrium may be the only abnormal finding.

Electrocardiography

The electrocardiogram is pathognomonic in the majority of patients. The P waves in lead 2 are tall and peaked, often being higher than the QRS complexes. The P–R interval may be prolonged. Right bundle branch block, complete or incomplete, is seen (Figure 9.10). Pre-excitation, as in the Wolff–Parkinson–White syndrome, occurs frequently and arrhythmias, particularly paroxysmal atrial tachycardia and atrial flutter, are common. In mild cases a right bundle branch block may be the only finding.

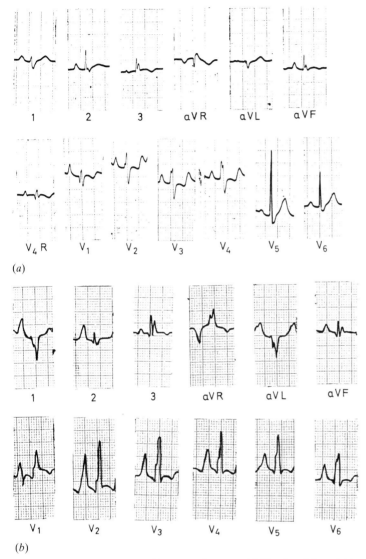

Figure 9.10 Ebstein's anomaly. Electrocardiograms. (*a*) Showing right atrial hypertrophy, slightly prolonged P–R interval and right bundle branch block pattern with small voltage QRS complexes. (*b*) Another patient, showing giant P waves

Echocardiography

Cross-sectional echocardiography shows the pathogenic anatomy of the tricuspid valve much more precisely than angiocardiography. The tricuspid valve is displaced into the right ventricular cavity and this is well seen in the four-chamber view. It is possible to see whether there is sufficient tissue in the anterior leaflet and that it is not severely tethered and will be suitable for a plastic reconstruction of a monocusp valve. If it is not then a valve replacement will be required.

Doppler studies will assess the degree of tricuspid regurgitation and from these studies the right ventricular pressure can be calculated. It must be remembered that in the normal newborn infant tricuspid regurgitation may be functional but disappears in the first few days of life. Serial studies will determine if the regurgitation is organic.

Cardiac catheterization

This is very rarely necessary now because of the excellent views at echocardiography. Furthermore, the investigation carries a greater risk than in other lesions because of the danger of arrhythmias.

Treatment

Asymptomatic children require no treatment but competitive sports are best avoided in view of the risks of arrhythmias. Rhythm disorders occur in about 20% of patients. They should be treated with drugs such as propranolol and verapamil. Till *et al.* (1987) reported that flecainide intravenously controlled attacks when other drugs had failed to do so. If there is a Wolff–Parkinson–White syndrome with pre-excitation and a re-entrant tachycardia which does not respond to medical treatment, then surgical division of the anomalous pathway should be considered.

Mair *et al.* (1985) have reported encouraging results from plastic reconstruction of the tricuspid valve. This reconstruction was possible in 81% of their cases, 15% had a prosthetic valve and the remainder had a Fontan operation. The atrial septal defect is closed, part of the large right atrium removed, the atrialized portion of the right ventricle plicated and the anterior leaflet of the tricuspid valve used to produce a monocusp valve. If an accessory conduction pathway is identified at surgery it is interrupted at the time of operation. Eighty-seven per cent of their patients improved following surgery and they now recommend operation for all patients who are significantly cyanosed and polycythaemic.

The problem of treatment is greatest in the young infant and child who have severe symptoms. Some who have heart failure improve with anti-failure treatment but *if* they do not, surgery should be considered. The risks are very high in this age-group and should be fully discussed with the parents.

Bibliography and references

Tetralogy of Fallot

Abbott, M. E. (1936) *Atlas of Congenital Heart Disease*, American Heart Association, New York, p. 46

Bertranon, E. G., Blackstone, E. H., Hazelrig, J. B., *et al.* (1978) Life expectancy without surgery in tetralogy of Fallot. *American Journal of Cardiology*, **42**, 458–466

Finnegan, P., Patel, R. G., Singh, S. P., *et al.* (1976) Total correction of tetralogy of Fallot: postoperative haemodynamic assessment. *British Heart Journal*, **38**, 315

Fuster, V., McGoon, D. C., Kennedy, M. A., *et al.* (1980) Long-term evaluation (12 to 22 years) of open heart surgery for tetralogy of Fallot. *American Journal of Cardiology*, **46**, 635–642

Gunteroth, W. G., Morton, B. C., Mullins, G. L., *et al.* (1968) Venous return with knee–chest position and squatting in tetralogy of Fallot. *American Heart Journal*, **75**, 313–318

Hegerty, A., Anderson, R. H. and Deanfield, J. E. (1987) Myocardial fibrosis in tetralogy of Fallot: effect of surgery or part of the natural history? *British Heart Journal*, **59**, 123

Martelle, R. R. and Linde, L. M. (1961) Cerebrovascular accidents with tetralogy of Fallot. *American Journal of Diseases of Children*, **101**, 206–209

Moulton, A. L., Brenner, J. I., Ringel, R., *et al.* (1985) Classic versus modified Blalock–Taussig shunts in neonates and infants. *Circulation,* **72,** Suppl. II, 35–44

Ramsay, J. M., Macartney, F. J. and Haworth, S. G. (1985) Tetralogy of Fallot with major aorto-pulmonary collateral arteries. *British Heart Journal,* **53,** 167–172

Taussig, H. B., Crocetti, A., Eshagpour, E., *et al.* (1971) Long-term observations of the Blalock–Taussig operation. *Johns Hopkins Medical Journal,* **129,** 243

Pulmonary atresia with ventricular septal defect

Fäller, K., Haworth, S. G., Taylor, J. F. N., *et al.* (1981) Duplicate sources of pulmonary blood supply in pulmonary atresia with ventricular septal defect. *British Heart Journal,* **46,** 263–268

Macartney, F. J., Scott, Olive and Deverall, P. B. (1974) Haemodynamics and anatomical characteristics of pulmonary blood supply in pulmonary atresia with ventricular septal defect – including a case of persistent fifth aortic arch. *British Heart Journal,* **36,** 1049–1060

Singh, S. P., Astley, R. and Rigby, M. (1980) Wider experience with pulmonary vein angiography and indirect measurement of pulmonary artery pressure. Abstract, *World Congress on Paediatric Cardiology*

Sullivan, I. D., Wren, C., Macartney, F. J., *et al.* (1988) Pulmonary atresia with ventricular septal defect and multifocal blood supply: results of a policy of surgical unifocalisation. *British Heart Journal,* **59,** 121

Pulmonary atresia with intact ventricular septum

Bull, C., de Leval, M. R., Mercanti, C., *et al.* (1982) Pulmonary atresia and intact ventricular septum. A revised classification. *Circulation,* **66,** 266–272

De Leval, M., Bull, C., Hopkins, R., *et al.* (1985) Decision making in the definitive repair of the heart with a small right ventricle. *Circulation,* **72** Suppl. II, 52–60

Hamilton, J. R. L., Fonseka, S. F., Wilson, N., *et al.* (1987) Operative balloon dilatation for pulmonary atresia with intact ventricular septum. *British Heart Journal,* **58,** 4

Moller, J. H., Girod, G., Amplatz, K., *et al.* (1970) Pulmonary valvotomy in pulmonary atresia with hypoplastic right ventricle. *Surgery St. Louis,* **68,** 630

Sideris, E. B. and Olley, P. M. (1982) Left ventricular function and compliance in pulmonary atresia with intact ventricular septum. *Journal of Thoracic and Cardiovascular Surgery,* **84,** 192–199

Zuberbuhler, J. R., Fricker, F. J., Park, S. C., *et al.* (1979) Pulmonary atresia with intact ventricular septum – morbid anatomy. In *Paediatric Cardiology* Vol. 2 (*Heart Disease in the Newborn*) (eds M. J. Godman and R. M. Marquis), London, Churchill Livingstone, pp. 285–295

Pulmonary valve stenosis with right-to-left shunt at atrial level

Ettedgui, J. A., Martin, R. P., Jones, O. D. H., *et al.* (1988) Balloon dilatation of the pulmonary valve in neonates: technical considerations and results. *British Heart Journal,* **59,** 118

Ebstein's anomaly

Mair, D. D., Seward, J. B., Driscoll, D. J., *et al.* (1985) Surgical repair of Ebstein's anomaly: selection of patients and early and late operative results. *Circulation,* **72,** Suppl. II, 70–76

Til, J. A., Rowland, E., Shinebourne, E. A., *et al.* (1987) Treatment of refractory supraventricular arrhythmias with flecainide acetate. *Archives of Disease in Childhood,* **62,** 247–252

Chapter 10

Cyanotic lesions with increased pulmonary blood flow

Transposition of the great arteries

Incidence

Transposition of the great arteries is the second commonest cyanotic lesion. In the Bristol series it comprised 4.1% of all congenital lesions. There is some suggestion that it may be less common than 10 or 20 years ago, but the difference is small, 3.8% in the last 12 years compared with 4.5% in the previous 12 years.

Definition

The aorta arises from the right ventricle and the pulmonary artery from the left ventricle (Figure 10.1). (This is sometimes called discordant ventriculo-arterial connection). The aorta therefore lies in front of the pulmonary artery, either directly or slightly to one or other side.

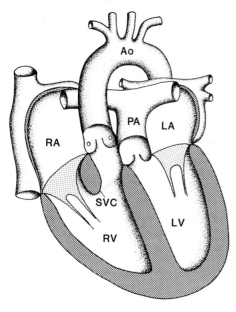

Figure 10.1 Complete transposition of the great arteries. The aorta (Ao) arises from the right ventricle (RV) above, anterior and to the right of the pulmonary artery (PA) which arises from the left ventricle (LV). LA, left atrium; RA, right atrium; SVC, supraventricular crest

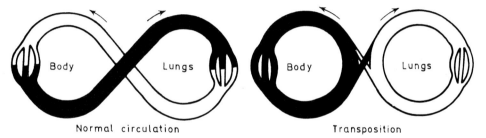

Figure 10.2 Complete transposition of the great arteries. In the normal circulation right and left sides of the heart are connected in series; in the transposition they are in parallel and the effective flow to the lungs for gas exchange is the small amount of cross-over at, for example, an atrial septal defect

The physiological effect of this is to produce effectively two separate circulations (Figure 10.2) rather than the normal 'figure-of-eight' circulation. Mixing of blood between the pulmonary circulation of arterialized blood and the systemic circulation of desaturated blood can occur initially through the ductus arteriosus and the foramen ovale. As soon as the ductus closes, which is usually within 24 hours, severe cyanosis becomes apparent.

Clinical presentation

In uncomplicated transposition, without a ventricular septal defect, the baby usually looks healthy at birth, but is noted to be, or to become, persistently cyanosed within the first day of life. This is usually the only finding initially, the baby is not breathless, there is no murmur and heart failure does not develop except as a terminal event if the condition is untreated. If prompt action is not taken, the baby becomes increasingly blue and develops a progressive metabolic acidosis.

Radiology is useful in that it usually shows normally filled lung vessels, unlike most other cyanotic lesions presenting early. The typical 'egg-on-its-side' shape to the heart (Figure 10.3) is due to a combination of a narrow vascular pedicle produced by the aorta remaining in front of and parallel with the pulmonary artery rather than crossing it as in the normal heart, and the enlargement of the right ventricle. The narrowness of the vascular pedicle may not, however, be apparent in the neonatal period due to the overlying thymus.

The electrocardiogram shows a normal axis for age and is usually within normal limits, although a proportion show some evidence of right ventricular hypertrophy, and this is always aparent later (Figure 10.4).

Echocardiography allows the diagnosis to be made rapidly in most patients. The intracardiac anatomy is normal, but the orientation of the great arteries and the two semilunar valves is abnormal. In the normal heart, the aorta and pulmonary artery take a half-turn about each other (Figure 4.11(d)) with the result that whichever plane is imaged one vessel is seen in cross-section and one in longitudinal section (known to echocardiographers as 'ball and sausage'). In transposition the two great arteries lie parallel to each other and in the long axis view both are seen in longitudinal section (Figure 10.5). In most cases it is possible to follow the anterior great artery and see that it gives off the aortic arch branches while the posterior one shows branching to form right and left pulmonary arteries. Even if this is not possible, the parallel relationship makes the diagnosis likely.

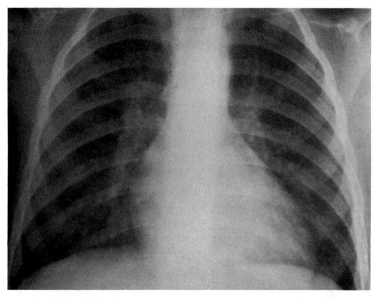

Figure 10.3 Radiograph of transposition of the great arteries. There is a narrow vascular pedicle and the shape of the heart resembles an egg on its side. Pulmonary vasculature is normal or slightly increased

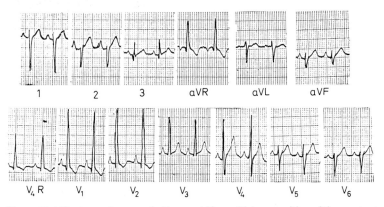

Figure 10.4 Electrocardiogram of a 2-year-old boy with transposition of the great arteries. (Balloon atrial septostomy in infancy.) There is right atrial and right ventricular hypertrophy. The electrical axis is $-160°$ (extreme right axis deviation in this case) and the q waves in V_4R to V_2 are due to right atrial enlargement

Cardiac catheterization is not usually necesssary for diagnostic reasons but, if the baby is being treated by balloon septostomy (see below) this will require the insertion of catheters and confirmation of the diagnosis is usually carried out at the same time, which can be done by making injections into both ventricles (Figure 10.6). The pressure in the two ventricles is usually the same in the first few days of life and it is often difficult to demonstrate much shunting of blood in either direction.

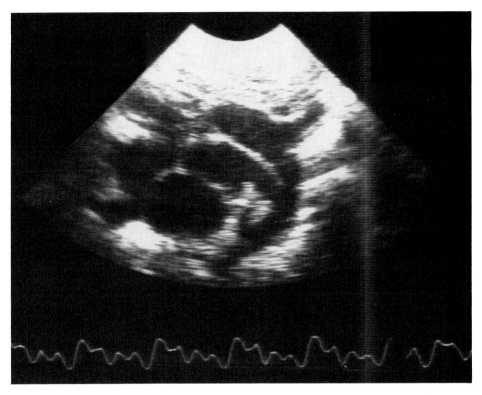

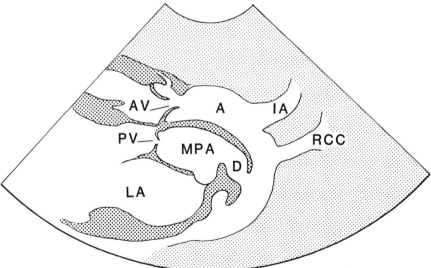

Figure 10.5 Transposition of great arteries. Parasternal, long-axis view. The characteristic findings are that the aorta arises anteriorly from the right ventricle and the two great arteries both appear in longitudinal section (see text). A, aorta; AV, atrioventricular valve; D, ductus arteriosus; IA, innominate artery; LA, left atrium; MPA, main pulmonary artery; PV, pulmonary valve; RCC, right common carotid artery

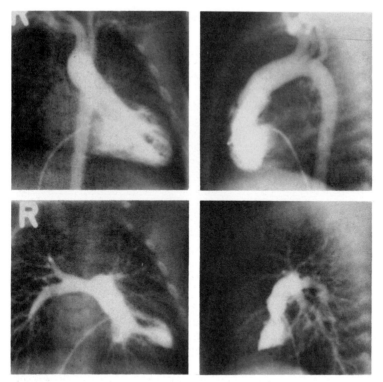

Figure 10.6 Transposition of the great arteries and no ventricular septal defect. Upper films are of a right ventricular injection, lower ones of a left ventricular injection. Anteroposterior films are on the left and lateral ones on the right

Treatment

As with any cyanotic condition, urgent transfer to a paediatric cardiology unit is mandatory. If the baby's condition is good and the journey only likely to last an hour or less, this can be done without any prior treatment. If the baby is severely cyanotic and acidotic, the metabolic acidosis should be corrected by intravenous sodium bicarbonate and a prostaglandin infusion started (see Chapter 2 for details). The problem with prostaglandin infusion is that it may induce apnoea so that prophylactic intubation and ventilation is sometimes recommended for the journey. However, apnoea is less common with the smaller doses now used and almost always responds to a brief period of face-mask ventilation. Paediatricians and their referral centre need to have a plan for transfer of such babies. The giving of oxygen is illogical and some cardiologists feel that it may actually do harm by speeding closure of the ductus.

Until about 5 years ago the subsequent management of uncomplicated transposition was uniform throughout most centres and consisted of early balloon septostomy (see below) to provide adequate mixing of saturated and desaturated blood, followed some months later by an operation to divert systemic and pulmonary venous blood to the opposite sides. More recently a few surgeons have carried out a direct arterial switch as the first and only operation.

Balloon atrial septostomy with delayed definitive surgery

At the time of diagnostic cardiac catheterization, once measurements and angiography have been done, a larger sheath is inserted into the femoral vein to accommodate the balloon catheter. This is either of the type recommended by Rashkind (who invented the technique) or one used for embolectomy (Figure 10.7(a)). The catheter is advanced under radiographic control until the balloon at the tip is in the left atrium, taking care that it does not enter the pulmonary veins or left ventricle. The balloon is then inflated with contrast medium (Figure 10.7(b)) and pulled by a sharp tug back into the right atrium and mouth of the inferior vena cava. Some cardiologists inflate initially to the maximum volume in the belief that this is more likely to rupture the septum, while some start with about 1 ml and repeat the procedure increasing gradually by 0.5 ml at a time to about 4 ml. The size of the hole produced can be estimated by seeing what volume in the balloon can easily be withdrawn without resistance.

In experienced hands the procedure rarely causes problems and is well tolerated by the baby. Further measurements are made to check that the oxygen saturation has risen (sometimes from as low as 20 or 30% when the ductus is closed) to 60 to 80%. The higher figures are obtained when there is a partially open ductus. The atrial pressures are also checked as abolition of a gradient confirms that the hole is adequate. The size of the hole is also checked by echocardiography. Failure to achieve an adequate septostomy is usually due to delay in carrying out the procedure, but a few babies have a relatively small fossa ovalis (the thin central part of the interatrial septum which ruptures easily), and this can be seen on the preseptostomy echo. One approach to this problem or to the subsequent reclosure of the hole is to make a larger hole using a catheter with a 'concealed blade' called a septome, which makes a slit in the thicker part of the atrial septum.

Prior to the development of balloon septostomy Blalock and Hanlon devised an operation to remove the posterior part of the interatrial septum without the use of cardiopulmonary bypass and this is occasionally used in infants past the neonatal period. There are other reasons for failure of the arterial saturation to rise adequately, including failure of pulmonary vessels to dilate normally in the first few days of life and careful evaluation of the infant with 'failed septostomy' is required. In particular, if cross-sectional echocardiography shows a good-sized hole, another explanation for persistently severe cyanosis should be sought.

If prostaglandins have been used they are stopped as soon as the septostomy has been carried out. Although it is tempting to continue their use for a while to keep the arterial oxygen saturation high, a persistently patent ductus can lead to heart failure and the need for surgical closure.

Usually the infant thrives following septostomy and can leave hospital 2–3 days later, at which time the oxygen saturation is usually about 70% at rest and no medical therapy is required. He is then followed in outpatients and reassessed at about 3–4 months, either by a repeat cardiac catheter or, more commonly now, by echocardiography, to check that the ductus is closed and ventricular function satisfactory. Definitive surgery is carried out shortly after this, usually between 6 and 9 months. The reason for this timing is that most surgeons are more confident about their results at this sort of age than earlier, and symptoms and complications (particularly polycythaemia and intravascular thrombosis) become more likely if operation is deferred beyond the first birthday. Most surgeons will, however, operate earlier if the baby is symptomatic and not thriving.

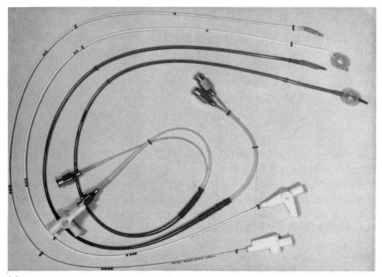

(a)

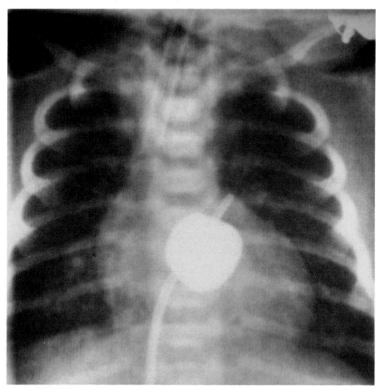

(b)

Figure 10.7 (a) Atrioseptostomy catheters. Outer pair: Fogarty catheters (by Edwards Laboratories). Inner pair: Rashkind double-lumen type (USCI). One of each pair has been partially inflated (*see also* (b)). (b) Double-lumen Rashkind catheter partially inflated in the left atrium

Arterial switch operation (Figure 10.10)

An anatomical, rather than a physiological correction, in which the aorta and pulmonary artery are 'switched' back to their proper connections, has always appealed to surgeons and cardiologists, but two important obstacles have been present. The first is that the left ventricle in uncomplicated transposition involutes during the first few months of life in the way the right ventricle does in the normal heart, so that the left ventricle becomes incapable of supporting the pressures in the systemic circulation. The second is that the coronary arteries arise from the aorta very near to the aortic valve and could not be moved with the aorta, necessitating freeing them from the aorta and then reanastomosing them after the great arteries have been switched. This was felt technically to be too difficult, and when it was originally attempted in neonates it led to a high incidence of coronary artery obstruction due to fibrosis around the anastomoses to the new aorta. In addition, the earliest attempts at switch operation required the insertion of a short conduit in the pulmonary artery, but this will not grow with the patient, again making early operation undesirable.

In an attempt to avoid operating early, but to maintain the high pressure in the left ventricle, banding of the pulmonary artery was tried. However, this produced a reduction in pulmonary blood flow and an unacceptably low arterial oxygen saturation, so that the operation had to be combined with a systemic to pulmonary artery shunt. This proved adequate to allow growth of the baby to about 2 years old, which was the age at which the switch operation was carried out. However, the combined procedures had a substantially higher mortality than Mustard or Senning operations.

More recently, alterations in technique have allowed direct reanastomosis of the pulmonary artery without an intervening conduit and excision of the coronary arteries is carried out with a larger circle of aorta. This has reduced the liability to subsequent fibrosis causing obstruction of the coronary arteries at the site of the anastomosis.

In a few centres the 'switch' operation is therefore now carried out within the first few days, and without preceding balloon septostomy, but with prostaglandin infusion to maintain the baby's oxygenation by keeping the ductus open.

Postoperative course

Following either a 'switch' or redirection of venous inflow (Senning or Mustard operation) the baby grows well and has little in the way of outward signs. Following the Senning and Mustard operations auscultation reveals a loud sound in the pulmonary area (due to the anteriorly placed aorta) and often a short systolic murmur due to a slight gradient between left ventricle and pulmonary artery caused by the thickened interventricular septum bulging into the lower-pressure, left ventricle. Following the arterial switch operation there should be no significant abnormality detectable. Long-term follow-up into adult life is essential following either type of operation. Arrhythmias are common following Mustard's operation and the ability of the right ventricle to continue indefinitely as the systemic ventricle must be suspect. There is currently no information on the long-term results of the 'switch' operation and this must be adequately documented by careful follow-up of all survivors. Overall about 75–80% of children born with uncomplicated transposition over the past 20 years survived into adult life, the mortality being partly from operation, partly from complications while awaiting surgery and partly from late complications such as stenosis of pathways or ventricular arrhythmias.

Transposition with ventricular septal defect

About 20% of patients with transposition have a large ventricular septal defect without pulmonary stenosis. This radically alters the presentation and treatment of the condition.

Clinical presentation

The baby seems well at birth, although careful examination reveals mild cyanosis, but within the first week breathlessness and progressive cardiac failure develop. Cyanosis remains minimal. The heart is clinically enlarged and there is a short ejection systolic murmur at the base due to high flow through the pulmonary valve and usually an apical short diastolic murmur, also due to high flow through the mitral valve. The heart failure is refractory to medical treatment, the infant fails to thrive and, unless treated, usually dies within the first 4–6 months. A small proportion develop an increased pulmonary vascular resistance, which leads to an improvement in failure but an increase in cyanosis, and by the age of a year the resistance is usually too high for surgery to be safe or beneficial.

Radiology

The heart is usually severely enlarged and there is marked pulmonary plethora. The characteristic narrow vascular pedicle is usually preserved.

Electrocardiography

The electrocardiogram shows biventricular hypertrophy, with right ventricular hypertrophy predominating.

Echocardiography

The large ventricular septal defect is identified and the abnormal connection of the great arteries. The pulmonary artery is large and frequently over-rides the ventricular septal defect. All cardiac chambers are enlarged and, unless there is an atrial septal defect, the left atrium is bowed to the right indicating raised left atrial pressure.

Cardiac catheterization

This shows equal systolic pressures in both ventricles and both great arteries. Blood in the pulmonary arteries is highly saturated, reflecting a very high pulmonary blood flow. Aortic saturation is lower, usually 80–85%. Left atrial pressure is high, often at levels likely to cause pulmonary oedema. Angiography indicates the abnormal arterial connections and the VSD (multiple defects may be seen).

Treatment

A decision has to be made on the choice between early definitive surgery, in which case an arterial 'switch' is usually the preferred operation, or early palliation with balloon atrial septostomy and initial banding of the pulmonary artery. (Although the arterial saturation is usually high enough to make balloon septostomy seem unnecessary, once the pulmonary blood flow has been reduced by banding it may fall precipitously. In addition, providing better communication lowers left atrial pressure and improves pulmonary congestion.) However, banding is often difficult to carry out tight enough to restrict pulmonary flow and lower pulmonary artery pressure without reducing arterial saturation unduly. Provided it is carried out before the infant is in severe cardiac failure or has pulmonary vascular disease, the arterial switch operation is the best option. Even though extra time is needed to close the ventricular septal defect as well, the child is bigger and therefore the results are the same as those in simple transposition.

If banding of the pulmonary artery is carried out, definitive surgery can usually be deferred for up to two years. There is then a choice of procedures:

1. Close the ventricular septal defect and carry out a modified arterial switch operation, removing the constricted segment of pulmonary artery.
2. Close the ventricular septal defect, reconstruct the banded pulmonary artery and carry out a Senning or Mustard operation.
3. Carry out a Rastelli operation (see Chapter 11) in which the left ventricular blood is diverted through the ventricular septum and into the aorta by a patch across the right ventricular outflow and place a conduit between the right ventricle and pulmonary artery, which is closed off from the left ventricle.

The procedure adopted depends on factors such as the position and size of the ventricular septal defect, the size of the pulmonary artery and the size and function of the two ventricles.

Overall, patients with transposition and ventricular septal defect have a higher mortality than those with uncomplicated transposition, but greater use of the arterial switch operation may counter this trend.

Transposition with large ventricular septal defect and coarctation of the aorta or interruption of the aortic arch

This combination occurs sufficiently frequently to warrant a brief mention (about 7% of all transpositions). Cardiac failure develops within the first few days. Usually the femoral pulses are reduced or absent, but the ductus may remain open allowing good perfusion of the abdomen and lower limbs. The diagnosis is made by echocardiography and confirmed by cardiac catheterization.

The need to operate on the coarctation as well usually means that a one-stage operation (arterial swtich) carries too high a risk and the usual procedure is to repair the coarctation and band the pulmonary artery after balloon atrial septostomy. Subsequent treatment is similar to that following banding for transposition with large ventricular septal defect, although the coarctation may need re-operation or balloon dilatation, in addition.

Transposition with ventricular septal defect and pulmonary stenosis

This is the rarest of the three complicated types of transposition (about 7% of all transpositions), although prior to satisfactory surgical treatment of transposition it was the type with the best chance of surviving the first year of life.

Presentation

Cyanosis is usually noted within the first few days of life but, unlike in simple transposition, it does not tend to increase and the infant may do well without any treatment. The degree of cyanosis depends on the severity of the pulmonary stenosis. If severe, the cyanosis is marked, if mild, the cyanosis is mild (but cardiac failure due to increased pulmonary blood flow may occur). Usually cyanosis is moderate and, although pulmonary blood flow is increased, this can be tolerated. As well as cyanosis the infant has a loud systolic murmur at the left sternal border so that the initial diagnosis is often tetralogy of Fallot, but the normal or increased pulmonary vasculature in the chest radiograph indicates a more complex lesion.

Diagnosis

The condition can only reliably be diagnosed by echocardiography and cardiac catheterization and the latter is necessary to obtain full information about the state of the pulmonary arteries. Pulmonary artery pressure is usually normal and systolic pressures in both ventricles and aorta are the same.

Treatment

A Blalock–Taussig shunt may be necessary in the first year or two if cyanosis is severe or becomes so. An arterial switch operation is not practicable because the stenotic pulmonary valve becomes the new aortic valve where its malfunction is much more important. It is sometimes possible to carry out a Senning or Mustard operation with simultaneous closure of the ventricular septal defect and pulmonary valvotomy, but it is often difficult to relieve the pulmonary stenosis accurately. The Rastelli operation then becomes the only practicable one, since the pulmonary valve can then be excluded from the circulation.

Bibliography and references

Transposition

Aberdeen, E., Waterston, D. J., Carr, I., et al. (1965). Successful 'correction' of transposed great arteries by Mustard's operation. *Lancet* **1**, 1233

Blalock, A. and Hanlon, C. R. (1950) The surgical treatment of complete transposition of the aorta and pulmonary artery. *Surgery, Gynecology and Obstetrics*, **90**, 1

Sillard, D. H., Mohri, H., Merendino, K. A., et al. (1969) Total surgical correction of transposition of the great arteries in children less than six months of age. *Surgery, Gynecology and Obstetrics*, **129**, 1258

Ferencz, C. (1968) Transposition of the great vessels; pathophysiological considerations based upon a study of the lungs. *Circulation*, **33**, 232

Gutgesell, H. P., Garson, A. and McNamara, D. G. (1979) Transposition of the great arteries; Longterm follow-up after balloon atrial septostomy in 112 patients. *Paediatric Cardiology*, **1**, 88–89

Haller, J. A., Crisler, C., Bawley, R., *et al.* (1969) Mustard operation for transposition of the great vessels. Technical considerations. *Journal of Thoracic and Cardiovascular Surgery,* **58,** 296.

Imamura, E. S., Morikawa, T., Tatsuno, K., *et al.* (1971) Surgical considerations of ventricular septal defect associated with complete transposition of the great arteries and pulmonary stenosis. *Circulation,* **44,** 914

Jatene, A.D., Fontes, V.F. and Pualista, P.P. (1976) Anatomic correction of transposition of the great arteries. *Journal of Thoracic and Cardiovascular Surgery,* **72,** 364–70

Jordan, S. C. and McCarthy, C. (1967) Haemodyanmic consequences of atrial septostomy in an infant with transposition of the great arteries. *Lancet,* **1,** 310

Mair, D. D., Rutter, D. G., Danielson, G. K., *et al.* (1976) The palliative Mustard operation: rationale and results. *American Journal of Cardiology,* **37,** 762–68

Mustard, W. T. (1964) Successful two-stage correction of transposition of the great vessels. *Surgery, St. Louis,* **55,** 469

Parsons, C. G., Astley, R., Burrows, F. G. O. *et al.* (1971) Transposition of great arteries. A study of 65 infants followed for 1 to 4 years after balloon septostomy. *British Heart Journal,* **33,** 725

Quaegebeur, J. M., Rohmer, J. and Brom, A. G. (1977) Revival of the Senning operation in the treatment of transposition of the great arteries. *Thorax,* **32,** 517–24

Quaegebeur, J. M., Rohmer, J., Ottenkamp, J., *et al.* (1986) The arterial switch operation: an eight year experience. *Journal of Thoracic and Cardiovascular Surgery,* **92,** 361–84

Rashkind, W. J. (1971) Transposition of the great arteries. *Pediatric Clinics of North America,* **18,** 1075

Rashkind, W. J. and Miller, W. W. (1966) Creation of an atrial septal defect without thoracotomy; a palliative approach to complete transposition of the great vessels. *Journal of the American Medical Association,* **196,** 991

Rastelli, G. C., McGoon, D. C. and Wallace, R. B. (1969) Anatomic correction of transposition of the great arteries with ventricular septal defect and subpulmonary stenosis. *Journal of Thoracic and Cardiovascular Surgery,* **58,** 545

Shumacker, H. B. Jr. and Girod, D. A. (1969) Transposition of the great vessels. Long-term follow-up of corrected case. *Journal of Thoracic and Cardiovascular Surgery,* **57,** 747

Singh, A. K., Stark, J. and Taylor, J. F. N. (1976) Left ventricle to pulmonary artery conduit in the treatment of transposition of great arteries, restrictive ventricular septal defect and acquired pulmonary atresia. *British Heart Journal,* **38,** 1213

Tynan, M. (1972) Haemodynamic effects of balloon atrial septostomy in infants with transposition of great arteries. *British Heart Journal,* **34,** 791

Venables, A. W. (1970) Balloon atrial septostomy in complete transposition of the great arteries in infancy. *British Heart Journal,* **32,** 61

Viles, P. H., Ongley, P. A. and Titus, J. L. (1969) The spectrum of pulmonary vascular disease in transposition of the great arteries. *Circulation,* **40,** 31

Yacoub, M. H., Radley-Smith, R. and MacLaurin, R. (1977) Two-stage operation for anatomical correction of transposition of the great arteries with intact interventricular septum, *Lancet,* **1,** 1275

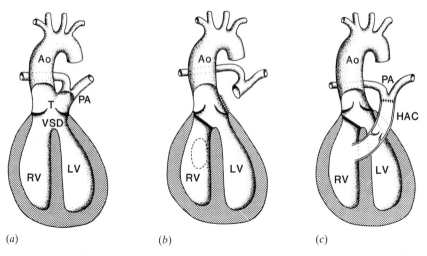

(a)   (b)   (c)

Figure 11.2 Rastelli operation for type 1 truncus, viewed from the left. (*a*) Preoperative. (*b*) The pulmonary trunk (PA) has been detached from the truncus (T) which is then repaired. Through a right ventriculotomy the ventricular septal defect (VSD) is patched to the base of the truncus so as to direct the left ventricular (LV) blood into aorta (Ao). (*c*) A homograft aortic conduit (HAC), bearing the aortic valve (which now becomes the recipient's pulmonary valve), is inserted to direct the blood from the right ventricle (RV) into the pulmonary artery

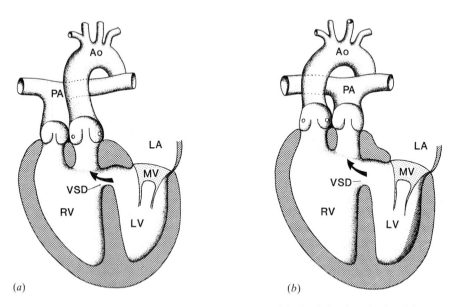

(a)   (b)

Figure 11.3 Origin of both great arteries from the right ventricle. Both the aorta (Ao) and the pulmonary artery (MPA) arise from the right ventricle (RV) and neither is contiguous with the mitral valve (MV). In (*a*) the ventricular septal defect (VSD) is directly below the aorta so that oxygenated blood from left atrium (LA) and left ventricle (LV) flows preferentially into the aorta and the patient is not cyanosed. Repair is more simple than in (*b*) (sometimes called the Taussig–Bing complex) where the pulmonary artery is close to the defect and the aorta receives mainly desaturated blood

Origin of one pulmonary artery from the aorta

This is a rare anomaly and may be thought of as a partial form of truncus arteriosus (the name 'hemi-truncus' has been used). Usually it is the right pulmonary artery which arises from the aorta and often there are other associated defects including ventricular septal defect, patent ductus arteriosus and tetralogy of Fallot.

Patients usually present with breathlessness and cardiac failure within the first two months of life. The pulses are bounding and there is a systolic or continuous murmur best heard in the aortic area and over the right lung. Chest radiographs show cardiac enlargement and plethora of the right lung field. Angiography is required to establish the diagnosis.

Surgical treatment is required and consists of re-anastomosing the anomalous pulmonary artery to the main pulmonary artery. Cardiopulmonary bypass is usually required as the main and left pulmonary arteries usually lie too far to the left and are too small to allow a side clamp to be placed without arresting the circulation. If a graft is required this will need replacing later, and an alternative approach is simply to band the right pulmonary artery and defer correction for a few years.

Origin of both great arteries from the right ventricle (double-outlet right ventricle)

An uncommon condition, origin of both great arteries from the right ventricle is best regarded as a partial form of transposition. As the term implies, both pulmonary artery and aorta arise from the right ventricle (Figure 11.3), each with its own outflow tract (or conus) and with neither valve being in continuity with the mitral valve (this distinguishes it from the extreme degrees of over-riding of the aorta sometimes seen in tetralogy of Fallot). In typical cases there is a normally developed left ventricle and an associated ventricular septal defect to allow emptying of the left ventricle. (Cases without a functioning left ventricle are dealt with under forms of primitive ventricle, page 202).

Four haemodynamic situations are possible:

1. Large ventricular septal defect with no pulmonary stenosis and the ventricular septal defect close to the aortic valve (Figure 11.3(a)). This simulates a ventricular septal defect with pulmonary hypertension. Cyanosis is absent and the infant presents with breathlessness and heart failure.
2. Large ventricular septal defect with no pulmonary stenosis and the ventricular septal defect close to the pulmonary valve (Figure 11.3(b)). This is similar to transposition with large ventricular septal defect. There is mild cyanosis and the early onset of cardiac failure (this condition is sometimes referred to as the Taussig–Bing malformation).
3. Large ventricular septal defect and pulmonary stenosis. The situation mimics tetralogy of Fallot (irrespective of whether the ventricular septal defect is subaortic or sub-pulmonary) and produces cyanosis but not heart failure.
4. The ventricular septal defect is (or becomes) small, leading to left ventricular outflow obstruction. Breathlessness and pulmonary oedema occur and the left ventricle becomes hypertrophied often to an extreme degree.

The definitive diagnosis is unlikely to be made on clinical grounds, as the presentation of each of the four groups mimics some other lesion. The chest radiograph reflects the variety of the condition and may show plethora or oligaemia. The electrocardiogram usually shows right ventricular hypertrophy (except with a closing ventricular septal defect) and frequently shows a QRS axis superiorly and to the right (-90 to -160 degrees). The condition and its associated abnormalities are shown by echocardiography and angiography. As with any complex anomaly, cardiac catheterization will also be needed to indicate the level of pulmonary vascular resistance in those without pulmonary stenosis.

Treatment

Those patients presenting with breathlessness and heart failure require frusemide and digoxin. If pulmonary stenosis is severe and cyanosis marked in the first day or so, a prostaglandin infusion is required to keep the ductus arteriosus open. A decision then has to be made on either an early attempt at correction or a palliative procedure – banding of the pulmonary artery if no pulmonary stenosis or a Blalock–Taussig shunt if severe cyanosis.

When the ventricular septal defect is subaortic, correction is possible, relatively simply by putting an intracardiac patch between the lower edge of the ventricular septal defect and anterior part of the subaortic conus so that the left ventricle drains only to the aorta and the right ventricle to the pulmonary artery, the pulmonary stenosis being dealt with at the same time.

Most patients with origin of both great arteries from the right ventricle, however, have the ventricular septal defect nearest to the pulmonary artery. Closing the defect as described above turns the condition into complete transposition of the great arteries. The second part of the operation is then to correct the transposition in one of the ways described in Chapter 10, either doing an 'arterial switch' operation (the most common approach) or a venous diversion of the Mustard or Senning variety.

Patients with small or closing ventricular septal defects present considerable problems. Enlargement of the defect may not be easy without damaging the conducting tissue, and the alternative operation of putting a conduit from the left ventricle to the aorta has proved not entirely satisfactory in either the short term or long term.

As with any complex condition, 'correction' should be regarded as a provisional term and follow-up throughout life is required to detect subsequent complications, not only the usual ones of arrhythmias but also late closure of the septal defect or obstruction to either ventricular outflow tract.

Total anomalous pulmonary venous connection

Definition

As the name implies, none of the pulmonary veins is connected to the left atrium and all drain by some route or other into the right atrium. Anomalous pulmonary venous drainage is the physiological result of the anatomical defect termed anomalous pulmonary venous connection.

Incidence

The condition is uncommon, accounting for just over 1% of all cases of congenital heart disease (1.2% in the Bristol series).

Table 11.1 Types of total anomalous pulmoanry venous connection

Type	Variety	Obstruction	Incidence*
Supracardiac	Left innominate vein	±	36
	Superior vena cava	−	11
Cardiac	Right atrium	−	15
	Coronary sinus	−	16
Infracardiac	Portal vein	+ +	6
	Ductus venosus	+	4
	Inferior vena cava	+	2
	Hepatic vein	+	1

*Data from Burroughs and Edwards, 1960.

Anatomy and physiology

The sites of anomalous venous drainage are usually divided into supracardiac, cardiac and infracardiac types anatomically and obstructed and non-obstructed types physiologically (see Table 11.1 and Figure 11.4) Mixed forms are also found with some veins draining via supracardiac channels and some directly into the right atrium or coronary sinus.

With the non-obstructed forms there is a large flow of arterialized blood into the right atrium which mixes with the systemic venous blood. Most of the mixed blood then flows into the right ventricle and pulmonary artery The amount which enters the left atrium depends upon the size of the interatrial communication (Burroughs and Edwards, 1960). With a large defect, about one-third to one-quarter of the total blood entering the right atrium is shunted into the left atrium; with a patent foramen ovale, as little as one-sixth to one-tenth. The right ventricle is greatly dilated and moderately hypertrophied and the pulmonary artery is large. The pulmonary arteries show mild hypertensive changes and the lungs are relatively normal histologically. The left side of the heart is normal-sized or small. When the drainage is into the coronary sinus the oxygenated blood streams preferentially through the tricuspid valve and the caval blood streams into the left atrium so that the arterial blood is less saturated than that in the pulmonary artery.

When there is pulmonary venous obstruction the pulmonary blood flow is not greatly increased and therefore the amount of oxygenated blood returning to the right atrium is small. Hence the patient is clearly cyanosed. The pulmonary venous hypertension produces secondary pulmonary arterial hypertension and the small pulmonary arteries show severe hypertensive vascular disease, the lungs are oedematous, and on section show dilatation of lymphatics and the presence of 'heart failure' cells (haemosiderin-laden macrophages) in the alveoli. The right ventricle is only slightly dilated but more hypertrophied than in the non-obstructed form.

Associated defects

About 40% of patients with total anomalous pulmonary venous connection have other cardiovascular defects, particularly dextrocardia, abnormalities of systemic venous return, ventricular septal defect and endocardial cushion defects.

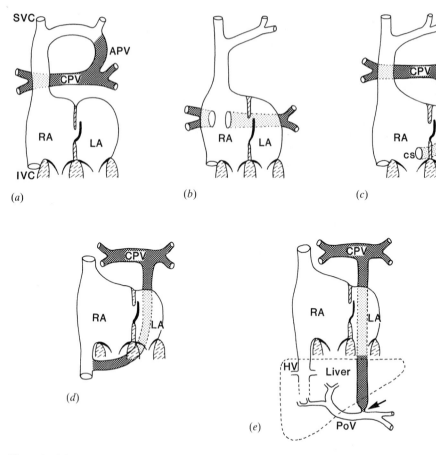

Figure 11.4 Types of total anomalous pulmonary venous connection. (*a*) Supracardiac via ascending pulmonary vein and left innominate vein. (*b*) Cardiac, direct to right atrium. (*c*) Cardiac into coronary sinus. (*d*) Infracardiac into inferior vena cava. (*e*) Infracardiac into portal vein. APV, ascending pulmonary vein; RA, right atrium; LA, left atrium; SVC, superior vena cava; CPV, confluence of pulmonary veins; IVC, inferior vena cava; CS, coronary sinus; PoV, portal vein; HV, hepatic vein

Transposition and pulmonary atresia have also been reported. Apart from dextrocardia the presence of other defects has a profound effect on the clinical presentation.

Clinical presentation

The infant with obstructed anomalous pulmonary venous connection presents in the first few days of life with cyanosis and evidence of pulmonary venous congestion – cough, respiratory difficulty and sometimes, frank pulmonary oedema. Clinical examination reveals obvious central cyanosis, poor pulses and a rapid respiratory rate with marked lower costal and intercostal incession. There are no murmurs but the second heart sound is loud and usually not audibly split. Fine râles may be heard over the lungs. The chest radiograph shows pulmonary venous obstruction

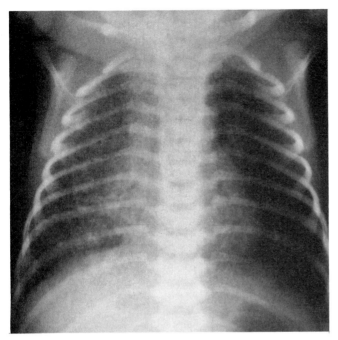

Figure 11.5 Radiograph showing miliary appearance of the lungs (particularly on right side) in patient with total anomalous pulmonary venous drainage to the portal vein

and often a miliary or reticular pattern due to pulmonary oedema (Figure 11.5). The electrocardiogram is normal or shows right ventricular hypertrophy.

Non-obstructed forms do not usually produce symptoms for the first two to three months of life and occasionally not until the second or third year. The symptoms are usually respiratory difficulty and failure to gain weight. A respiratory infection may precipitate referral to hospital. Examination typically reveals an undernour-ished infant with a tinge of cyanosis on feeding or crying but little or none at rest. The respiratory rate is raised and there is moderate lower costal incession. The heart rate is fast, the right ventricular pulsation easily palpable at the left sternal border and a fairly loud systolic ejection murmur is heard in the pulmonary area, due to the high right ventricular output. The second heart sound is usually clearly split without obvious variation over the different phases of respiration and there is usually a diastolic murmur due to high tricuspid blood flow. This murmur is usually best heard at the lower left sternal border but may be heard further laterally when right atrial enlargement rotates the heart in a clockwise direction, displacing the tricuspid valve laterally.

Radiology

The chest radiograph shows right atrial and right ventricular enlargement (best seen on lateral views) and obvious pulmonary plethora (Figure 11.6). The characteristic 'cottage loaf' appearance of the type with connection via the left innominate vein is rarely seen in infancy.

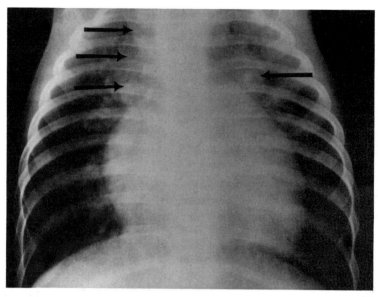

Figure 11.6 Radiograph of 3-month-old patient with supracardiac type of total anomalous pulmonary venous connection. The right ventricle is enlarged and the lungs pleonaemic. The ascending pulmonary vein is faintly seen on the left of the upper mediastinum and the superior vena cava is prominent on the right

Electrocardiography

The standard leads show right axis deviation and usually right atrial hypertrophy. In precordial leads there is evidence of right ventricular hypertrophy with either a qR or an rsR′ pattern in leads V_1 and V_2.

Diagnosis

The obstructed form of total anomalous pulmonary venous connection should be suspected in any newborn infant with cyanosis and severe respiratory difficulty when there is little or no response to oxygen, particularly if the chest radiograph shows a normal-sized heart. Other causes of pulmonary venous hypertension, such as hypoplastic left heart syndrome or myocardial disease, may present similarly but the heart is much larger on radiography. The main problem is to distinguish the condition from respiratory distress syndrome and the absence of any marked response to oxygen makes investigation by echocardiography mandatory.

In the unobstructed form the clinical picture may resemble left-to-right shunting through a septal defect but the mild cyanosis, fixed splitting of the second heart sound and prominent tricuspid diastolic murmur are not seen in simple septal defects. Furthermore, the electrocardiogram, which shows right axis deviation and right ventricular hypertrophy rules out atrioventricular septal defect. In older children the auscultatory signs resemble those of atrial septal defect, but there is mild, but definite, cyanosis and more cardiomegaly in total anomalous pulmonary venous connection.

Although the usual presentation of the non-obstructed form is with cardiac failure at 4–6 weeks, cardiologists are increasingly seeing patients referred in the first day or so of life. These are babies who are well but are noted or suspected to be mildly blue and 'fail' the hyperoxia test. Within a few days the cyanosis becomes less obvious as the pulmonary blood flow increases, but by this time the diagnosis will already have been made by echocardiography. For similar reasons cardiologists are often asked to see and investigate 2- or 3-day-old babies with persistent tachypnoea and diffuse pulmonary opacities in case they have obstructed total anomalous pulmonary venous connection rather than primary lung disease. That this is a wise precaution is shown by the increase in the number of cases of obstructed total anomalous pulmonary connection both in absolute terms and in relative frequency compared with the non-obstructed form. Ten years ago only 20% of all cases were the obstructed form; now they constitute 40%.

Echocardiography

The right atrium and ventricle and the pulmonary artery are all enlarged, particularly in the non-obstructed forms. Pulmonary veins are not seen entering the left atrium and no Doppler signal of pulmonary venous flow is detected at the back of the left atrium. When the foramen ovale is small the atrial septum is conspicuously bowed to the left, indicating the higher right atrial pressure. Doppler flow through the atrial septal defect or foramen ovale is right to left and often has a high velocity. Once these findings are apparent, the operator is alerted to look for the confluence of pulmonary veins behind the left atrium and the anomalous channel or channels. When the drainage is to the coronary sinus this structure is large and easily identified in a central position, and can be traced to its opening in the right atrium.

Cardiac catheterization

Although the diagnosis can reliably be made by echocardiography, cardiac catheterization is necessary if all the pulmonary veins cannot be shown on echocardiography, since mixed types of drainage do occur. In the rare cases which present in older children it is also necessary to check on the level of pulmonary vascular resistance as this may be high enough to preclude operation.

The characteristic finding in the *non-obstructed* form is a large shunt of oxygenated blood into the right atrium. The exact site of the shunt can be determined by careful sampling in the venae cavae and in different parts of the atrium, coupled with samples, if necessary, from both innominate veins. There is moderate elevation of right ventricular and pulmonary artery pressures. The pulmonary wedge pressure is normal or slightly elevated. The left atrial pressure is lower than the right atrial if there is only a patent foramen ovale. Arterial blood is nearly fully saturated except when the pulmonary venous return is through the coronary sinus, when the arterial saturation is usually only about 80%, whereas it may be 90% in the pulmonary artery.

In the *obstructed* form the right atrial blood is less highly saturated but the shunt can still be readily detected. The right ventricular and pulmonary artery pressures are markedly elevated and the wedge pressure, if it can be obtained, is elevated.

The catheter can usually be passed into the confluence of the pulmonary veins in the supracardiac and cardiac forms, and angiography can be performed either from

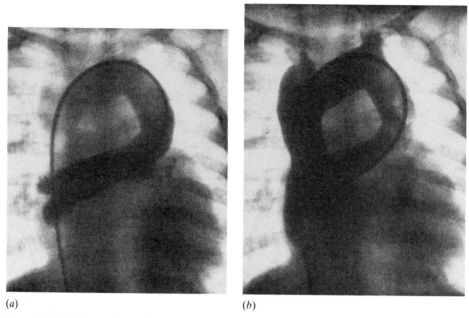

(a)   (b)

Figure 11.7 Total anomalous pulmonary venous drainage to superior vena cava. The catheter has been passed into the collecting vein. (a) The radio-opaque dye demonstrates the dilated vein which causes the 'cottage loaf' appearance in the upper mediastinum on the plain radiograph. (b) The dye has entered the superior vena cava and right atrium

this site or by injecting into the right ventricle or pulmonary artery and following the contrast round into the pulmonary veins (Figure 11.7).

Confusion may occur with the types of anomalous pulmonary venous connection draining into the right atrium or coronary sinus where the findings resemble those of an uncomplicated atrial septal defect, but infants and small children with uncomplicated atrial septal defect are virtually never symptomatic and the presence of desaturated blood in the left atrium and left ventricle, together with a right atrial pressure a little higher than left, should make the true diagnosis clear.

Prognosis

In the *obstructed* type, death usually occurs any time from the first day to the end of the second month. Without surgery, most patients with the *unobstructed* form have symptoms in infancy and even in those who survive the first year of life the prognosis is poor.

Treatment

Medical therapy is generally ineffective in the obstructed form. It is tempting to give repeated doses of frusemide to reduce pulmonary oedema, but the only result is to produce a low-output state and hyponatraemia without altering the clinical or radiological picture. Intubation and artificial ventilation may be required pending surgery. In the non-obstructed types treatment with frusemide should be started to reduce cardiac failure and the tendency to pulmonary oedema. Operation is required urgently in obstructed forms and most cases with non-obstructed drainage. This is carried out under cardiopulmonary bypass, usually with preliminary surface cooling.

When the anomalous pulmonary venous connection joins the coronary sinus operation is carried out within the heart to open the coronary sinus widely into the left atrium (along whose posteroinferior border it runs). The opening of the coronary sinus into the right atrium and the atrial septal defect (if present) are then closed with a patch. (This leaves the coronary sinus blood draining into the left atrium but the small right-to-left shunt so produced is not symptomatically important.) In patients with pulmonary veins draining directly into the right atrium, a patch of pericardium or Teflon is used to divert the pulmonary veins through the atrial septal defect, which is enlarged if necessary. In all other forms a wide, direct anastomosis is made between the confluence of pulmonary veins and the posterior wall of the left atrium. Usually this is performed behind the heart but occasionally through an incision opening both atria. The anomalous venous connections are then ligated.

The results of surgery on non-obstructed forms are good, with an operative mortality less than 10% but between 25 and 50% for obstructive forms, the higher risk being due to the need for operation within the first few days of life and the intense pulmonary venous obstruction and oedema preoperatively. Subsequent progress is usually excellent but occasionally stenosis develops at the site of the anastomosis. This seems to be an idiosyncracy of individual patients and tends to recur after reoperation.

Congenital absence of pulmonary venous connection

Occasional cases have been described in which pulmonary veins connect neither to the left atrium nor any other part of the circulation. These patients present within the first day of life, as extremely dyspnoeic, blue and with poor cardiac output. In many, the ductus arteriosus remains patent, so that a persistent fetal circulation occurs. Since the flow through the lungs is very poor, it is almost impossible to diagnose the condition angiographically, but it is suspected in an infant with radiological features of obstructed total anomalous pulmonary venous obstruction. If time permits, surgical exploration is worthwhile as there is usually a confluence of pulmonary veins suitable for anastomosis to the left atrium, but occasionally there are no pulmonary veins at all to be found.

Single or primitive ventricle (univentricular heart)

Incidence

Single ventricle appears to have become more common than earlier reports suggest and accounted for 3.6% in the Bristol series (including tricuspid atresia), which makes it about as common as transposition of the great arteries.

Definition

Much has been written recently on the definition of single ventricle and the classification of its various forms. We use the term 'single ventricle' to indicate a heart which has only one complete ventricle with an inlet valve and an outlet portion, even though the outlet valve is atretic. As will be seen, this means that tricuspid atresia is included as a form of single ventricle, whereas pulmonary atresia with ventricular septal defect is not. The reason for this apparently arbitrary ruling is that in pulmonary atresia with ventricular septal defect the right ventricle receives and ejects blood as an independent chamber while in tricuspid atresia the right ventricle, if present, receives blood from the left ventricle and does not therefore act independently of the main ventricle.

Anatomy and physiology

With the advent of extended palliation using the modified Fontan operation, many patients with single ventricle will be suitable for operation and it is more important to discuss the various anatomical types and their physiological importance. Four main types are described, each of which may have the great arteries in the normal or transposed position (unimportant in terms of the type or blood which they receive) and a normal or obstructed pulmonary valve (which determines the types of symptoms). It is important that any individual form of single ventricle is described in full, rather than relying on eponyms or types. The parts which need to be described are:

1. The anatomy of the main ventricle, whether it has the structure resembling a left or a right ventricle. The left ventricular type has a rounded apex, small trabeculae on its inner wall and two (at least) well-formed papillary muscles.
2. The number and type of inlet valves. If there are two there will always be one mitral and one trucuspid valve, but if only one it may be either type or a composite valve with elements of both mitral and tricuspid tissue.
3. The nature and position of any other ventricular elements. A ventricular element with an outlet valve but no inlet, filling from the main chamber, is called an outlet chamber; one with neither inlet nor outlet is called a trabecular pouch.
4. The type and size of communication between the main ventricle and any outlet chamber needs to be defined, in particular noting whether the communication is small enough to produce obstruction to the flow of blood.
5. The position and connection of the great arteries, whether to the main ventricle or to the outlet chamber.
6. Whether the aortic valve or the pulmonary valve is obstructed, either at the valve itself or by subvalve muscular tissue.
7. Other abnormalities such as coarctation or abnormalities of venous return must also be identified.

It would appear that there is an infinite variety of types of single ventricle, but in practice only four of them are common. Although many of the features described do not affect the physiology of the heart, they are important when it comes to planning treatment and explaining the prognosis to parents.

Double-inlet left ventricle

The most common type has a main ventricle with the morphology of a normal left ventricle, that is with relatively small muscle trabeculae, and two inlet valves (Figure 11.8(a)). The right ventricle is usually represented by an outflow chamber which in 80% gives rise to the aorta, so that, technically, transposition also exists. About 30% have pulmonary stenosis or atresia and coarctation of the aorta occurs

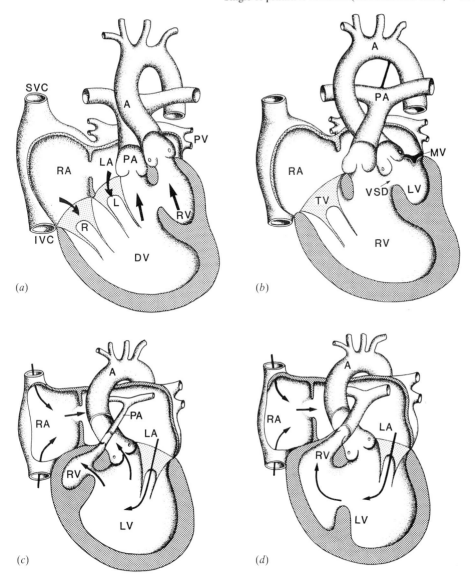

Figure 11.8 Some types of primitive ventricle. (*a*) Double inlet ventricle. The interatrial septum is present and both mitral and tricuspid valves drain into the main ventricular cavity, which has the morphology of a left ventricle. One of the great arteries, usually the pulmonary artery, arises from the main ventricle and the other, usually the aorta, from an outlet chamber with right ventricular morphology. This communicates with the main ventricle by a ventricular septal defect, which may be small and restrict the flow of blood. (*b*) Mitral atresia (primitive ventricle with absent left-sided atrioventricular valve). The main ventricle is of right ventricular morphology. There is either an outflow chamber giving rise to the aorta, as shown, or both great arteries arise from the main (right) ventricle. (*c*) Tricuspid atresia (primitive ventricle with absent right-sided atrioventricular valve). The main ventricle has left ventricular morphology and the pulmonary artery arises from an outflow chamber with right ventricular morphology. The ventricular septal defect or the pulmonary valve is restrictive. (*d*) As (*c*) but with unobstructed flow to the lungs. A, aorta; DV, double inlet ventricle; IVC, inferior vena cava; LA, left atrium; LV, left ventricle; MV, mitral valve; PA, pulmonary artery; RA, right atrium; RV, right ventricle; SVC, superior vena cava; TV, tricuspid valve; VSD, ventricular septal defect.

in about 40% of those without pulmonary stenosis. Mixing of blood occurs in the ventricle, and in the absence of pulmonary stenosis pulmonary blood flow increases rapidly in the first few weeks of life, this tendency being accentuated if there is aortic stenosis or coarctation.

Single ventricle with absent right atrioventricular valve (tricuspid atresia)

This type, the second most common overall and the commonest form to present with cyanosis, used to be described simply as tricuspid atresia and accounted for about 1.5% of all cases of congenital heart disease. There is no direct communication from right atrium to right ventricle and all the right atrial blood passes from the right atrium via an atrial septal defect or patent foramen ovale to the left atrium where mixing with pulmonary venous blood occurs. The left atrium drains through a mitral valve into the ventricle which has the morphology of a normal left ventricle. The right ventricle is usually represented by an outflow chamber into which blood flows through a ventricular septal defect and thence into the pulmonary artery. Usually there is obstruction to flow into the pulmonary artery at either the ventricular septal defect or the pulmonary valve (Figure 11.8(c)). This obstruction may be mild initially and increase either due to closure of the ventricular septal defect (which may become complete) or to the development of muscular obstruction below the pulmonary valve (analogous to the infundibular stenosis that develops in tetralogy of Fallot). Occasionally there is no obstruction at either ventricular septal defect or pulmonary valve (Figure 11.8(d)), in which case pulmonary flow is high.

Sometimes there is also transposition, with the pulmonary artery arising from the main ventricle, in which case pulmonary blood flow is high and the physiological situation similar to a double-inlet left ventricle.

Single ventricle with absent left atrioventricular valve (mitral atresia)

The mitral valve is atretic and blood from the left atrium has to pass into the right atrium, against the valve action of the foramen ovale. In the right atrium pulmonary and systemic venous blood mix and pass through the tricuspid valve into a ventricle with the morphology of a normal right ventricle, that is the apex is pointed, there are large trabecular muscles and only small papillary muscles. There is a ventricular septal defect which communicates with a rudiment of left ventricle (Figure 11.8(b)). Sometimes the aorta arises from this rudiment, which is then termed an outflow chamber, and sometimes both great arteries arise from the right ventricle, in which case it is called a trabecular pouch. Coarctation occurs in about half of cases and the ascending aorta may be hypoplastic with most of the systemic flow coming through a patent ductus. Because of the difficulty in blood getting out of the left atrium there is high pulmonary venous pressure with the early development of pulmonary oedema.

Rarely pulmonary stenosis coexists in which case the picture is similar to tricuspid atresia with cyanosis the dominant symptom.

Single ventricle with single atrioventricular valve

This is a rare condition but is seen particularly with abnormalities of venous drainage and cardiac situs (see Chapter 12). The atrial septum is also deficient, either in the form of large ostium primum type of defect or represented just by a narrow rim of tissue. The single atrioventricular valve has elements of both mitral and tricuspid tissue as in a complete atrioventricular septal defect. The single ventricle is usually of indeterminate type with some elements suggesting both right and left ventricles. The atrioventricular valve (again, as in atrioventricular septal defect) may show varying degrees of regurgitation. There are usually two great arteries with or without pulmonary stenosis.

Presentation

Irrespective of the exact anatomy, the presentation of patients with single ventricle depends almost entirely on the presence or absence of pulmonary valve obstruction. Without obstruction cyanosis is minimal and breathlessness and heart failure due to a high pulmonary blood flow develop early, within the first few weeks.

With pulmonary stenosis cyanosis is the presenting symptom or sign and its severity depends on the degree of pulmonary stenosis. Patients with mitral atresia and only a foramen ovale present with, or develop, pulmonary oedema. Chest radiographs reflect the presence or absence of pulmonary stenosis. The electrocardiogram is often helpful in alerting clinicians to the possibility of a complex abnormality. In tricuspid atresia there is usually conspicuous left axis deviation and absence of the expected degree of right ventricular dominance normally found in the neonatal period (and common in other cyanotic conditions such as transposition and tetralogy of Fallot) (Figure 11.9). In double-inlet left ventricle there is also absence of right ventricular hypertrophy, but the axis may be normal or leftward.

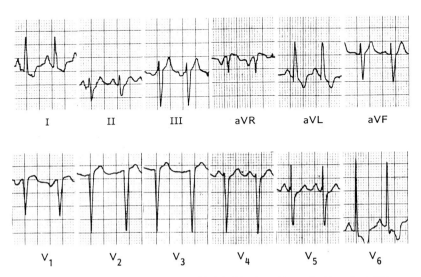

Figure 11.9 Electrocardiogram of 8-year-old girl with tricuspid atresia. Note the tall P waves, left axis deviation ($-40°$) and left ventricular hypertrophy

Echocardiography

Most of the details of the anatomy of single ventricle can be shown, in many cases more easily than by angiography (Figure 11.10). The most important finding is of only one ventricular chamber with an inlet valve. The presence of one or two atrioventricular valves is then sought. The type of valve present is inferred from the atrium to which it is attached rather from its actual anatomy. Search is then made for other ventricular structures – trabecular pouch or outflow chamber – and for a great artery arising from it or from the main chamber.

Cardiac catheterization

This is not usually necessary, if good quality echocardiograms have been obtained. When definitive surgery is being considered, a full haemodynamic study is required to assess, in particular, pulmonary artery size and vascular resistance.

Treatment

When treatment is first considered it is important that parents understand that the condition is not correctable. It should be possible from the echocardiogram, with or without cardiac catheterization, to have a good idea about the possibilities of palliation, particularly extended palliation by the Fontan procedure (see below) and this needs careful discussion with the parents. Regrettably some varieties of primitive ventricle are not, either because of the intrinsic anatomy or because of additional associated abnormalities, going to be suitable for such operations and parents may feel that they do not want operations which are unlikely to do more than extend life for a few years to be carried out. Equally it is important that parents understand the management plan and that it may need to be varied according to developments.

Initial treatment depends upon whether cyanosis or heart failure is the presenting problem. If cyanosis is severe, due to pulmonary stenosis or atresia, a palliative Blalock–Taussig shunt is carried out to provide symptomatic improvement. This must be done with particular care to avoid kinking the pulmonary artery or allowing the shunt to perfuse one side at the expense of the other, as this may make subsequent operation more hazardous. If pulmonary flow is high, leading to heart failure, banding of the pulmonary artery is carried out both to control the heart failure and also to prevent hypertensive pulmonary vascular disease. Coarctation, if present, can be dealt with at the same operation. Provided these aims are met, or if the infant naturally has just enough pulmonary stenosis to prevent either severe cyanosis or heart failure (usually this means a pulmonary flow between one and two times the systemic flow), the infant usually grows well and develops normally up to a year or so, but inevitably thereafter becomes more blue due to either relative tightening of the band or relative reduction in the size of the Blalock–Taussig shunt. In either case a (repeat) shunt may be necessary.

The next objective is to get the patient to the age of about 5 years, which is the time when most surgeons prefer to carry out definitive surgery.

Although attempts have been made to partition single ventricles with two inlet and two outlet valves, as the most physiological solution, the mortality has proved high even in the most favourable cases, and most surgeons prefer to consider patients for Fontan's operation. In principle, this operation takes advantage of the

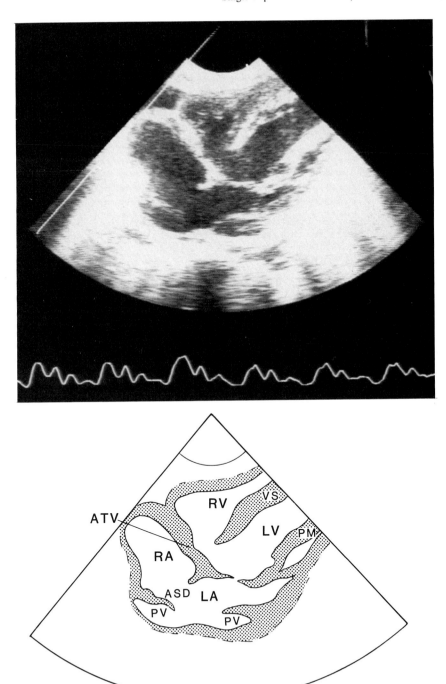

Figure 11.10 Echocardiogram of single ventricle with absent right atrioventricular valve (tricuspid atresia). ASD, atrial septal defect; ATV, atretic tricuspid valve; LA, left atrium; LV, left ventricle; PM, papillary muscle; PV, pulmonary vein; RA, right atrium; RV, right ventricle; VS, ventricular septum

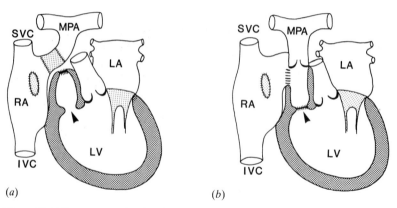

Figure 11.11 Fontan operation for tricuspid atresia. (*a*) The right atrium is connected to the main pulmonary artery (MPA). (*b*) Patient's own pulmonary valve is normal; the right atrium is connected to the outflow chamber and the ventricular septal defect (arrowed) closed. IVC, inferior vena cava; LA, left atrium; LV, left ventricle; RA, right atrium; SVC, superior vena cava

fact that the pulmonary artery pressure in normal hearts is only marginally higher than in the right atrium and that experimental work in animals showed that the right ventricle could be excluded from the circulation and blood would still flow without undue difficulty from the right atrium to the pulmonary artery. In the Fontan operation the surgeon does just that, closing the atrial septal defect (and the tricuspid valve orifice in patients with two atrioventricular valves) and joining the right atrial appendage to the main pulmonary artery (Figure 11.11). The pulmonary artery is disconnected from the ventricular system. A modification has also been described which allows the operation to be performed when there is a single atrium or in mitral atresia, the common atrium being partitioned to provide two atria, one of which has blood directed through the atrioventricular valve into the single ventricle and the other is connected to the pulmonary artery.

The success of the operation depends on selecting patients who satisfy a number of criteria. The most important ones are the size of and pressure in the pulmonary arteries. The main pulmonary artery must be at least 80% of the normal for the age and size, and there must be no stenosis or kinking of the main branches. The pulmonary artery pressure must be essentially normal. The other important factor is the function of the main ventricle, which becomes the left ventricle, since left ventricular failure will lead to passive pulmonary hypertension, which the right heart without a ventricle is unable to overcome. These criteria impose important restrictions on the suitability of patients for operation, and if they cannot be met the patient is best left in the palliated condition with additional shunt procedures if cyanosis is severe, sometimes allowing later review of operability if the original criteria for advising against Fontan's operation was small size of pulmonary arteries. Additionally, they mean that it is important that palliative procedures in early infancy do not produce complications such as stenosis of pulmonary arteries from Blalock shunts, or pulmonary hypertension or ventricular failure from excessive shunts or failure to band the pulmonary artery early enough or tight enough.

Operation is carried out under cardiopulmonary bypass and through a midline incision. The details are shown in Figure 11.11. The postoperative course is frequently complicated by high venous pressure and severe water retention, which may take up to two weeks to resolve. Thereafter the patient is pink but may remain with raised venous pressure and the need for long-term diuretic therapy. Exercise tolerance is improved, but does not become normal. In essence the patient has exchanged central cyanosis for a restriction in cardiac output imposed by the lack of a functioning right ventricle. Late complications from stenosis of anastomoses may occur but are less common since surgeons stopped inserting homo- or heterograft valves in the right atrial–pulmonary artery anastomosis and in the IVC–right atrial junction in an attempt to make the right atrium function more like a ventricle.

Single atrium

Definition and anatomy

Single atrium is best looked at as a form of atrioventricular septal defect. The reasons for this are, first that there is usually a rim of septal tissue posteriorly and superiorly, so that the deficiency appears as a huge ostium primum defect, and secondly because there is always depression of the crest of the inlet septum and deformity of the atrioventricular valves, ranging from a cleft in the anterior mitral valve leaflet to a common atrioventricular valve and single ventricle. The condition is frequently associated with abnormalities of systemic and pulmonary venous connection, absence of the coronary sinus and rhythm disturbances (nodal rhythm and atrioventricular block). It is also associated with abnormalities of cardiac situs.

Clinical presentation

When there are two ventricles and a reasonably competent mitral valve the presentation is similar to that of an incomplete atrioventricular septal (ostium primum) defect, breathlessness occurring from four months onwards, and the baby is only minimally cyanosed. The right ventricle is enlarged, there is a systolic murmur due to the mitral regurgitation and also a pulmonary systolic murmur due to high flow, often with an additional tricuspid diastolic murmur. The chest radiograph shows a large heart, mainly involving the right ventricle, and pulmonary plethora. The electrocardiogram shows left axis deviation and right ventricular overload. The p waves are often abnormal in morphology and there may be first, second or complete atrioventricular block. When associated with more complex lesions, the presentation is that of the dominant lesion and the single atrium is only detected by echocardiography.

Diagnosis

Echocardiography allows the diagnosis to be made with little difficulty. The connections of coronary sinus and systemic and pulmonary veins must also be defined and the mitral valve studied for evidence of cleft anterior leaflet and regurgitation.

Treatment

Provided that there are no other major cardiac anomalies, the condition is suitable for surgical correction. Surgical repair should be carried out within the first few years, since pulmonary hypertension and hypertensive pulmonary vascular disease usually make the patient inoperable by the age of 10. A large patch of Dacron is sutured into the common atrium to make an interatrial septum. If there are associated anomalies of pulmonary or systemic venous drainage these are corrected by suitable orientation of the patch, which then ends up as a serpiginous structure. Before the patch is complete the cleft mitral valve is repaired by direct suture as in an ostium primum defect. Other complicating lesions can usually be corrected at the same time and if the patient has complete heart block a permanent pacing system is usually implanted at the same time, using epicardial leads.

Bibliography

Truncus arteriosus

Wallace, R. B., Rastelli, G. C., Ongley, P. A., et al. (1969) Complete repair of truncus arteriosus defects. *Journal of Thoracic and Cardiovascular Surgery*, **57**, 95

Origin of both arteries from right ventricle

Hightower, B. M., Barcia, A., Bargeron, L. M., et al. (1969) Double-outlet right ventricle with transposed great arteries and subpulmonary ventricular septal defect. The Taussig–Bing malformation. *Circulation*, **39**, Suppl. 1, 207

Neufeld, H. N., DuShane, J. W. and Edwards, J. E. (1961) Origin of both great vessels from the right ventricle. II. With pulmonary stenosis. *Circulation*, **23**, 603

Neufeld, H. N., Wood, E. H., Kirkin, J. W., et al. (1961) Origin of both great vessels from the right ventricle. I. Without pulmonary stenosis. *Circulation*, **23**, 399

Total anomalous pulmonary venous connection

Bonham Carter, R. E., Capriles, M. and Noe, Y. (1969) Total anomalous pulmonary venous drainage: a clinical and anatomical study of 75 children. *British Heart Journal*, **31**, 45

Burroughs, J. T. and Edwards, J. E. (1960) Total anomalous pulmonary venous connection. *American Heart Journal*, **59**, 913

Clarke, D. R., Stark, J., De Leval, M., et al. (1977) Total anomalous pulmonary venous drainage in infancy. *British Heart Journal*, **39**, 436

Dillard, D. H., Mohri, H., Jessel, E. A., et al. (1967) Correction of total anomalous pulmonary venous drainage in infancy utilizing deep hypothermia with total circulatory arrest. *Circulation*, **36**, Suppl. 1, 105

Duff, D. F., Nihill, M. R. and McNamara, D. G. (1977) Infradiaphragmatic total anomalous pulmonary venous return. Review of clinical and pathological findings and results of operation in 28 cases. *British Heart Journal*, **39**, 619

Gatham, G. E. and Nadas, A. S. (1970). Total anomalous pulmonary venous connections. Clinical and physiologic observations of 75 pediatric patients. *Circulation*, **42**, 143

Primitive ventricle

Barber, G., Hagler, D. J., Puga, F. J., et al. (1984) Surgical repair of univentricular heart (double inlet left ventricle) with obstructed subaortic chamber. *Journal of the American College of Cardiology*, **4**, 771–8

DeLeon, S. Y., Ilbawi, M. N., Idriss, F. S., et al. (1986) Fontan operation for complex lesions. Surgical considerations to improve survival. *Journal of Thoracic and Cardiovascular Surgery*, **92**, 1029–37

Driscoll, D. J., Danielson, G. K., Puga, F. J., et al. (1986) Exercise tolerance and cardiorespiratory response to exercise after the Fontan operation for tricuspid atresia and functional single ventricle. *Journal of the American College of Cardiology*, **7**, 1087–94

Ebert, P. A. (1984) Staged partitioning of single ventricle. *Journal of Thoracic and Cardiovascular Surgery*, **88**, 908–13

Fontan, F. and Baudet E. (1971) Surgical repair of tricuspid atresia. *Thorax,* **26,** 240–8

Gale, A. W., Danielson, G. K., McGoon, D. C., *et al.* (1979) Modified Fontan operation for univentricular heart and complicated congenital heart disease. *Journal of Thoracic and Cardiovascular Surgery,* **78,** 831–8

Gale, A. W., Danielson, G. K., McGoon, D. C., *et al.* (1980) Fontan procedure for tricuspid atresia. *Circulation,* **62,** 91–6

Girod, D. A., Rice, M. J., Mair, D. D., *et al.* (1985) Relation of pulmonary artery size to mortality in patients undergoing the Fontan operation. *Circulation,* **72,** Suppl. II, 93–6

Hagler, D. J., Seward, J. B., Tajik, A. J., *et al.* (1984) Functional assessment of the Fontan operation: combined M-mode, two-dimensional and Doppler echocardiographic studies. *Journal of the American College of Cardiology,* **4,** 756–64

Kirklin, J. K., Blackstone, E. H., Kirklin, J. W., *et al.* (1986) The Fontan operation. Ventricular hypertrophy, age and date of operation as risk factors. *Journal of Thoracic and Cardiovascular Surgery,* **92,** 1049–64

Lee, C-N., Schaff, H. V., Danielson, G. K., *et al.* (1986) Comparison of atriopulmonary versus atrioventricular connections for Modified Fontan/Kreutzer repair of tricuspid atresia. *Journal of Thoracic and Cardiovascular Surgery,* **92,** 1038–42

Mayer, J. E., Helgason, H., Jonas, R. A., *et al.* (1986) Extending the limits for modified Fontan procedures. *Journal of Thoracic and Cardiovascular Surgery,* **92,** 1021–8

Ottenkamp, J., Wenick, A. C. G., Quaegebeur, J. M., *et al.* (1985) Tricuspid atresia. Morphology of the outlet chamber with special emphasis on surgical implications. *Journal of Thoracic and Cardiovascular Surgery,* **89,** 597–603

Warnes, C. A. and Somerville, J. (1986) Tricuspid atresia in adolescents and adults: current state and late complications. *British Heart Journal,* **56,** 535–43

Double-outlet right ventricle

Kanter, K. R., Anderson, R. H., Lincoln, C., *et al.* (1985) Anatomic correction for complete transposition and double-outlet right ventricle. *Journal of Thoracic and Cardiovascular Surgery,* **90,** 690–9

Macartney, F. J., Rigby, M. L., Anderson, R. H., *et al.* (1984) Double-outlet right ventricle. Cross-sectional echocardiographic findings, their anatomical explanation and surgical relevance. *British Heart Journal,* **52,** 164–7

Mazzucco, A., Faggian, G., Stellin, G., *et al.* (1985) Surgical management of double-outlet right ventricle. *Journal of Thoracic and Cardiovascular Surgery,* **90,** 29–34

Chapter 12

Complex lesions, malposition and malconnection

With improved knowledge of cardiac anatomy and function and newer surgical techniques, it has become possible to correct or palliate many complex defects. A complete determination of the cardiac anatomy is necessary before radical surgery can be contemplated and, since with complicated lesions no part of the anatomy can be assumed, detailed investigation by echocardiography and cardiac catheterization is required.

Most patients with complex lesions present within the first few days of life and a detailed, but not necessarily complete, evaluation is required then, both to allow the long-term possibilities to be discussed with parents and to allow planning of palliative operations which will alleviate immediate symptoms while not interfering with later, definitive surgery. In practice, the palliative surgical options are usually confined to establishing systemic to pulmonary artery shunts in those patients who have a severely reduced pulmonary blood flow and banding the pulmonary artery in those in whom it is excessive.

It has become important to establish definitions and nomenclature which allow detailed and full descriptions of the anatomy to be passed between physicians and surgeons in different centres, so that results of different methods of treatment can be compared. This has led to a comprehensive terminology (Tynan *et al.*, 1979) which is generally accepted throughout the world. Essentially this is based on the *connections* between the different parts of the heart, to which are added the *positions* and *additional lesions*. This avoids the confusion that arises with such terms as dextrocardia (which can mean displacement of a normal heart into the right chest by pulmonary disease, rotation of the heart or a mirror image of the normal), or the use of eponyms such as 'Holmes Heart' for a variety of single ventricle.

Malposition of the heart

It is unfortunate, in this context, that we have for centuries used such terms as right and left ventricle. In the normal heart there is no problem, as the ventricle on the right always has the same morphology – a tricuspid inlet valve, small papillary muscles, a heavily trabeculated septum and a prominent ridge of muscle (the conus septum) separating inlet and outlet portions, while the ventricle to its left has a bicuspid (mitral) inlet valve, large papillary muscles, a finely trabeculated septal surface and continuity between inlet and outlet valves. However, in complex hearts the ventricles may occupy unusual positions, and we have to decide whether we define a ventricle as a 'right ventricle' if it occupies a position to the right of the other ventricle or if it has the anatomical features of a normal right ventricle. The agreed convention is to use the latter terminology and thus define a right ventricle as a ventricle with the anatomy of a normal right ventricle, irrespective of the position it occupies. Right and left atria are similarly defined.

Position of the viscera and atria

The position of the viscera is important in complex heart disease, mainly because the right atrium nearly always occupies the same side (*situs*) as the liver.

The terms used are first defined:

Solitus: usual or normal.
Situs solitus: normal place.
Situs solitus of the viscera: the viscera are in their normal place.
Situs solitus of the atria: the atria are in their normal place.
Inversus: the opposite side to normal.
Situs inversus of the viscera: the viscera are on the opposite sides to normal, i.e. liver on the left, stomach on the right.
Situs inversus of the atria: the atria are on the opposite sides to normal, i.e. right atrium on left.
Ambiguous: not clearly related to one side or other.
Situs ambiguous of viscera: liver and stomach not clearly related to one side (midline liver).
Atrial situs ambiguous: either a common atrium or two identical atria (usually right) one on either side.

Clinical and radiological determination of visceral and atrial situs

It may be possible to determine the side of the liver clinically, but nearly always a radiograph showing not only the chest but the upper abdomen is necessary. A small amount of swallowed contrast is useful in demonstrating the stomach, but often the gastric air bubble is sufficient.

Although the liver is a good guide to atrial situs, a more accurate method is to study the bronchial anatomy (Van Mierop, Eisen and Schiebler, 1970). Usually a slightly penetrated film will be adequate, but occasionally tomograms will be required. The right main bronchus is more vertical than the left, and the distance to its first (eparterial) bronchus is shorter. If it can be determined which is the right bronchus, then the right atrium will lie on that side. If there is ambiguous atrial situs with two right atria, then there will be two equally short ('right') main bronchi.

Asplenia is usually associated with 'right-sided isomerism', that is to say that normal right-sided structures are found in a mirror image condition on the left side as well. There are then two right lungs (with three lobes) and bilateral superior venae cavae, usually with a single atrium.

A similar, but rarer syndrome of polysplenia, associated with left-sided isomerism and complex anomalies is also described (Moller *et al.*, 1967).

Attempts have been made to explain the various abnormalities of position and connection in complex anomalies on an embryological basis (Van Praagh, Vlad and Keith, 1964), in particular with reference to the early looping of the primitive cardiac tube. The normal loop is towards the right (D- or dextrolooping). Looping to the left (L- or laevolooping) is thought to cause 'corrected' transposition, while failure to develop any loop is associated with the syndromes of asplenia and polysplenia.

Abnormalities of connection of the cardiac chambers

While the positions of the various chambers may indicate something of the overall cardiac abnormality it is the connection of the various parts of the heart which is fundamental in determining the physiological result and in determining surgical treatment. Connections are said to be *concordant* if they follow the normal pattern, e.g. right atrium to right ventricle and left atrium to left ventricle, and *discordant* if they follow any other pattern, such as left atrium to right ventricle or right ventricle to aorta. In addition, there may be a *double* connection to or from one chamber, such as a double-*inlet* ventricle, where both atria drain through separate mitral and tricuspid valves into one ventricle or a double-*outlet* right ventricle giving rise to both aorta and pulmonary artery. If there is no connection from one atrium direct to a ventricle this is described as *absent* connection so that tricuspid atresia may, in most circumstances, be described as absent right atrioventricular connection. In some hearts, usually those with only one ventricle or atrium, it may be impossible to describe the connection according to these rules and the term *ambiguous* is used.

In theory one should start with the pulmonary and systemic veins and work through the heart in a sequential fashion until the connections of the great arteries have been described. In practice, it is usual to start with the position of the atria, and describe any abnormal connections of the systemic and pulmonary veins separately.

The rule for describing a complex abnormality is as follows (Table 12.1): first, describe the atrial situs, second the atrioventricular and ventriculo-arterial connections, thirdly describe where cardiac chambers and great arteries lie in relation to each other and fourthly describe associated defects such as septal defects and valvular abnormalities (a fifth section, describing the cardiac rhythm, is sometimes added, where appropriate).

The value of such a system is that it allows complex abnormalities to be described in a way which is recognizable to cardiologists and surgeons. In less complex anomalies it is more usual to retain the pre-existing names. For example, simple

Table 12.1 Types of connection

Atrial situs	Solitus
	Inversus
	Ambiguous
Atrioventricular connection	Concordant
	Discordant
	Absence of one AV valve
	Double-inlet ventricle
	Ambiguous
Ventriculo-arterial connection	Concordant
	Discordant
	Double-outlet ventricle
	Single outlet

transposition, in which the aorta is connected to the right ventricle and the pulmonary artery to the left, would be described as: 'normal atrial situs with concordant atrioventricular and discordant ventriculo-arterial connection' or in shortened version 'solitus, concordant, discordant (s,c,d)' but the diagnosis of transposition implies all of this.

Principles of treatment

Each patient with a complex abnormality is considered individually, since there are few patients who will 'match' any individual in anatomy and function. In any patient five possibilities have to be considered in terms of definitive treatment and three for palliative treatment. Since the definitive objectives often influence decisions on palliation, these are considered first, although in many patients palliation will be the first event chronologically.

Definitive possibilities
1. No treatment is necessary as the physiological result of the abnormality is nil or minimal. This includes the occasional patient with corrected transposition (see below) but only minor associated abnormalities.
2. Correction may be possible. This includes most conditions in which there are two ventricles with atrioventricular valves and a normal or near-normal aortic valve. (Absence or atresia of the pulmonary valve is not a contraindication since it is possible to manage with no pulmonary valve, provided one can insert an adequate conduit from the heart to the pulmonary artery.)
3. Extended palliation may be possible with operations such as the Fontan procedure. This applies to many patients with a single ventricle, provided that it has a normal inlet valve and there is a normal aortic valve.
4. Limited palliation may be possible, but no definitive operation can be envisaged. Clearly there are social and ethical problems in palliating an infant in whom no definitive procedure seems possible.
5. No definitive or palliative procedure is possible. Cardiac or cardiopulmonary transplantation may be a possibility in some of these patients.

Palliative operations
1. Associated conditions may be corrected. This particularly applies to patients with coarctation of the aorta with primitive ventricle.
2. Banding of the pulmonary artery in patients with excessive pulmonary blood flow. This not only reduces the overall load on the heart and improves heart failure, but can prevent the development of hypertensive pulmonary vascular disease. Since many patients will later be considered for a Fontan procedure (where a normal pulmonary vascular resistance is a prerequisite) it is important that banding is carried out early, within the first few months of life. Unfortunately, this usually means that, with growth, the child becomes unacceptably cyanosed, necessitating further surgery within one to two years.
3. When there is severe cyanosis, a systemic to pulmonary artery shunt (classical Blalock or central shunt) will improve cyanosis and also encourage pulmonary arteries to grow to a size suitable for the Fontan procedure. Care must be taken not to overload a single ventricle, causing failure, or to distort the pulmonary artery anatomy.

Atrial anomalies

Besides abnormal position (situs) of the atria in patients with situs inversions and situs ambiguous, other anomalies of the atria may occur.

Bilateral right atria occur with asplenia as part of the right-sided isomerism. The condition is recognized by angiography as both atria have short wide appendages. The corresponding condition of *bilateral left atria* occurs with greater rarity.

Juxtaposition of the atrial appendages usually occurs on the left side and the morphologically right one is superior to the left. The condition is only diagnosed at angiography (or autopsy) and its only real importance is that it implies complex malformation of atria, ventricles and atrioventricular valves.

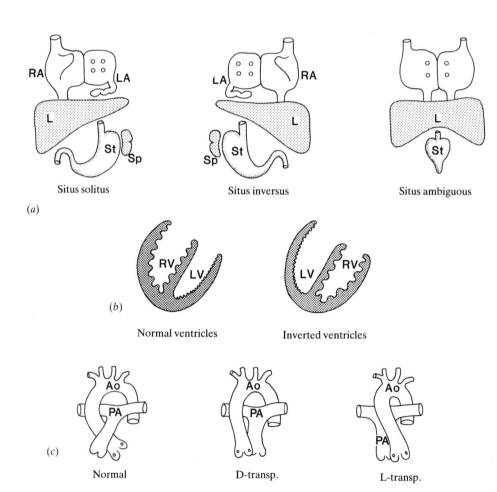

Figure 12.1 Varieties of dextrocardia. In row (*a*) are shown the three types of visceral and atrial situs. Note that the anatomical 'right atrium' (RA) is always on the same side as the liver. Row (*b*) shows the ventricular situs. RV and LV refer to ventricles which have the anatomical characteristics of the normal right and left ventricles respectively. Row (*c*) represents the three possible arrangements of the great arteries. In theory, 18 different combinations are possible. Ao, aorta; L, liver; LA, left atrium; LV, left ventricle; PA, pulmonary artery; RA, right atrium; RV, right ventricle; Sp, spleen; St, stomach

Diagnosis of complexes associated with malposition

It will be clear that a complete diagnosis cannot be made without cardiac catheterization. Echocardiography prior to catheterization is helpful in establishing whether there is a single ventricle and whether one or two atrioventricular valves are present (Solinger, Elbi and Minhas, 1975). The diagnosis is then built up in a sequential fashion, as indicated in Figure 12.1 or by determining the connections as described earlier in this chapter.

Corrected transposition (or L-transposition) of the great arteries

Definition

As in complete transposition, the great arteries have changed places so that the aorta lies anterior and the pulmonary artery posterior, but in addition the aorta and pulmonary artery have changed places in a right-to-left direction so that the aorta lies to the left of the pulmonary artery instead of to the right of it and the pulmonary artery is to the right of the aorta instead of to its left. The primitive heart tube has looped to the left instead of the right and the aorta occupies the left or laevo-position, that is, L-transposition (Figure 12.2).

The ventricles with their appropriate atrioventricular valves do not occupy their normal positions. The anatomical right ventricle lies on the left and the anatomical left ventricle lies on the right.

In the terminology described previously, this condition represents 'atrioventricular discordance with ventriculoarterial discordance' – that is connection of right

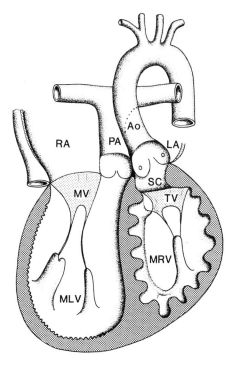

Figure 12.2 Corrected or L-transposition. The aorta arises from the systemic ventricle (MRV) which resembles the normal right ventricle, having a tricuspid valve (TV) and crista supraventricularis (SC) separating the tricuspid and aortic valves. The pulmonary artery (PA) arises behind and to the right of the aorta (Ao) from the pulmonary ventricle (MLV) which has a mitral valve (MV) which is in direct continuity with the pulmonary valve. The right atrium (RA) and left atrium (LA) are normally situated

atrium to anatomical left ventricle (with left atrium to right ventricle) and anatomical left ventricle to pulmonary artery (with right ventricle to aorta).

The result therefore in corrected transposition is that systemic venous blood enters the normal right atrium and then passes through a *mitral* valve into the smooth walled, morphological 'left' ventricle, which supplies the pulmonary artery lying posterior and to the right of the aorta. The pulmonary venous blood comes back to a normal left atrium and passes through a *tricuspid* valve into a trabeculated, morphological 'right' ventricle which supplies the aorta which lies anterior and to the left of the pulmonary artery. Clearly, then, the oxygenated blood reaches the aorta and the deoxygenated blood reaches the lungs. If there were no other defects the only functional abnormality would be that the morphological right ventricle supplied the aorta and the morphological left ventricle supplied the pulmonary artery.

It is, however, very rare for corrected transposition to occur without associated abnormalities. Ventricular septal defect and pulmonary stenosis are the most common abnormalities and frequently the left atrioventricular valve (the tricuspid) is abnormal and allows regurgitation into the left atrium. Heart block of all degrees is common, and other arrhythmias may occur.

Natural history

The overall prognosis without surgery is poor. Infants may die from arrhythmias or congestive heart failure. The patients most likely to survive without therapy are those with ventricular septal defects and pulmonary stenosis.

Clinical presentation

It is the associated defects which determine the way in which the lesion presents. The ventricular septal defects are usually large and the symptoms and signs are like those described for this lesion in its uncomplicated form. Corrected transposition is suspected, however, if there is atrioventricular block or paroxysmal atrial tachycardia, and is also likely if there is clinical evidence of 'mitral' regurgitation. When there is a ventricular septal defect and pulmonary stenosis the presentation is similar to a tetralogy of Fallot.

Radiology

There is a long bulge on the left cardiac border formed by the aorta, which is not visible in the usual place (Figure 12.3). The lung fields may be plethoric or oligaemic, depending on whether ventricular septal defect or pulmonary stenosis is the dominant lesion.

Electrocardiography (Figure 12.4)

Atrial arrhythmias are common. In 75% of the patients there is a qR pattern in leads V_4R and V_1 and an absence of the normal q wave in V_5 and V_6. This is due to the fact that the interventricular septum is depolarized in the opposite direction to that of the normal heart. Heart block varying from first to third degree occurs in at least one-third of the patients.

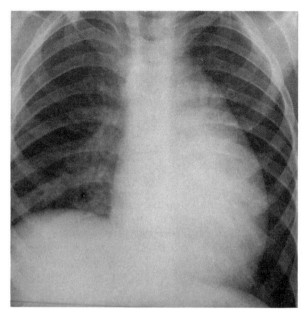

Figure 12.3 Corrected transposition. Plain radiograph. The upper part of the left border of the heart is made up of the ascending aorta. A right-sided Blalock operation has been performed which accounts for the increased vasculature and elevations of the diaphragm on the right side

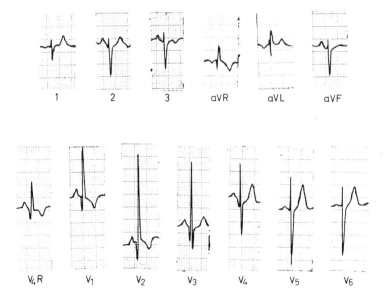

Figure 12.4 Electrocardiograph of patient with corrected transposition, ventricular septal defect and pulmonary stenosis. There are q waves in V_4R to V_3 but not in V_{5-6} and also (not due to corrected transposition) left axis deviation and right ventricular hypertrophy

Echocardiography

The anatomy and associated defects can usually be determined accurately by echocardiography. The diagnosis is usually suspected when the subcostal or apical four-chamber views fail to show the aorta arising in continuity with the atrioventricular valve from the posterior and lateral ventricle. In practice the aorta is often so far lateral that it is difficult to visualize due to the overlying lung, but in a parasternal view the pulmonary artery can be seen more posteriorly than normal and in direct continuity with the atrioventricular valve, rather than separated by the conus septum. The two papillary muscles of the anatomical left ventricle are usually the most obvious anatomical feature which enables its position, medially and posteriorly, to be determined.

Investigation

Cardiac catheterization and angiography show the abnormal position of the aorta and confirm the associated lesions. It is easier to enter the aorta through a ventricular septal defect than to enter the pulmonary artery from the venous ventricle. Arrhythmias, both heart block and tachycardia, are common during catheterization.

Treatment

Surgeons were formerly hesitant to operate inside the heart of patients with corrected transposition because of uncertainties about the position of the conducting tissue and the risks of producing heart block. The likely position of the atrioventricular bundle is now known and, where doubt exists, it can be mapped intra-operatively. In addition, pacemakers are now used more readily and with better results in patients with postoperative block. The indications for operation are therefore similar to those in patients with the equivalent lesions but normal connections, but intracardiac surgery is best avoided under the age of 2 years, as there is less room to define the anatomy, and pacemakers present more problems in the very young.

The likely associated lesions requiring surgery are:

1. Ventricular septal defect. Banding is preferable to direct closure if operation is required in the first year for uncontrollable symptoms or increasing pulmonary vascular resistance.
2. Pulmonary stenosis with ventricular septal defect. If the situation is 'balanced', i.e. there is not severe cyanosis or severe heart failure, definitive repair is undertaken from the age of 2 years onwards.
3. Left atrioventricular valve regurgitation. This is treated as for mitral regurgitation, i.e. conservatively in the first year, and then by valve replacement, if there are symptoms or progressive cardiac enlargement.
4. Complex lesions. Usually the corrected transposition element is unimportant in relation to the other anomalies, such as primitive ventricle, which are treated on their merits.
5. Heart block. First-degree block requires no specific treatment, but may progress to higher degrees later. Second- and third-degree block on their own do not usually produce either syncope or impaired exercise tolerance to require pacing, but if associated with lesions causing heart failure, the slow rate may be a

disadvantage. If pacing is required and the child is under 2 years, or if surgery is being carried out for an associated lesion, epicardial leads can be attached for pacing. Using atrial and ventricular leads for sequential atrioventricular pacing has physiological advantages but in young children requires pacemaker generators with larger bulk and shorter battery life. Over the age of about 2 years it is usually possible to maintain pacing using transvenous wires, although the relatively smooth interior of the left ventricle, into which the transvenous wire will pass, requires some form of active fixation to ensure that the wire does not become displaced.

6. Supraventricular tachycardia. This can usually be managed by drug treatment, but surgery is occasionally necessary.

Asplenia

Congenital heart disease may be associated with asplenia, when the spleen is absent, or polysplenia, when there are multiple small spleens. The heart lesion is usually a complicated one, causing cyanosis. There is often pulmonary atresia, a functionally common atrium and a common atrioventricular valve. The ventricular septum is always defective. Anomalies of systemic and pulmonary venous drainage are common. There is often malposition of the abdominal viscera.

Examination of the peripheral blood is helpful in diagnosing the condition and should be carried out in cyanotic infants. There is an increase in the number of nucleated red cells and target cells, and Howell–Jolly bodies are seen. Infants with asplenia are prone to infections. Many die early in life from severe infections. Otherwise the prognosis is that of the congenital heart lesion which is of a complex nature.

Anomalies of systemic venous connection

Anomalous systemic venous connections are comparatively unimportant in cardiology except for the technical problems which they introduce in investigation and surgery. They may be divided into those where the return is to the right atrium, where there is no physiological disturbance, and those in which there are one or more systemic veins draining into the left heart, which produces mild or moderate cyanosis without any other physical signs (Table 12.2). Usually there are associated

Table 12.2 Anomalies of systemic venous connection

Physiologically normal
Left superior vena cava – coronary sinus with or without right SVC
Inferior vena cava – azygos vein
Inferior vena cava – hemi-azygos vein – left SVC – coronary sinus
Coronary sinus – left SVC – left innominate vein – right SVC
Coronary sinus – IVC

Producing cyanosis
Left SVC – left atrium with or without right SVC
Coronary sinus – left atrium
IVC – left atrium
IVC + SVC – left atrium

severe defects, including common ventricle, which are responsible for the clinical picture; the anomalous venous drainage is an incidental finding. Asplenia is commonly associated.

Bibliography

Malposition and malconnection

Anderson, R. H., Becker, A. E., Freedom, R. M., *et al.* (1985) Sequential segmental analysis of congenital heart disease. *Paediatric Cardiology*, **5**, 281–288

Moller, J. H., Nakib, A., Anderson, R. C., *et al.* (1967) Congenital cardiac disease associated with polysplenia. A developmental complex of bilateral 'left sidedness'. *Circulation*, **36**, 789

Ruttenberg, H. D., Neufield, H. N., Lucas, R. L., Jr, *et al.* (1964) Syndrome of congenital cardiac disease with asplenia. *American Journal of Cardiology*, **13**, 387

Solinger, R., Elbi, F. and Minhas, K. (1975) Deductive echocardiographic analysis of infants with congenital heart disease. *Circulation*, **50**, 1072

Tynan, M. J., Becker, A. E., Macartney, F. J., *et al.* (1979) Nomenclature and classification of congenital heart disease. *British Medical Journal*, **41**, 544

Van Mierop, L. H. S. (1986) Diagnostic code for congenital heart disease, supplement. *Paediatric Cardiology*, **7**, 31–34

Van Praagh, S., Vlad, P. and Keith, J. D. (1964) Anatomic types of contenital dextrocardia. Diagnostic and embryologic implications. *American Journal of Cardiology*, **15**, 510

Van Mierop, L. H. S., Eisen, S. and Schiebler, E. S. (1970) The radiographic anatomy of the tracheobronchial tree as an indication of visceral situs. *American Journal of Cardiology*, **26**, 432

Corrected transposition

de la Cruz, M. V., Anselmi, C., Cisneros, F., *et al.* (1959) An embryologic explanation for corrected transposition of the great vessels: additional description of the main anatomic features of this malformation and its varieties. *American Heart Journal*, **57**, 104

Dekker, A. (1965) Corrected transposition of the great vessels with Ebstein malformation of left atrioventricular valve. *Circulation*, **31**, 119

Fernandez, F., Laurichesse, J., Seebat, L., *et al.* (1970) Electrocardiogram in corrected transposition of the great vessels of the bulboventricular inversion type. *British Heart Journal*, **32**, 165

Gerlis, L. M., Wilson, N. and Dickenson, D. F. (1986) Abnormalities of the mitral valve in congenitally corrected transposition (discordant atrioventricular and ventriculo-arterial connection). *British Heart Journal*, **55**, 475–479

King, H., Kilman, J. N., Petry, F. L., *et al.* (1964) Surgical correction for 'mitral' incompetence in corrected transposition of the great vessels. *Journal of Thoracic and Cardiovascular Surgery*, **47**, 769

Van Praagh, R. and Van Praagh, S. (1966) Isolated ventricular inversion with a consideration of the morphogenesis, definition and diagnosis of non-transposed and transposed great arteries. *American Journal of Cardiology*, **17**, 395

Vargas, F. J., Kreutzer, G. D., Schlichter, A. J., *et al.* (1985) Repair of corrected transposition associated with ventricular septal defect and pulmonary stenosis. *Annals of Thoracic Surgery*, **40**, 509–511

Abnormalities of systemic veins

Buirski, G., Jordan, S. C., Joffe, H. S., *et al.* (1986) Superior vena caval abnormalities: their occurrence rate, associated cardiac abnormalities and angiographic classification in a paediatric population with congenital heart disease. *Clinical Radiology*, **37**, 131–138

Huhta, J. C., Smallhorn, J. F., Macartney, F. J., *et al.* (1982) Cross-sectional echocardiographic diagnosis of systemic venous return. *British Heart Journal*, **48**, 288–401

Chapter 13

Miscellaneous congenital abnormalities

Diseases of the coronary arteries

Anomalous coronary artery

The commonest abnormality is when one of the coronary arteries arises from the pulmonary trunk and the other arises normally from the aorta.

When the right coronary artery arises from the pulmonary trunk there are no symptoms. Flow occurs from the aorta (via anastomoses between the left and right coronary arteries) to the pulmonary artery. There is no ischaemia of the muscle supplied by the anomalous artery and the lesion is usually discovered at autopsy.

When the left coronary artery arises from the pulmonary trunk, it is of clinical importance because symptoms occur. Three different haemodynamic situations may develop depending on the pressure in the pulmonary artery:

1. If the pulmonary artery pressure is low, blood from the normal coronary artery will flow through anastomoses with the anomalous vessel and a left-to-right shunt will develop into the pulmonary artery, producing a 'steal' of blood from the territory of the normal coronary artery.
2. If the pulmonary artery pressure is moderately raised, blood flows from the collateral vessels into the anomalous coronary but there is only a small retrograde flow into the pulmonary artery and no significant 'steal' of blood from the territory of the normal coronary artery.
3. If the pulmonary artery pressure is high, then the anomalous coronary artery perfuses the myocardium with desaturated blood.

Clinical presentation
Children who have developed a good collateral circulation with only a small amount of steal of blood into the pulmonary artery, may survive without symptoms in infancy. Others, with myocardial ischaemia, present in the third or fourth weeks of life with screaming attacks on exertion, followed by pallor and sweating and sometimes loss of consciousness. These attacks may become more frequent and then heart failure occurs; most of this group die in a few weeks but a few improve and the attacks lessen. Others present a chronic picture of mitral regurgitation and borderline congestive heart failure.

The size of the heart varies with the severity of the symptoms and in those who have suffered areas of infarction, there may be paradoxical pulsation due to ventricular aneurysm. About one-third of patients have functional mitral regurgitation due to left ventricular dilatation and papillary muscle dysfunction. In older children who have a high flow through anastomotic vessels, there is a continuous murmur usually to the left of the sternum.

Electrocardiogram

This classically shows deep Q waves and inverted T waves over the territory supplied by the anomalous vessel. Occasionally there is only the pattern of left ventricular hypertrophy.

Echocardiography

This may show only one coronary artery arising from the aorta and a coronary artery arising from the pulmonary artery. Aneurysm of the ventricular wall is seen if present and mitral regurgitation will also be demonstrated.

Aortography

This may be necessary to show retrograde filling of the anomalous vessel (Figure 13.1). In Group 3 an injection of contrast into the pulmonary artery may be necessary to demonstrate the anomalous origin.

Treatment

Infants having anginal attacks are at risk of sudden death and require surgery to implant the anomalous vessel into the aorta. Infants with heart failure will often improve after treatment with digoxin and diuretics and surgery can be deferred in

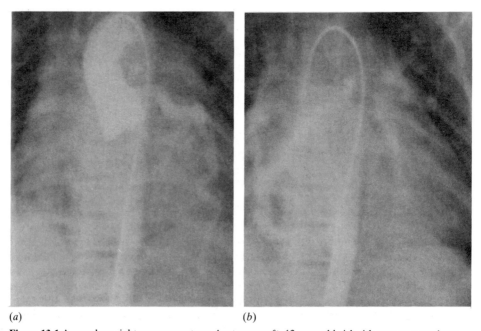

(a)   (b)

Figure 13.1 Anomalous right coronary artery. Aortogram of a 12-year-old girl with no symptoms but a continuous murmur. (a) Early phase showing a large left coronary artery arising normally from the aorta. (b) Later phase. The anomalous right coronary artery has filled through collateral channels and is seen draining upwards into the pulmonary artery, the left branch of which is clearly opacified

the hope that a collateral circulation will develop and myocardial perfusion improve. If there is deterioration after treatment for cardiac failure, then surgery has to be considered.

Children who have survived without symptoms require no treatment.

Ligation of the anomalous artery as it enters the pulmonary trunk has been suggested but the outcome of this is difficult to predict because some patients still need the supply of blood from the pulmonary artery.

Undoubtedly now the best operative procedure is the excision of a cuff of the pulmonary artery containing the ostium of the anomalous artery and anastomosing it to the side of the ascending aorta. The pulmonary artery is then repaired by sutures.

Coronary artery fistula

A rare anomaly consists of a fistula from one of the coronary arteries into a chamber of the heart or into a coronary vein. Patients do not usually have symptoms in childhood and the lesion is suspected when a soft continuous murmur is heard along the left or right sternal edge. It must be differentiated from other causes of continuous murmurs and is demonstrated by aortography. Attempts at resection may damage the blood supply to the part of the heart supplied by the affected vessel and are not generally advised unless there is evidence of important haemodynamic abnormality, such as cardiac enlargement, or a large shunt on cardiac catheterization. Now that surgeons are experienced in using grafts to bypass coronary artery disease in adults, they can use this technique to place a graft into the coronary artery distal to the fistula and then ligate the artery proximally.

Coronary artery aneurysm

A rare lesion, coronary artery aneurysm is only detected clinically if it is large enough to cause a continuous or diastolic bruit. The aneurysm may develop a secondary communication with a coronary vein or rupture into a cardiac chamber and then act as a coronary artery fistula. Treatment is the same as for coronary artery fistula.

Coronary artery narrowing

The coronary arteries may be narrowed by arterial disease such as fibromuscular hyperplasia, generalized arterial calcification and as part of the hypercalcaemia syndrome. In Japan, Kawasaki disease or mucocutaneous lymph node syndrome (Kawasaki et al., 1974) (see Chapter 21) produces an intense coronary arteritis with occlusion and aneurysm formation; Landing and Larson (1977) reported a similar syndrome in North America under the name of infantile periarteritis nodosa. They are also involved in systemic diseases such as xanthoma tuberosum, progeria and Friedreich's ataxia and, in adolescence, in familial hypercholesterolaemia. Symptoms of heart failure are more common than chest pain and are usually progressive. Successful surgical treatment has not yet been reported.

Aneurysm of a sinus of Valsalva

A congenital weakness of one or more sinuses of Valsalva can lead to progressive dilatation with two important consequences. First, an aneurysm develops which eventually bursts either, rarely, into the pericardial cavity or, more commonly, into one of the cardiac chambers, usually the right atrium. A large shunt is produced which causes cardiac failure. Irrespective of the site of communication the pulse is collapsing and a loud murmur is heard. This is diastolic only when the rupture is into the left ventricle, but continuous when it is into any other cavity. Aortography demonstrates the lesion which can be repaired under cardiopulmonary bypass. This situation is more common in adult life. Bacterial endocarditis is a frequent complication.

The second consequence of aneurysmal dilatation of the sinus of Valsalva is the production of aortic incompetence by depriving the aortic valve of its support. Although repair is theoretically possible, in practice it is difficult and replacement of the aortic valve is frequently required. For this reason attempts at repair should be postponed, if at all possible, until the patient is fully grown.

Aorto–left ventricular tunnel

This is a rare lesion presenting as aortic regurgitation. The tunnel arises at right-angles from the aorta (unlike a sinus of Valsalva aneurysm) and enters the left ventricle. Surgical repair is possible once the condition has been demonstrated by angiography (Somerville, English and Ross, 1974) but older patients with the condition frequently have additional valvar aortic regurgitation.

Arteriovenous aneurysm of the lung

In arteriovenous aneurysm of the lung, a branch of the pulmonary artery containing desaturated blood communicates with a pulmonary vein without passing through the alveoli. Hence desaturated blood reaches the left side of the heart, and the patient becomes cyanosed. Patients present with cyanosis, clubbing of fingers and toes and polycythaemia. There are usually no murmurs over the heart but a continuous murmur is audible over the aneurysm in the lung. It is important to listen over the whole of the chest routinely or this condition may be overlooked.

Lesions may be single or multiple, and occur in one or both lungs. Shadowing in the lung may be seen on a plain radiograph and pulmonary angiography will demonstrate the abnormal communication. Treatment is to remove the affected lobe or segment and is then curative, but when there are multiple aneurysms this may not be possible.

Sequestrated segment of the lung

During the development of the lung, vessels in the lung parenchyma join up to the developing pulmonary trunks. Occasionally a segment of lung fails to develop a vascular connection with the pulmonary artery, but retains instead a major communication with the systemic arterial circulation. This sequestrated segment of

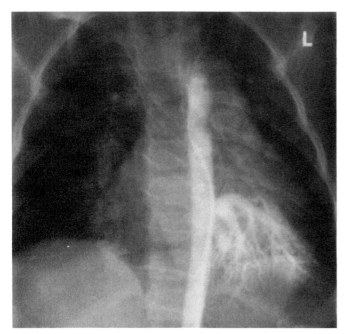

Figure 13.2 Sequestrated segment of lung. A large branch from the aorta supplies a segment of the left lower lobe

lung is usually overvascularized and does not expand properly. It tends to be the seat of recurrent infection and on the plain radiograph appears collapsed. There is often a continuous murmur over the affected area, almost always in one or other of the lower lobes (usually the right), but if this is not heard the usual clinical diagnosis is basal bronchiectasis. If there is doubt, an arteriogram will settle the diagnosis. Removal of the segment is advised because of the risk of recurrent infection, but care is necessary to secure the supplying artery, which usually enters the segment from below and frequently originates from the aorta below the diaphragm.

A similar condition, sometimes called an intralobar sequestration, may occur in which there are both normal pulmonary arteries and an anomalous supply to a segment of lung (Figure 13.2). If the condition is diagnosed early and the segment of lung otherwise healthy, the anomalous artery can be ligated and the lung segment left in place.

Scimitar syndrome

This is a type of anomalous pulmonary venous drainage in which the veins from the right lung drain to the inferior vena cava. The right lung is hypoplastic and this results in dextrocardia because the heart moves over to the right side. The arterial supply to the lung is from branches from the descending aorta with or without a normal pulmonary artery. The single pulmonary vein which descends to the right cardiophrenic angle and resembles a scimitar in shape can be clearly seen on the frontal view of a chest radiograph (Figure 13.3). There may be stenosis on this vein

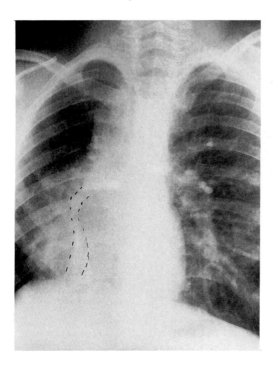

Figure 13.3 Plain radiograph of a patient with scimitar syndrome showing dextrocardia and anomalous vein outlined with dashes

as it enters the inferior vena cava. Children with the abnormality frequently have chest infections in the small right lung, but they tend to improve as they get older. Most children do not require surgery. Those that do usually have some stenosis on the collecting vein; surgery is then necessary to implant the vein into the right atrium and then construct a tunnel so that the vein drains into the left atrium. Some patients have symptoms which cannot be explained solely on the anomalous venous connection. It is likely that the right lung itself is grossly abnormal and that the only treatment is right pneumonectomy.

Pulmonary artery sling

In this rare anomaly the left pulmonary artery arises from the right pulmonary artery (Figure 13.4) and winds backwards round the trachea and right bronchus. The ductus (or ligamentum) keeps it pulled tight around the trachea. It may occur on its own or in association with other anomalies, mainly tetralogy of Fallot. Although not producing any haemodynamic abnormality it causes constriction of the trachea or right main bronchus and presents as a stridor or right-sided obstructive emphysema (Figure 13.5). Surgical treatment consists usually of reimplantation into the main pulmonary artery, but sometimes division of the ligament of the ductus provides relief of symptoms.

Dupuis *et al*. (1988) describe 8 patients with pulmonary artery sling in whom the abnormality followed a benign course. There was spontaneous improvement in two of their patients who had stridor, wheezing and respiratory distress in infancy.

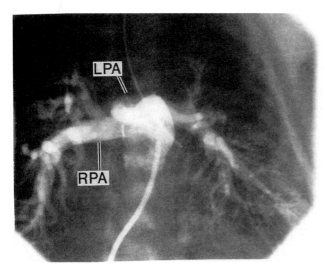

Figure 13.4 Angiogram from patient with pulmonary artery sling. Injection of dye into the main pulmonary artery shows the left pulmonary artery (LPA) arising from the right pulmonary artery (RPA) and then crossing to the left side

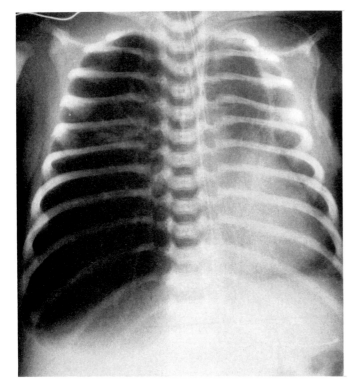

Figure 13.5 Plain radiograph from patient with pulmonary artery sling, shows over-inflation of right lung with herniation over to the left side due to compression of the right main bronchus

Bibliography and references

Diseases of the coronary arteries

Kawasaki, T., Kokasi, F., Okawa, S., *et al.* (1974) A new infantile acute muco-cutaneous lymph node syndrome (MLNS) prevailing in Japan. *Pediatrics, Springfield,* **54**, 271

Landing, B. H. and Larson, E. J. (1977) Are infantile periarteritis nodosa with coronary artery involvement and fatal mucocutaneous lymph node syndrome the same? Comparison of 20 patients from North America with patients from Hawaii and Japan. *Pediatrics, Springfield,* **59**, 651

Scimitar syndrome

Neill, C. A., Ferencz, C., Sabiston, D. C., *et al.* (1960) The familial occurrence of hypoplastic right lung with systemic arterial supply and venous drainage: scimitar syndrome. *Bulletin of the Johns Hopkins Hospital,* **107**, 1

Pulmonary artery sling

Dupuis, C., Vaksmann, G., Pernot, C., *et al.* (1988) A symptomatic form of left pulmonary artery sling. *American Journal of Cardiology,* **61**, 177–181

Aorto–left ventricular funnel

Somerville, J., English, T. and Ross, D. N. (1974) Aorto-left ventricular tunnel. Clinical features and surgical management. *British Heart Journal,* **36**, 321

Part 3

Special problems

Chapter 14

Heart disease in the newborn infant

Introduction

Over the past 20 years there has been an increasing awareness of the importance of early referral of newborn infants with heart disease to special centres. The ease and safety of transport in new ventilator incubators has encouraged this transfer and early referral itself has been an important factor in the life expectancy of these babies.

There has been continuing improvement in diagnostic methods, medical management and surgical treatment which have further improved the outlook for them.

Transport

It is important that the baby arrives at the referral centre in as good a condition as possible. Complications must be prevented; if they are allowed to occur it may be impossible to resuscitate the baby satisfactorily. The following complications must be avoided before and during transport.

1. Hypothermia
Cyanosed infants will readily become hypothermic and if hypothermia is allowed to occur, it is extremely difficult to correct and increases the hazards of investigation. The baby must be transported in an incubator with extra layers of cotton wool and aluminium foil to prevent heat loss.

2. Acidosis
Metabolic acidosis occurs rapidly in cyanosed infants and must be corrected by intravenous bicarbonate before transfer (see page 272).

3. Metabolic disturbances
Hypoglycaemia, hypocalcaemia and hypovolaemia should be corrected.

4. Severe hypoxia
If this can be improved by ventilation then it should be established before the journey begins. In ductus-dependant conditions prostaglandin infusion may be necessary.

Echocardiography

This investigation has become more reliable and new developments yield an increasing amount of information. Cross-sectional echocardiography gives a clear anatomical picture of the structure of the heart; the application of Doppler echocardiography helps to assess gradients across valves and blood flows between the chambers of the heart, and now the application of colour Doppler flow imaging adds a new dimension by providing what in effect is 'ultrasonic angiocardiography'. The latter helps in diagnosing anomalous pulmonary venous drainage with obstruction in the newborn and helps to determine the precise anatomy in various forms of single ventricle. The confidence in echocardiography is now so high that it no longer seems justifiable to subject sick newborn infants to cardiac catheterization and angiography. This often caused a deterioration in their condition and certainly the risks of invasive investigation are higher in the newborn period than at any other time. The risks of the investigation outweigh any increase in the information obtained.

Prostaglandins

There are some heart lesions in the newborn which are incompatible with survival if the ductus arteriosus closes. These are pulmonary atresia, severe coarctation of the aorta and simple transposition of the great arteries without any septal defect. An intravenous infusion of prostaglandin will ensure patency of the ductus which then provides an adequate pulmonary or systemic blood flow and in the case of transposition provides mixing between the two circulations (see Chapter 2).

If surgery is necessary in the newborn, the baby can now be referred for surgery in a much better state than previously. The cardiologist can ensure that he is warm, well oxygenated, has no acidosis or metabolic upset and has a good cardiac output. Consequently the results of surgery have improved; severe coarctation of the aorta is a good example of this (see Chapter 7).

Surgery

If necessary most newborn infants can now be helped by surgery even though the operation may be palliative. At open heart surgery new methods of cardioplegia give better protection to the myocardium and the use of continuous positive airway pressure helps to wean babies off the ventilator, in the postoperative period, with greater safety.

Anatomical correction of transposition using Jatene's operation (1976) is now possible and may become the procedure of choice in transposition of the great arteries if the risks and complications diminish (see Chapter 10). Late follow-up studies are still awaited. Caval obstruction following the Mustard operation and arrhythmias following both Mustard and Senning procedures cause concern and early operation in the neonatal period to correct the abnormality may be advised in the future. Norwood is using a palliative procedure for babies with hypoplasia of the left heart (see below) but the mortality is high and the long-term results not yet known.

The results of surgery for total anomalous pulmonary venous drainage with obstruction have not improved despite earlier diagnosis and treatment. This may be because there are abnormalities of the veins in the parenchyma of the lungs (de Leval, 1986).

Balloon valvuloplasty

The most severe forms of valve stenosis are seen in the newborn period. They need help the most, but the procedure is extremely difficult in these tiny babies and the valves are often dysplastic, making it difficult to achieve a good result. Ettedgui *et al.* (1988) found that balloon valvuloplasty in the newborn in pulmonary stenosis does not yield uniformly good results and is technically difficult. Wren *et al.* (1987) attempted valvuloplasty in 8 newborn infants with critical aortic stenosis, 5 died and 3 were improved. There is a high mortality rate from surgery in critical aortic stenosis but de Leval has had better results by performing aortic valvotomy using inflow occlusion, and approaching the valve either through the aorta or through the apex of the ventricle.

Diagnosis

The clinical diagnosis of heart disease is more difficult in the newborn period than at any other time, yet a correct diagnosis without delay is essential for effective treatment. It is important to stress that the absence of a heart murmur does not rule out heart disease; there may be no heart murmurs in some of the most severe, yet operable, cyanotic lesions (see page 243).

If an infant is cyanosed in the first few days of life and if that cyanosis does not improve with oxygen, it is useless to adopt a wait and see attitude. Nowadays, with the help of echocardiography, the problem of whether there is heart disease or not can be easily solved and if a peripheral unit does not have facilities for echocardiography the baby should be referred. If heart disease is not present no harm will result as long as care is taken during transport. The condition which used to give the greatest difficulty in diagnosis was symptomatic heart disease in the newborn without a structural lesion, i.e. persistent fetal circulation and transient myocardial ischaemia (see page 246). Echocardiography has been invaluable in ruling out structural heart disease in these very sick infants.

Severe heart disease usually presents with cyanosis or heart failure – or both.

Cyanosis
In deciding whether cyanosis is due to heart disease, the following other causes of cyanosis have to be excluded.

Peripheral cyanosis of the hands and feet is commonly observed in the newborn and must be differentiated from true central cyanosis.

Mechanical purpura. If there is delay in delivery of the body after the birth of the head, mechanical purpura on the face may make the infant appear cyanotic, but the lips are pink.

Polycythaemia. Some infants may have polycythaemia due to delayed clamping of the cord or the fetal transfusion syndrome.

Racial. Apparent cyanosis of the lips is seen in infants with pigmented skin.

Respiratory diseases causing cyanosis may cause difficulty, but in the respiratory distress syndrome, dyspnoea develops in the first 6 hours of life and the child has an expiratory grunt; cyanosis occurs only when the dyspnoea is severe and is usually promptly relieved by oxygen. The chest radiograph shows bilateral diffuse reticulogranular pattern and a well-defined tracheobronchogram.

Lung disease can cause cyanosis and dyspnoea but there may be localizing signs in the chest and a good chest radiograph will show neonatal pneumonia, the massive aspiration syndrome, pneumothorax, lobar emphysema, pleural effusion or diaphragmatic hernia. The oxygen test (Jones *et al.*, 1976) is helpful in differentiating primary lung disease from cyanotic heart disease. If the arterial oxygen tension rises over 150 mm when the infant is breathing 80% oxygen, primary lung disease is likely and cardiac catheterization can be avoided.

Persistent fetal circulation, see p. 245.

Myocardial ischaemia in the newborn, see p. 246.

Choanal atresia, when bilateral, causes severe cyanosis and respiratory distress but it is obvious that the infant can breathe only through his mouth. Symptoms are present from birth and the diagnosis is confirmed by the inability to pass a catheter through either nostril into the nasopharynx.

Brain damage, with or without haemorrhage, often causes cyanosis but there are usually periods of apnoea rather than dyspnoea and there may be twitching or convulsions, a high-pitched cry, changes in muscle tone and reflexes and a bulging fontanelle.

Sepsis may cause peripheral cyanosis but is then accompanied by evidence of peripheral circulatory collapse.

Heart failure

In recognizing the early signs of heart failure in the newborn, frequent and careful observation is more valuable than anything else. The signs are:

tachycardia	heart rate more than 180/min at rest
tachypnoea	respiratory rate more than 60/min persistently when the infant is at rest
excessive weight gain	gain of more than 1 oz/day even though feeding is poor
liver enlargement	liver palpable 2 or more cm below the right costal margin in the midclavicular line
wheezing respirations and a dry cough	occur when there is left ventricular failure and moist sounds can be heard over both lungs

There may be no cyanosis and no murmurs at this stage, but heart disease may be suggested by feeling abnormal or unequal peripheral pulses. The earlier in life the signs of heart failure develop, the more serious is the lesion causing it. *Any infant developing heart failure in the first month of life should be referred for investigation immediately*. Heart failure in the first month of life can rarely be treated medically for any length of time. Simple lesions such as patent ductus arteriosus and ventricular septal defect rarely cause heart failure as early as the first month of life (Figure 14.1) except in premature babies. It is usually caused by a lesion requiring surgery or is due to a complex inoperable lesion.

Diagnosis of individual lesions

Having established that heart disease is present because of the existence of cyanosis or heart failure, or both, it then remains to diagnose the precise lesion. The classic

Cyanosis

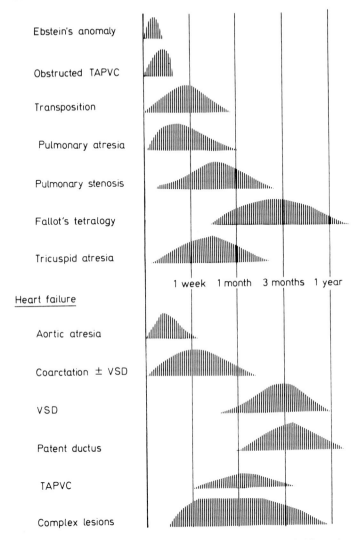

Ebstein's anomaly

Obstructed TAPVC

Transposition

Pulmonary atresia

Pulmonary stenosis

Fallot's tetralogy

Tricuspid atresia

1 week   1 month   3 months   1 year

Heart failure

Aortic atresia

Coarctation ± VSD

VSD

Patent ductus

TAPVC

Complex lesions

Figure 14.1 Onset of symptoms during the first year of life. TAPVC, total anomalous pulmonary venous connection; VSD, ventricular septal defect. The shaded areas represent the variation in onset of symptoms, not the duration of symptoms

signs found in older children are often absent in the newborn. Auscultation is surprisingly unhelpful unless diastolic murmurs are present or unless one can be certain whether the second heart sound is single or split. Diastolic murmurs are heard in absent pulmonary valve (p. 146) and with the systolic murmur gives a to-and-fro rhythm. An early diastolic murmur occurs in some infants with Type I persistent truncus arteriosus due to an incompetent truncal valve. A scratchy diastolic murmur is heard at the lower left sternal edge in Ebstein's anomaly. It is helpful for the paediatrician to know what time in life individual lesions most

Table 14.1 Differential diagnosis of heart disease in the newborn infant – main findings

Lesion	Cyanosis	Heart failure	Heart shape	Pulmonary vascularity	Electrocardiogram
Pulmonary atresia with VSD	Severe	None		Reduced	RAD RVH
Pulmonary atresia with intact septum	Severe	Occurs when RV very small	Hollow pulmonary arc; uptilted apex. RA +	Reduced	Normal axis LVH or decreased right ventricular activity for age
Tricuspid atresia	Severe	None	Square heart. RA + Pulmonary arc hollow	Reduced	LAD LVH RAH
Tricuspid atresia with high pulmonary flow	Slight or moderate	Frequently	RA + Pulmonary arc +	Increased	LAD LVH RAH
Severe pulmonary stenosis with ASD	Slight initially, gradually increasing	Rare in first month	Large RA	Reduced	RAH + + RVH
Ebstein's disease	Moderate	Rare in first month	Large RA	Reduced	RAH Right bundle branch block
Transposition with intact septum	Rapidly becomes severe	Second to fourth week		Normal or increased	RVH

Total anomalous PVD with obstruction	Rapidly becomes severe	Liver enlarged if drainage below diaphragm		Pulmonary venous congestion	RAH RVH
Hypoplasia of left heart	Slight at first, increasing by third day	First few days of life and is severe	Normal size	Increased + pulmonary venous congestion	RVH RAD
Coarctation of aorta	Slight	In first week; left heart failure frequent	General enlargement	Increased + pulmonary venous congestion	RVH RAD
Truncus	Slight or moderate	In first few weeks	Pulmonary arteries high up or not seen	Increased	RVH but may be LVH or combination of RV + LV
Atrioventricular canal	None	In first few weeks	RA + PA + RV + LV +	Increased	LAD, rsR pattern in $V_3R + V_1$. Usually combined ventricular hypertrophy
Normal heart with enlarged thymus	None	None	Broad pedicle	Normal	Normal

commonly cause severe distress. Lambert, Canent and Hohn (1966) and Varghese and co-workers (1969) found that the commonest *in the first week of life* are:
1. Hypoplasia of the left heart
2. Transposition of the great arteries
3. Coarctation of the aorta syndrome
4. Multiple major cardiac defects

In making a diagnosis it is simplest first to consider the group which present primarily with *severe cyanosis* and, secondly the group which present primarily with *heart failure* – although clearly there is some overlap between these two groups. *It is valuable to remember that patients who have lesions associated with a reduced supply of blood to the lungs, rarely develop heart failure.*

Group 1: Patients presenting with severe cyanosis
1. Transposition of the great arteries (with inadequate mixing between the two circulations).
2. Pulmonary atresia or severe pulmonary valve stenosis with intact ventricular septum.
3. Pulmonary atresia or severe pulmonary stenosis with ventricular septal defect.
4. Total anomalous pulmonary venous drainage *with obstruction* to the venous return.
5. Tricuspid atresia.
6. Ebstein's anomaly of the tricuspid valve.

Group 2: Patients presenting with heart failure
1. Hypoplasia of the left heart.
2. Coarctation of the aorta syndrome.
3. Severe aortic stenosis.
4. Persistent truncus arteriosus.
5. Double-outflow right ventricle without pulmonary stenosis.
6. Complete atrioventricular defect.
7. Cor triatriatum.
8. Complex, combined lesions.
9. Large arteriovenous fistula.

After clinical examination, it is valuable to have a radiograph and an electrocardiogram. The classic findings are listed in Table 14.1. It is important in assessing the heart shape that the film is straight and taken during inspiration and is of the correct penetration to assess the pulmonary vascularity. It is well to remember that the classic shape of the heart in a particular lesion may be masked by an enlarged thymus gland or an abnormal vessel such as a left superior vena cava. A film taken early in life may fail to show an increase in pulmonary vascularity which will become obvious later and, similarly, pulmonary venous congestion in total anomalous pulmonary venous drainage with obstruction may not be obvious initially.

If taking a radiograph and electrocardiogram is going to cause much delay and if the paediatrician thinks heart disease is present, it is better to transfer the baby without them. *It is unwise to wait for the classic findings to develop while the baby's condition deteriorates. It is better to make the wrong diagnosis and refer the infant for investigation than to make the correct diagnosis when the infant is moribund.*

It is important to stress that although ventricular septal defect and patent ductus arteriosus are very common causes of heart failure, they rarely cause heart failure in the first three weeks of life except in premature infants where the fall in pulmonary vascular resistance is more rapid than in the full-term baby (see Patent ductus arteriosus in premature infant, Chapter 6). One should always suspect a more complex lesion or a combination of defects when symptoms occur in the newborn infant. A simple atrial septal defect does not give rise to symptoms in infancy unless there is another lesion such as obstruction at the mitral valve or the aortic valve.

Many of the lesions which commonly present in the newborn period are discussed elsewhere in this book. It remains to discuss hypoplasia of the left heart, interruption of the aortic arch and the problems of persistent fetal circulation, all of which present in the first week of life. Arteriovenous malformations, when large, present in the newborn period and, although rare, must always be remembered.

Hypoplasia of the left heart

As the name suggests, in hypoplasia of the left heart there is underdevelopment of the whole of the left side of the heart. In the most severe form there is atresia of the aortic valve, the left ventricle is rudimentary and represented by a mere slit, and there is atresia or severe hypoplasia of the mitral valve. The left atrium empties through a foramen ovale or atrial septal defect to the right atrium and right ventricle (Figure 14.2). If there is a small communication between the two atria, the left atrial pressure and consequently the pulmonary venous pressure become markedly elevated and pulmonary oedema results. The only way that blood can reach the aorta is by retrograde flow through the patent ductus arteriosus. The ascending aorta is markedly hypoplastic, as are the coronary arteries arising from it, and blood flows down the aorta in a retrograde manner from the patent ductus.

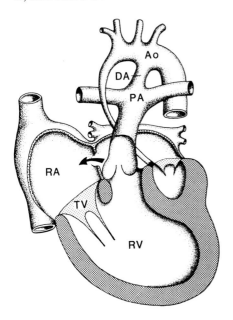

Figure 14.2 Aortic atresia. DA, ductus arteriosus; Ao, aorta; PA, pulmonary artery; RA, right atrium; RV, right ventricle; TV, tricuspid valve

In the less severe form the aortic valve is narrowed and the ascending aorta and its arch are small and form an obstruction to outflow from the left ventricle. The mitral valve ring is also small so there is a high left atrial pressure which predisposes to pulmonary hypertension.

Natural history

Patients with this condition become critically ill in the first few hours or days of life. The symptoms occur earlier than with any other heart lesion and it is the commonest cause of heart failure in the first two to three *days* of life. The majority die in the first week of life although, surprisingly, a few patients survive for two or three months on medical treatment.

Clinical presentation

The baby usually appears normal at birth but during the first day of life becomes breathless and slightly blue. When the patent ductus arteriosus begins to close, the baby suddenly worsens. The pulses are difficult to feel but are easier to feel in the legs because of preferential flow through the ductus to the descending aorta. The respirations become more rapid and heart failure develops. There may be no systolic murmur or only a faint one along the left sternal border. The second heart sound is single (only pulmonary valve closure is heard). There is oliguria or anuria because of the low renal blood flow. Babies with this condition often deteriorate quite suddenly and when the paediatrician first sees the baby, the clinical picture resembles that of a baby with severe septicaemia – pale, collapsed and pulseless. This clinical appearance during the first 3 days of life should always suggest the possibility of hypoplasia of the left heart; the enlarged liver suggests a cardiac cause.

Radiology

Radiology shows generalized cardiac enlargement in the first 24–48 hours and there is evidence of pulmonary venous congestion or frank oedema.

Electrocardiography

The electrocardiogram usually shows right axis deviation and right ventricular hypertrophy with very little left ventricular activity.

Echocardiography

The appearances on the cross-sectional echocardiogram are diagnostic (Figure 14.3). The tiny left ventricle and hypoplastic ascending aorta are seen and there is enlargement of the right ventricle and pulmonary artery. Cardiac catheterization is no longer necessary.

Treatment

The efficacy of surgical treatment has not yet been proved and in most centres no treatment is advised for this lesion. Norwood, Lang and Hansen (1983) recommend

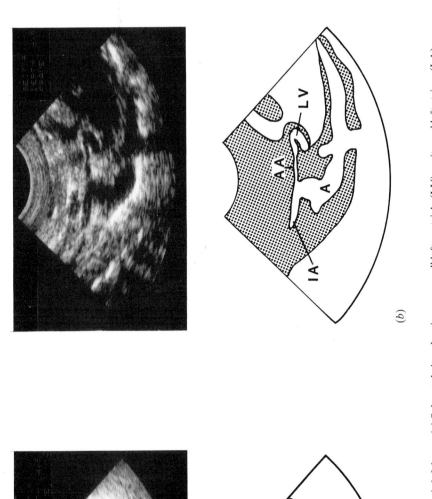

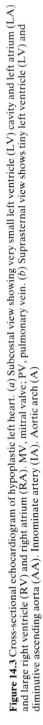

(a)

(b)

Figure 14.3 Cross-sectional echocardiogram of hypoplastic left heart. (a) Subcostal view showing very small left ventricle (LV) cavity and left atrium (LA) and large right ventricle (RV) and right atrium (RA). MV, mitral valve; PV, pulmonary vein. (b) Suprasternal view shows tiny left ventricle (LV) and diminutive ascending aorta (AA). Innominate artery (IA). Aortic arch (A)

giving the baby prostaglandins and then proceeding with a palliative operation in which the main pulmonary artery is detached from its two branches and, with a Teflon gusset, is used to reconstruct the new aorta and aortic arch; then a modified Blalock–Taussig shunt is carried out to restore blood flow to the lungs through the branches which were removed from the main pulmonary artery trunk. The mortality of this procedure is high and the heart functions as a single ventricle. It is hoped to carry out a Fontan procedure subsequently in such patients but it is not yet known how many patients will be suitable for this, nor what the long-term results will be.

Interrupted aortic arch

This is a rare abnormality and it is usually associated with a ventricular septal defect as well as a patent ductus arteriosus through which a right-to-left shunt is essential for survival. If the ductus closes the baby will die. In about 10% of patients the condition is associated with the di George syndrome (see below); in another 10% it is associated with a common arterial trunk (truncus arteriosus). The three common types of interruption are shown in Figure 14.4. In Type (a) the right subclavian artery arises from the ascending aorta whereas the left subclavian artery arises from the descending aorta opposite the ductus and distal to the interruption. In Type (b) both subclavian arteries arise from the ascending aorta and in Type (c) both subclavian arteries arise from the descending aorta distal to the interruption, so that the only pulses palpable are those in the neck.

Clinical presentation

The baby's condition may be satisfactory until the ductus begins to close; this usually happens in the first few days of life, and the baby becomes pale and shocked and develops severe heart failure. The onset resembles that of severe coarctation of the aorta or hypoplasia of the left heart. The pulses vary with the type of atresia. In Type (a) the right arm pulses will be felt but the left arm and leg pulses will be weak or absent; in Type (b) the arm pulse will be felt but the leg pulses will be weak or

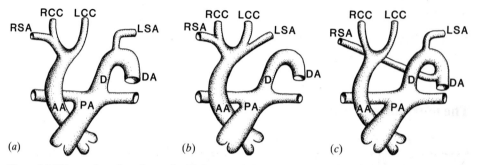

Figure 14.4 Types of aortic arch atresia. (*a*) Between left common carotid (LCC) and left subclavian artery (LSA). (*b*) Beyond left subclavian. (*c*) Between left common carotid and left subclavian with anomalous right subclavian artery (RSA). AA, ascending aorta; D, ductus; DA, descending aorta; PA, pulmonary artery; RCC, right common carotid

absent; in Type (c) pulses will be felt only in the neck and all limb pulses will be weak or absent. This lesion illustrates the importance in cardiology of *always palpating the pulses in all four limbs and in the neck*. Type (c) resembles a hypoplastic left heart, unless the carotids or temporal arteries are palpated. There are no heart murmurs and the second heart sound is single. The babies develop severe intractable heart failure which is resistant to medical treatment.

Radiology

The radiograph shows an enlarged heart with pulmonary congestion.

Electrocardiography

The electrocardiogram may be normal or show combined ventricular hypertrophy.

Echocardiography

This is the most useful investigation initially. In the suprasternal view the lesion may resemble a coarctation and it may be necessary to delineate the anatomy by angiocardiography. It is likely though that colour Doppler flow imaging will help in diagnosis. A large ventricular septal defect and two good-sized ventricles are seen.

Di George syndrome

There is hypoplasia or aplasia of the thymus and parathyroid glands in association with aortic arch anomalies. The baby often has hypertelorism and unusually-shaped ears and may also have a cleft lip and palate. Neonatal fits occur. The syndrome should be considered in all babies with interrupted aortic arch and parathyroid function and cell immunity tested.

Treatment

The only effective treatment is surgical. In Type (b) if the atretic segment is not too long, the left subclavian artery can be used in an anastomosis with the descending aorta after the ductus has been divided. This is done using deep hypothermia and a short period of cardiopulmonary bypass. Even though grafts can be used in Types (a) and (c), the operation is technically difficult and the long-term results are not good. Banding of the pulmonary artery is also necessary when there is a large ventricular septal defect.

The murmurless heart

One of the greatest problems with the sick newborn infant is deciding whether heart disease is present or not. There are a surprising number of lesions which may not produce a heart murmur in the newborn period, and these are listed in Table 14.2. They are divided into acyanotic and cyanotic groups, but it must be remembered that when heart failure and respiratory difficulty occur, the patient may appear cyanotic even though the underlying lesion is an acyanotic one.

Table 14.2 Murmurless heart in the newborn infant

Lesion	Radiology		Electrocardiography
	Vascularity of lungs	*Heart shape*	
A. Cyanotic			
Transposition of great arteries	Normal or increased	Narow pedicle and 'egg-shaped' heart	RAD RVH
Total anomalous pulmonary venous drainage with obstruction	Reticular appearance of pulmonary venous congestion	Normal size and shape	RAD RAV RVH
Hypoplasia of left heart	Increased and pulmonary venous congestion	General cardiac enlargement with broad pedicle	RAD RVH
Pulmonary atresia with VSD	Decreased	Boot shape with long left cardiac border and uptilted apex	RAD RVH
Pulmonary atresia with intact ventricular septum	Decreased	Large right atrium; left cardiac border normal	Normal axis. LVH or diminished right ventricular activity for age
Tricuspid atresia ± pulmonary atresia	Decreased	Square shape with prominent right atrium	LAD RAH LVH or poor RV activity
B. Acyanotic			
Normal heart and pulmonary disease	Normal or pulmonary venous congestion	Normal	Normal or RVH
Coarctation of aorta syndrome	Increased and pulmonary venous congestion	General cardiac enlargement	RAD RVH
Cor triatriatum	Pulmonary venous congestion	Normal	LAH RAD RVH
Myocarditis	Pulmonary venous congestion	General cardiac enlargement	Low voltage record with abnormal T waves
Endocardial fibroelastosis	Normal	General cardiac enlargement	LVH T waves in LV leads usually inverted
Common ventricle with L-transposition	Increased	Prominent left cardiac border	S waves in all precordial leads. q waves in V_4R and V_1
Anomalous coronary artery	Pulmonary venous congestion	General cardiac enlargement	Inverted T waves in leads 1, 2, 3. Deep Q waves in leads 1 and aVL. QS or QR waves in leads V_{2-4}

Persistence of the fetal circulation (transitional circulation)

This refers to a situation in which the haemodynamics of the fetal circulation persist after birth. There is constriction of the pulmonary vascular bed and if the pulmonary vascular resistance is higher than the systemic resistance then shunting will take place from the pulmonary artery through a persistent ductus arteriosus to the aorta and through the foramen ovale from the right atrium to the left atrium. The infant will then be cyanosed. Pulmonary vascular resistance may be high, secondary to some congenital heart lesion, but the term persistence of the fetal circulation refers to the primary form unassociated with any anatomical cardiac defect. The cause is unknown but it has been shown that the small pulmonary arteries have an abnormally thick muscular coat (Haworth and Reid, 1976).

Clinically the infant presents within 24 hours of birth with respiratory distress and cyanosis and there is usually a history of perinatal hypoxia or difficulty in resuscitating the baby after birth. The mother may be a diabetic. Examination shows a sick, distressed baby with marked heaving of the right ventricle which can be seen as well as felt. A systolic murmur due to tricuspid regurgitation is often heard at the lower left sternal edge. The baby remains cyanosed even after 100% oxygen (because of the right-to-left shunting) and cyanotic heart disease is suspected.

A radiograph shows cardiomegaly often with diminished pulmonary vascularity. An electrocardiogram shows right atrial and right ventricular hypertrophy.

Echocardiography

Cross-sectional echocardiography shows a normally formed heart with four chambers and normal atrioventricular valves. The right atrium and right ventricle are dilated, the interatrial septum bows to the left and a right-to-left shunt is demonstrated by Doppler echocardiography. A right-to-left shunt through a ductus may also be shown on Doppler studies. Suprasternal views must always be carried out to exclude coarctation of the aorta and interrupted aortic arch. Colour Doppler studies are valuable in excluding total anomalous pulmonary venous drainage with obstruction. Cardiac catheterization is not usually necessary now.

Treatment

These babies are often very sick and treatment is urgent. They need to be kept well oxygenated and ventilatory support may be necessary. Acidosis and hypoglycaemia must be corrected and if there is severe polycythaemia some blood should be removed and replaced with plasma. Unless treatment is given promptly a vicious circle of events ensues, the baby becomes increasingly blue, the pulmonary vascular resistance rises further and myocardial dysfunction results.

Tolazoline has been used with some success to dilate the pulmonary vascular bed (Goetzman *et al.*, 1976). Abbott *et al.* (1978) used nitroprusside for its direct vasodilator effect. Tolazoline does cause haemorrhagic and renal complications which limit its use.

Dopamine given into a central venous line in a medium dose of 2–10 μg/kg/min has a direct effect on the beta-adrenergic cardiac receptors causing an increase in cardiac output. It gives immediate inotropic support to the hypoxic failing myocardium and by dilating peripheral vascular beds it reduces some of the after-load on the heart. Renal function improves and the effectiveness of giving digoxin and diuretics is increased (Fiddler *et al.*, 1980). There is a significant mortality in this condition; Levin *et al.* (1976) quotes 25–30%. The sooner it is recognized and treated the better the outcome.

Myocardial ischaemia in the newborn

It has been recognized that some infants with transient tachypnoea and heart failure in the neonatal period show electrocardiographic (and sometimes echo or angiographic) evidence of myocardial ischaemia (Rowe and Hoffman, 1972; Rowe *et al.*, 1979).

Incidence and aetiology

Minor degrees with rapid resolution are probably fairly common but symptoms severe enough to warrant treatment or raise suspicion of more serious disease are uncommon. Even in severe cases the coronary arteries are structurally normal (Rowe *et al.*, 1979). Most infants have a history of perinatal distress and asphyxia which may cause myocardial damage. Myocardial glycogen may be reduced when there is fetal hypoxaemia (Dawes *et al.*, 1960), and the myocardium of the newborn is dependent on glucose.

Clinical picture

Seventy per cent of affected infants have a history of fetal distress or asphyxia. Tachypnoea, a variable degree of cyanosis and enlargement of the liver are the most constant signs. A murmur due to mitral regurgitation is occasionally heard and râles may be heard over the back of the chest. In severe cases there is a 'shock' syndrome with diminished peripheral pulses and metabolic acidosis. The chest radiograph shows mild or moderate cardiac enlargment and, in severe cases, venous congestion and pulmonary oedema.

Electrocardiography

The electrocardiographic changes are still the subject of debate, but are generally regarded as indicative of myocardial ischaemia, with ST depression and T wave inversion mainly in left ventricular leads V_5–V_6 but sometimes seen in inferior leads (III and aVF) or anterior leads V_2–V_3 (Rowe *et al.*, 1979). Usually the abnormalities regress over a period of a week or two but some persist for up to 6 months.

Treatment and prognosis

Mild cases require no specific treatment. Digoxin, diuretics and oxygen, with the correction of hypoglycaemia and acidosis usually produce prompt improvement in those with more obvious signs and symptoms. Death has been reported but is rare in mature infants with no other problems. Most survivors make a complete recovery, although persistent mitral regurgitation may occur and it has been postulated that late onset arrhythmia from myocardial fibrosis may be a cause of 'cot death' (Keeton *et al.*, 1977).

Neonatal hypocalcaemia

Low serum calcium concentration is an uncommon, but treatable cause of heart failure in the newborn. Usually there are other, central nervous system signs of hypocalcaemia but it is worth checking the serum calcium of any newborn baby with unexplained heart failure or cardiomegaly. The condition responds to elevation of serum calcium by intravenous infusion followed by parathormone and vitamin D analogues. Ideally, the diagnosis should be made and treatment started before digoxin has been given, as there is a risk of arrhythmias when intravenous calcium is given to a digitalized patient. Electrocardiographic monitoring should, in any case, be employed.

Systemic arteriovenous fistulae

These lesions are rare but when they are large, they cause problems in the first two or three days of life. They most commonly occur in the brain or the liver and may be accompanied by telangiectasia or cutaneous angiomas. The lesions are often missed because they are not looked for.

Since there is a large shunt from an artery to a vein, the heart has to increase its stroke volume and output and heart failure usually results. Initially the pulses are collapsing but will become less so as the child's condition deteriorates. There is cardiac enlargement clinically and on the radiograph, which also shows pulmonary plethora. Heart murmurs are unimpressive, there being only a soft systolic murmur in the pulmonary area. The patient may become cyanosed because of the increased venous return to the right side of the heart and a right-to-left shunt developing through the foramen ovale and the ductus.

If the lesion is in the brain a continuous murmur may be heard over the occiput; if in the liver a continuous murmur is heard there.

The electrocardiogram shows either right ventricular hypertrophy or combined ventricular hypertrophy. Ultrasound scans of the brain or liver will suggest the abnormality.

Although the outlook is poor when the lesion is very large, patients have been helped by clipping the feeding vessel in the brain or by ligating the afferent vessel in the liver, or by resecting the area of the fistula if it is localized. Although good results have been obtained in individual cases, in the majority it is impossible to treat the fistula without interfering with the blood supply to the rest of the organ.

Arrhythmias in the newborn

The commonest are supraventricular tachycardia and complete heart block.

Supraventricular tachycardia

This may nowadays be diagnosed *in utero* by fetal echocardiography. If it causes heart failure *in utero*, it can be treated by giving digoxin to the mother. If sustained supraventricular tachycardia is present at birth or in the newborn period, it is best treated by D.C. cardioversion and digoxin then given. These babies quickly become acutely ill and the sooner normal rhythm is restored, the better.

Complete heart block (see page 289)

This may also be diagnosed *in utero* but no action is necessary unless the baby develops heart failure and then early delivery is advised. Most babies with heart block do not develop heart failure and thrive normally when the heart rate is 50/min or more. If, however, the rate is lower than that and ventricular ectopic beats occur, or symptoms of heart failure develop, then a pacemaker is necessary.

Bibliography and references

Abbott, T. R., Rees, G. J., Dickinson, D., *et al.* (1978) Sodium nitroprusside in idiopathic respiratory distress syndrome. *British Medical Journal*, **1**, 1113–1114

Dawes, G. S., Jacobson, H. N., Mott, J. C. *et al.* (1960) Some observations on fetal and newborn rhesus monkeys. *Journal of Physiology*, **152**, 271

Ettedgui, J. A., Martin, R. P., Jones, O. D. H., *et al.* (1988) Balloon dilatation of the pulmonary valve in neonates: technical considerations and results. *British Heart Journal*, **59**, 118

Fiddler, G. I., Chatrath, R., Williams, G. J., *et al.* (1980) Dopamine infusion for the treatment of myocardial dysfunction associated with a persistent transitional circulation. *Archives of Disease in Childhood*, **55**(3), 194–198

Goetzman, B. W., Sunshine, P., Johnson, J. D., *et al.* (1976) Neonatal hypoxia and pulmonary vascular response to tolazoline. *Journal of Paediatrics*, **89**, 617–621

Haworth, S. G. and Reid, L. (1976) Persistent fetal circulation; newly recognized structural features. *Journal of Paediatrics*, **88**, 614–620

Jatene, A. D., Fontes, V. F., Paulista, P. P., *et al.* (1976) Anatomic correction of transposition of the great arteries. *Journal of Thoracic and Cardiovascular Surgery*, **72**, 364–370

Jones, R. W. A., Baumer, J. H., Joseph, M. C., *et al.* (1976) Arterial oxygen tension and response to oxygen breathing in differential diagnoses of congenital heart disease in infancy. *Archives of Diseases in Childhood*, **51**, 667–673

Keeton, B. R., Southall, E., Ruttern, N., *et al.* (1977) Cardiac conduction disorders in six infants with 'near-miss' sudden deaths. *British Medical Journal*, **2**, 600–601

Lambert, E. C., Canent, R. V. and Hohn, A. R. (1966) Surgical management of the neonate with congenital heart disease. *British Heart Journal*, **55**, 1–3

Levin, D. L., Heyman, M. A., Ketterman, J. A., *et al.* (1976) Persistent pulmonary hypertension of the newborn infant. *Journal of Paediatrics*, **89**, 626

Norwood, W. I., Lang, P. and Hansen, D. D. (1983) Physiologic repair of aortic atresia-hypoplastic left heart syndrome. *New England Journal of Medicine*, **308**, 23–26

Report of New England Regional Infant Cardiac Program (1980) *Pediatrics, Springfield*, **65**, 2 part 2. Supplement

Rowe, R. D. and Hoffman, T. (1972) Transient myocardial ischaemia of the newborn infant. A form of severe cardiorespiratory distress in full term infants. *Journal of Paediatrics*, **81**, 243

Rowe, R. D., Finley, J. P., Gilday, D. L., *et al.* (1979) Myocardial ischaemia in the newborn. In *Paediatric Cardiology*, Vol. 2, Heart Disease in the Newborn (eds M. J. Godman and R. M. Marquis), Churchill Livingstone, London

Varghese, P. J., Celermajer, J., Izukawa, T., *et al.* (1969) Cardiac catheterization in the newborn. *Pediatrics, Springfield*, **44**, 24

Wren, C., Sullivan, I., Bull, C., *et al.* (1987) Percutaneous balloon dilatation of aortic valve stenosis in neonates and infants. *British Heart Journal*, **58**, 608–612

Chapter 15

Heart failure in infancy and childhood

Heart failure occurs more commonly in the first three months of life than in any other period of childhood; the earlier in life it occurs, the worse the prognosis. The abnormal loads on the heart produced by congenital cardiac abnormalities may prevent medical management alone being effective. It must be stressed that in congenital heart disease, the treatment of heart failure is only a first step in management and the infant must be referred to a paediatric cardiologist to establish the diagnosis and decide whether surgical treatment is indicated. Heart failure in the first four weeks of life *demands urgent investigation,* as does heart failure at any age which does not repsond *promptly* to digoxin and frusemide.

After 1 year of age, heart failure due to congenital heart disease is rare and the possibility that it has been precipitated by bacterial endocarditis or anaemia must be considered.

Assessment of symptoms and signs

It is often difficult to separate the symptoms and signs of the underlying cardiac disease from those due to heart failure but assessment of the following signs is helpful:

Restlessness

The baby is restless and fretful and looks anxious.

Tachycardia

When the rate is greater than 180/min in infants and 150/min in older children, heart failure is usually present. (If the rate is greater than 200/min in infants, or 180/min in older children, supraventricular tachycardia is probably present and should be looked for on the electrocardiogram.)

Gallop rhythm

A third heart sound is frequently heard at the cardiac apex in a normal heart in childhood but it is faint and not easy to hear. If there is a very obvious third sound causing a gallop rhythm, heart failure is likely.

Tachypnoea and dyspnoea

The respiratory rate in heart failure is greater than 60/min in infants and greater than 40/min in older children. Such rapid rates, however, and difficult breathing may occur when there is respiratory disease alone and they are not of value in differentiation.

Enlargement of the liver

This is a very valuable sign of heart failure. If the liver of an infant is more than 2 cm or more below the right costal margin in the midclavicular line, then failure is present.

Cardiomegaly

This is usually present in heart failure but the heart can be enlarged without failure. The only time that the heart remains small in the presence of heart failure is when there is obstructed pulmonary venous return.

Cough

A persistent, dry, irritating cough is common in left heart failure.

Sweating

This is a frequent and overlooked sign of early heart failure. Mothers will often comment that the baby's pillow is always moist. There is profuse sweating at inappropriate ambient temperatures. It particularly occurs in infants with large left-to-right shunts such as ventricular septal defect and patent ductus arteriosus. This is because such infants have a high metabolic rate and a diminished peripheral blood flow and the only way they can maintain a normal body temperature is by excessive sweating. Kennaird (1970) has shown that sweating is associated with overt heart failure or that the infant is on the verge of developing heart failure.

Pulmonary signs

Moist sounds in the chest may be due to infection or, alternatively, to left ventricular failure. Differentiation is difficult but when there is associated wheezing and the râles are bilateral, left ventricular failure must be considered. If the patient improves and the râles disappear after an intramuscular dose of frusemide, they are likely to have been due to left ventricular failure. A chest radiograph will show pulmonary venous congestion in left ventricular failure.

Oedema

This is a late manifestation of heart failure, but a gain in weight in an infant who is not taking an adequate amount of feed suggests fluid retention due to heart failure.

Treatment

It is most important to determine the cause of the heart failure and if there is a mechanical cause, to decide whether surgery is indicated.

Heart failure occurs when the heart fails to pump blood in sufficient quantity to satisfy the metabolic requirements of the body's tissues. The general aims of treatment are to increase cardiac performance, improve peripheral perfusion and decrease systemic and pulmonary venous congestion. Prompt treatment is essential.

1. *Position and oxygen.* The baby should be propped up as comfortably as possible and oxygen given in a concentration of 30%.
2. *Negative inotropic factors.* It is important to determine whether there are any negative inotropic factors operating such as acidosis, hypoglycaemia, hypocalcaemia and anaemia. These must all be corrected or they will aggravate the circulatory failure.
3. *Sedation.* This should be given if the child is restless. Phenobarbitone is best. Respiratory depressants must be avoided, particularly in cyanosed infants.
4. *Respiratory infection.* Any associated respiratory infection must be treated with antibiotics.
5. *Feeding.* Clear fluids should be given initially by oesophageal tube in young infants. As improvement occurs, milk feeds by bottle can be introduced.
6. *Temperature control.* Infants who have large shunts and high metabolic rates must be nursed in a relatively cool environment.
7. *Medication.* There are three groups of drugs used in the treatment of heart failure – inotropic drugs, diuretics and vasodilators.

Inotropic drugs
Undoubtedly in paediatric practice the most important inotropic drug is still digoxin. It acts on the heart muscle and is most effective when there is generalized depression of myocardial contractility. Infants who have a high pulmonary blood flow and severe left ventricular overload, have a high cardiac output and there is now doubt as to whether the use of digoxin in such infants provides any significant benefit. The work of Nyberg and Wettrell (1978) suggests that lower doses of digoxin than those previously used are effective and a regime based on their studies is shown in Table 15.1. The aim is to achieve a serum digoxin level of 1–3 ng/ml. Hypoxia and acidosis as well as hypokalaemia increase the tendency for digoxin toxicity to occur. Digoxin should not be used when there is obstruction to the outflow tract in lesions such as tetralogy of Fallot.

Dopamine is a powerful inotropic drug given in a central line in a dose of 5 µg/kg/min. It is mainly used in acute failure and in acute myocarditis.

Table 15.1 Digoxin dosage: Oral doses

Age of patient	Digitalizing dose over 24 h given in 3 doses ½, ¼, ¼ at 8-hourly intervals	Maintenance dose over 24 h given 12-hourly
Premature	15 µg/kg/day	5 µg/kg/day
Newborn to one month	40 µg/kg/day	10 µg/kg/day
One month to two years	50 µg/kg/day	15 µg/kg/day
Two years to 10 years	40 µg/kg/day	10 µg/kg/day

Oral digoxin is usually satisfactory but if the intravenous route is being used, the dose must be reduced to ¾ of the oral dose.

Diuretics

The most commonly used diuretic is frusemide. It is safe and is easily given either orally, intramuscularly or intravenously. Blood electrolytes should always be measured when it is used and if hypokalaemia is found, potassium supplements should be given orally (potassium chloride 2 mmol/kg/day). Frusemide is given in a starting dose of 1 mg/kg intravenously or orally, twice daily, increasing if necessary. Spironolactone can be combined with a diuretic to prevent potassium loss but if there is poor renal function hyperkalaemia may occur. The dose is 1–2 mg/kg 8-hourly. Chlorothiazide is a milder diuretic but is useful as a maintenance diuretic. In babies less than 6 months old the dose is 20–30 mg/kg/day orally. Over that age the dose is 10–20 mg/kg/day orally with a maximum dose of 1 g/day. Care must always be taken to avoid excessive diuresis which will cause hypovolaemia and make a low cardiac output worse.

Vasodilators

These have been used in children relatively recently. They have been found particularly useful in mitral incompetence and aortic incompetence and when there is myocardial ischaemia. When there is myocardial failure ventricular dilatation occurs which results in a high end-diastolic volume and pulmonary and peripheral oedema follow. Vasodilator drugs lower the systemic resistance and remove the load from the left ventricle. Captopril acts as a competitive inhibitor of angiotensin-converting enzyme. The oral dose is 0.1–0.5 mg/kg orally 6-hourly. Hydralazine is an arteriolar vasodilator and is given orally in a dose of 0.5–1.0 mg/kg 8-hourly.

Cardiogenic shock

Patients are sometimes admitted in a state of severe cardiogenic shock. This is most commonly due to excessive blood loss or to profound hypovolaemia following an excessive diuresis or diarrhoea and vomiting. A central line should be inserted and intravenous plasma or dextrose saline given. The child is ventilated with 50% oxygen. Acidosis, hypocalcaemia and hypoglycaemia are corrected and sodium and potassium levels must be checked and corrected. If the heart lesion is a duct-dependent one, prostaglandins are given (see page 123). Blood pressure and the electrocardiogram should be monitored. If the shocked state is associated with a high venous pressure, intravenous frusemide should be given with an inotropic agent such as dopamine.

If supraventricular tachycardia causes cardiogenic shock, cardioversion is the best treatment because most anti-arrhythmic agents have a marked negative inotropic effect.

Digoxin toxicity

This may occur from overdosage but is also seen when a child takes tablets prescribed for a parent or grandparent. The presence of a low potassium level in the blood potentiates the arrhythmogenic (but not the inotropic) action of digoxin. Care must be taken, therefore, when diuretics which cause potassium depletion are being given, or when the patient has diarrhoea and vomiting or is given steroids.

Although nausea, vomiting and diarrhoea are early symptoms of toxicity, they do not always occur and a cardiac arrhythmia may be the first evidence of toxicity.

There may be ventricular ectopic beats or pulsus bigeminus or bradycardia and atrioventricular dissociation. In newborn infants bradycardia, supraventricular arrhythmias and second- and third-degree heart block are the commonest. Paroxysmal atrial tachycardia with atrioventricular block may occur and if this is not recognized more digoxin may be administered to correct the rapid rate with disastrous results. If in doubt, further doses of digoxin should be withheld, an electrocardiogram recorded and the serum digoxin estimated.

Treatment of intoxication

1. Stop the digoxin. In many cases this may be sufficient and, after two or three days, treatment can be resumed using a lower dosage.
2. Check serum electrolytes.
3. Check digoxin levels in blood. Values more than 5 ng/ml are found in digoxin toxicity, levels between 3 and 5 ng/ml may be toxic in some circumstances.
4. If intoxication is severe, the potassium levels must be measured and constant electrocardiographic monitoring is essential. If the potassium level is low, older children can be given 1 g of potassium chloride orally every 8 hours. Intravenous potassium is only used in desperate cases and when the potassium level is known to be low and when there is a good urinary output. It should be given slowly over 1 hour using a solution of 40 mmol of potassium chloride in 500 ml of dextrose in water. The total dose should not exceed 2 mmol/kg body weight and it should be discontinued when the arrhythmia disappears or peaked T waves appear on the electrocardiogram (Neill, 1965).

An important development recently is the use of Fab digoxin-specific antibody fragments (Digibind). Their use has resulted in a significant reduction in mortality due to digoxin poisoning. They are, however, very expensive and supplies are limited and they should be reserved for serious cases. The dose is related to the serum digoxin concentration and the body weight.

References

Kennaird, D. L. (1970) Measurement of oxygen consumption and evaporative water loss in infants with congenital heart disease. *Archives of Disease in Childhood*, **45**, 818

Neill, C. A. (1965) Recognition and treatment of congestive heart failure in infants. *Progress in Cardiovascular Diseases*, **7**, 399

Nyberg, L. and Wettrell, G. (1978) Digoxin dosage schedules for neonates and infants based on pharmacokinetic considerations. *Clinical Pharmacokinetics*, **3**, 453–461

Chapter 16

Pulmonary hypertension, cor pulmonale and the Eisenmenger syndrome

Pulmonary hypertension

The term 'pulmonary hypertension' (strictly, pulmonary arterial hypertension) refers to an elevation of the pressure above the normal in the pulmonary artery. *In utero* and in the few days following birth pulmonary hypertension is normal. At other times it may take one of three forms.

1. *Passive pulmonary hypertension* is due simply to a back pressure transmitted through the pulmonary capillaries from raised pulmonary venous and left atrial pressure.
2. *Hyperdynamic pulmonary hypertension* is caused by high flow of blood in the pulmonary system. The pulmonary vessels can normally dilate to take an increase of 100–200% in flow without any actual increase in pulmonary artery pressure, as occurs in exercise and in uncomplicated atrial septal defects.
3. *Reactive pulmonary hypertension* represents an increase in the vascular resistance of the lungs, brought about by constriction of the small, muscular pulmonary arteries. The rise in resistance may in some circumstances be temporary and reversible, in others permanent. The only physiological stimulus which consistently produces a rise in pulmonary vascular resistance is hypoxia, and the sensing area of the lungs appears to be the pulmonary venous system. A rise in carbon dioxide tension or a fall in pH in the pulmonary venous system may also have an effect on pulmonary vascular resistance, particularly when occurring with hypoxia.

Although three types of pulmonary hypertension are described, it is unusual to find either passive or hyperdynamic forms in isolation. Patients with raised left atrial pressure from left heart obstruction usually have both passive and reactive pulmonary hypertension, and patients with large ventricular septal defects have both hyperdynamic and reactive components, and, if associated with left ventricular failure, all three types.

Hypertensive pulmonary vascular disease

Patients with pulmonary hypertension which has been present since birth have main pulmonary arteries which are similar in structure to the aorta, showing a thick medial coat with abundant elastic tissue. This is never seen in acquired pulmonary hypertension.

In both congenital and acquired forms, the small muscular pulmonary arteries show the most striking changes, which have been classified by Heath and Edwards (1958) into six grades of severity.

Grade 1 Muscular hypertrophy of the media and development of longitudinal muscle fibres.
Grade 2 Cellular intimal proliferation.
Grade 3 Intimal fibrosis, with narrowing of the lumen.
Grade 4 Dilatation, with thinning of the vessel wall.
Grade 5 Plexiform vascular lesions (possibly due to thrombosis and recanalization or to attempts at formation of anastomotic vessels).
Grade 6 Fibrinoid necrosis of the intima and media.

Muscular hypertrophy is regarded as a result of the stimulus causing the arterial constriction and the other lesions are the result of the high intravascular pressure. Grade 1 lesions are reversible. Grade 2 and 3 lesions are associated with reversible pulmonary hypertension and may themselves regress. Grades 4, 5 and 6 are uncommon but in general indicate irreversible pulmonary hypertension (as in primary pulmonary hypertension).

In addition to the arterial lesions the pulmonary arterioles develop a muscle coat which in health they do not possess.

Much has been written about the value of assessment of pulmonary vascular disease by lung biopsy in the selection of patients for surgery of ventricular septal defect and other lesions. Although patients with grade 4–6 lesions are not suitable for surgery, this is usually clear from their clinical state, and in most cases careful clinical and haemodynamic assessment is at least as reliable.

Signs of pulmonary hypertension
In severe pulmonary hypertension, not associated with intracardiac defects, the pulse has a small volume and there is peripheral and frequently slight central cyanosis, the latter being due to ventilation – perfusion inequality in the lungs. The jugular venous pressure shows a large 'a' wave when the condition is chronic and the mean level of pressure may be raised when the condition is acute or subacute. The right ventricular pulsation to the left of the sternum is increased and the second heart sound is very loud and palpable. Pulmonary artery dilatation gives rise to an ejection click and a soft ejection systolic murmur and there may be a pulmonary diastolic murmur due to functional pulmonary regurgitation.

Radiology, electrocardiography and echocardiography
Chest radiographs (Figure 16.1) show dilatation of the main pulmonary artery and its left and right branches, but the peripheral branches are small ('pruned' or 'pollarded' pulmonary arteries). The electrocardiogram in chronic pulmonary hypertension shows right ventricular hypertrophy, but in acute forms may show a right bundle branch block pattern or deep inversion of T waves in right ventricular leads (3, aVF and V_{2-3}). P waves are usually peaked in leads 2 and V_1 in either acute or chronic forms, due to right atrial hypertrophy.

Echocardiography shows an absence of the usual presystolic opening movement of the pulmonary valve and prolongation of the right ventricular ejection time. The hypertrophy of the right ventricular wall can also be demonstrated.

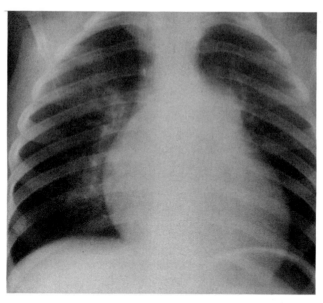

Figure 16.1 Pulmonary hypertension. Chest radiograph of a 4-year-old girl who had had a Pudenz valve inserted for infantile hydrocephalus. The tip of the valve is seen in the superior vena cava. Note the right atrial and right ventricular hypertrophy, the prominent main pulmonary artery and the 'pruning' of the pulmonary vessels peripherally

Causes of pulmonary hypertension
Passive (±reactive) pulmonary hypertension:
  Left ventricular failure
  Mitral valve disease
  Cor triatriatum
  Pulmonary veno-occlusive disease
  Obstructed total anomalous pulmonary venous connection

Hyperdynamic (±reactive) pulmonary hypertension:
  Patent ductus arteriosus
  Ventricular septal defect
  Atrial septal defect (rarely in childhood)
  Total anomalous pulmonary venous connection (non-obstructed)
  Transposition of the great arteries
  Truncus arteriosus
  Common or single ventricle
  High output states
  Carcinoid syndrome

Pure reactive pulmonary hypertension:
  Cor pulmonale
  Eisenmenger syndrome
  Primary pulmonary hypertension

Most of the conditions mentioned are dealt with in other sections of the book. The remainder are discussed in this chapter.

Pulmonary veno-occlusive disease

In this condition the pathological changes are in the pulmonary veins and venules and the changes in the pulmonary arteries are secondary to that. There is venous intimal fibrosis and in the majority of cases there has been thrombosis and recanalization in pulmonary veins. The aetiology is obscure. Repeated chest infections predisposed to the onset of pulmonary hypertension in the case described by Heath, Scott and Lynch (1971). Specific therapy is not available and the condition is fatal.

Thromboembolic pulmonary hypertension

Embolization to the lungs is a complication of ventriculo-atrial drains used in the treatment of hydrocephalus and the emboli may be infected. Embolization from the heart occurs in endomyocardial fibrosis, myxoma of the right atrium and right-sided endocarditis. Embolization from systemic veins is rare in childhood but has been reported from hepatic veins in patients with liver disease.

Thrombosis *in situ*

Thrombosis *in situ* occurs in patients with a generalized clotting tendency, in those with a low pulmonary flow (as in Fallot's tetralogy) and in those with pre-existing pulmonary hypertension.

Schistosomiasis

In Africa and South America schistosomiasis is the commonest cause of pulmonary hypertension but is unusual in those under the age of 10 years since emboli of the ova do not reach the lungs until hepatic involvement has produced portal hypertension and collateral channels bypassing the liver.

Primary pulmonary hypertension

Pulmonary hypertension occurring with no detectable cause is rare at any age and particularly so in children. The condition usually progresses to right heart failure and death within a year from diagnosis, but occasional patients remain static for many years. No specific therapy is known to affect the disease. There have been encouraging results using epoprostenol (prostacyclin), but this has to be given intravenously and long-term therapy has led to complications such as ascites and septicaemia (Jones, Higenbottam and Wallwork, 1987).

High altitude pulmonary hypertension

Inhalation of air with a low oxygen tension causes acute or chronic elevation of pulmonary artery pressure. In people living constantly at moderate altitude this is well tolerated but at very high levels or in subjects brought rapidly to moderate levels, right heart failure may occur. Restoration to sea level produces cure in acute cases and amelioration in chronic cases but the latter are then unable to return to the higher levels since rapid deterioration occurs.

Cor pulmonale

Heart disease due to malfunction of the lungs is known as pulmonary heart disease or cor pulmonale. The condition is recognized either because of symptoms and signs of right heart failure or from clinical or electrocardiographic evidence of right ventricular hypertrophy. The basic cause of cor pulmonale, irrespective of the underlying disease, is pulmonary hypertension caused by constriction of pulmonary arteries due to hypoxia.

Hypoventilation (Pickwickian syndrome)

Chronic hypoventilation, from severe obesity, central nervous system disease or from respiratory paralysis, causes pulmonary hypertension and right heart failure. In addition, the rise in arterial carbon dioxide tension is responsible for the drowsiness which is characteristic of the condition.

Kyphoscoliosis

Children with severe chest deformities become hypoxic partly due to pure ventilatory difficulty and partly due to ventilation–perfusion inequalities. The condition rarely causes heart failure before adult life.

Fibrocystic disease

Of all the chronic respiratory diseases, fibrocystic disease (mucoviscidosis) is most likely to produce pulmonary hypertension and right heart failure, although usually not before the early teens. When right heart failure does occur it is a bad prognostic sign and few patients survive much more than two years from its occurrence.

Asthma

In severe episodes some degree of acute right heart failure may occur, but chronic cor pulmonale is most unusual in childhood.

Upper airways obstruction

Choanal atresia, or stenosis, in infancy usually causes obvious respiratory obstruction but occasional patients present with unexplained right heart failure. Large tonsils and adenoids have also been described as a cause of acute and subacute cor pulmonale. Characteristically the patients are under 2 years of age and present with somnolence and right heart failure. Respiration may be obviously obstructed but sometimes is shallow and not always noisy, and cyanosis is moderate or severe. Examination of the heart shows evidence of pulmonary hypertension. Chest radiographs show considerable cardiomegaly and the electrocardiogram indicates right heart strain (Macartney, Panday and Scott, 1969.) This situation is also seen in achondroplasia when the postnasal space is particularly small.

Treatment is urgent and intubation is usually required. The blood gases and metabolic changes must be corrected. When the child is in a stable condition he should be referred for tonsillectomy.

The Eisenmenger syndrome

The Eisenmenger syndrome has been mentioned in the sections on ventricular septal defect, patent ductus arteriosus and atrial septal defect and is now described in further detail.

Eisenmenger in 1897 described a patient who gave a history of cyanosis and breathlessness since infancy and who developed heart failure at 32 years and died following a large haemoptysis. A large ventricular septal defect was found at autopsy and the aorta 'overrode' both ventricles. Eisenmenger stated that the pulmonary vascular resistance had been increased but did not realize that this caused the right-to-left shunt and cyanosis. Since his description, patients with large ventricular septal defects with right-to-left shunts producing cyanosis have been said to have 'the Eisenmenger complex'.

Paul Wood (1958) rightly pointed out that there were other lesions in which an increase in pulmonary vascular resistance to a level greater than the systemic vascular resistance resulted in a right-to-left shunt and cyanosis. He noted that such cases were often indistinguishable from one another if they were first seen when the patient had a right-to-left shunt. He therefore redefined the condition and called it 'the Eisenmenger syndrome'. Any condition in which there is 'pulmonary hypertension at systemic level, due to a high pulmonary vascular resistance, with a reversed or bidirectional shunt at aortopulmonary, ventricular or atrial level' may be given this name. It may occur in patent ductus arteriosus, aortopulmonary window, ventricular septal defect and atrial septal defect. The term has also been applied to other more complex defects when a very high pulmonary vascular resistance causes a dominant right-to-left shunt, such as persistent truncus, transposition (D- or L-) with ventricular septal defect and without pulmonary stenosis, single ventricle, single atrium, atrioventricular defect and total anomalous pulmonary venous connection.

When the Eisenmenger syndrome occurs the *defect between the two circulations is large*. Yet some patients with large defects do not develop a high pulmonary vascular resistance. There is still argument as to whether in some cases the high resistance is present from birth. Certainly in the majority of patients there is evidence of a large left-to-right shunt prior to the development of the Eisenmenger syndrome. It is rarely seen before 2 years of age in ventricular septal defect alone but occurs earlier, often by 1 year of age, when there is associated transposition of the great arteries. Children with Down's syndrome and ventricular septal defect or common A–V canal are particularly liable to develop pulmonary hypertension and reversal of shunt at an early age. The probable reason is that they tend to hypoventilate and become hypoxic. The Eisenmenger syndrome occurs much later in life in atrial septal defect than in patent ductus arteriosus and ventricular septal defect.

Natural history and prognosis

There is a gradual increase in cyanosis over many years and ultimately heart failure develops. Many patients die suddenly from haemoptysis associated with pulmonary artery thrombosis or dilated angiomatous lesions arising from small pulmonary arteries. Other complications are chest infections, bacterial endocarditis and cerebral abscess. Death usually occurs in the fourth of fifth decade (Wood, 1958).

Clinical picture

In patients who are minimally cyanosed, symptoms are few, and breathlessness and fatigue are noted only on strenuous exertion. Apart from cyanosis and finger clubbing, the signs are those of pulmonary hypertension. The pulse is generally of normal volume, but the jugular venous pulse shows an exaggerated 'a' wave. Increased right ventricular pulsation is palpable at the left sternal border, and closure of the pulmonary valve is palpable. Auscultation reveals a short ejection systolic murmur (due to ejection of blood into the dilated pulmonary artery), often preceded by an ejection click, and a very loud second heart sound in the pulmonary area. Splitting of the second heart sound is close or undetectable when the communication is at ventricular or aortopulmonary level, but may be wide when the communication is at atrial level. There may also be a soft early diastolic murmur in the pulmonary area and at the left sternal border, due to functional pulmonary incompetence. This is rather more common when the underlying defect is a patent ductus arteriosus.

Radiology

The heart shows little or no overall enlargement but the right ventricle is prominent in the lateral view. The main pulmonary artery and its branches are dilated, but the peripheral vessels are small ('pruning' of the pulmonary artery) (Figure 16.2). The radiograph may also be helpful in indicating the site of the intracardiac communication. With an atrial septal defect the pulmonary artery and its main branches are usually greatly enlarged; with a ventricular septal defect they are only slightly or moderately so. With a patent ductus arteriosus not only is the main pulmonary artery considerably dilated but the aortic arch may also be dilated.

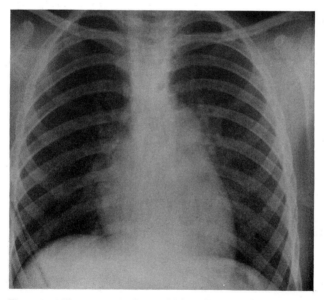

Figure 16.2 Eisenmenger sydrome. Plain radiographs showing normal-sized heart, prominent main pulmonary arteries and peripheral 'pruning', which is less marked than in Figure 16.1

Electrocardiography

Standard leads usually show strong right axis deviation. The P waves are peaked, indicating right atrial hypertrophy. Moderate or marked right ventricular hypertrophy is indicated by tall R waves in leads V_4R and V_1.

Cardiac catheterization

Cardiac catheterization carries more risk than usual in Eisenmenger's syndrome and angiocardiography is contraindicated because it may be followed by a severe rise in pulmonary vascular resistance and cause death. In the past cardiac catheterization was undertaken to be sure the diagnosis was correct. Fortunately, echocardiography can now demonstrate any structural disease of the heart and rule out any operable lesion. Also when tricuspid regurgitation can be detected, the pulmonary artery pressure can be estimated by applying the Bernouilli equation to the regurgitant jet of blood. In many patients therefore the pulmonary artery pressure can be estimated without catheterization. Doppler studies will also detect a right-to-left shunt through a ventricular septal defect or patent ductus arteriosus. Colour flow mapping will also demonstrate this, so although pulmonary vascular resistance cannot yet be measured non-invasively, the amount of information which can be obtained non-invasively makes cardiac catheterization unnecessary.

Treatment

Surgical closure is not possible when there is a right-to-left shunt and there is no known medical treatment which will influence the pulmonary vascular resistance. Anoxia from any cause should be avoided. Chest infections must be treated early and enthusiastically, and care must be taken to avoid anoxia during any anaesthesia. Pregnancy carries a high risk and should be avoided or terminated if it occurs. Oral contraceptives have been reported to cause rapid deterioration. Recently it has been suggested that excessive physical exertion in those patients with few symptoms, may cause rapid deterioration. Heart–lung transplantation is the only possible surgical treatment.

References

Pulmonary hypertension and cor pulmonale
Heath, D. and Edwards, J. E. (1958) The pathology of hypertensive pulmonary vascular disease. A description of six grades of structural changes in pulmonary arteries with special reference to congenital cardiac septal defects. *Circulation,* **18,** 533
Heath, D., Scott, Olive and Lynch, J. (1971) Pulmonary veno-occlusive disease. *Thorax,* **26,** 663–674
Jones, D. K., Higenbottam, T. W. and Wallwork, J. (1987) Treatment of primary pulmonary hypertension with intravenous epoprostenol (prostacyclin). *British Heart Journal,* **57,** 270–278
Macartney, F. J., Panday, J. and Scott, O. (1969) Cor pulmonale as a result of chronic naso-pharyngeal obstruction due to hypertrophied tonsils and adenoids. *Archives of Disease in Childhood,* **44,** 585–592

The Eisenmenger syndrome
Eisenmenger, V. (1897) Die angeborenen Defekte der Kammerschedewand des Herzens. *Zeitschrift Klinische Medizin,* **32,** Suppl. 1–28
Wood, P. (1958) The Eisenmenger syndrome. *British Medical Journal,* **2,** (i) 701–709; (ii) 755–762

Chapter 17

Complications of congenital heart disease

Thrombosis and embolism

Thrombosis is a common complication of cyanotic congenital heart disease. It is most often seen in the early years of life, particularly when the oxygen saturation of the arterial blood is less than 50%. It is the polycythaemia and high haematocrit which make clotting more likely, rather than the actual haemoglobin content of the blood. Indeed, the cyanotic infant who has an iron-deficiency anaemia and normal, or lowered, haemoglobin level but a high haematocrit, is most at risk from thrombosis. Dehydration from any cause such as gastroenteritis or sweating following pyrexia will further aggravate the tendency for thrombosis to occur.

Thrombosis is most serious when it occurs in the cerebral circulation. Its onset is often insidious and in young children the presence of malaise and headache may be overlooked. Vomiting often occurs and there may be visual defects. Often the first realization that something is wrong is the occurrence of monoplegia or hemiplegia. The hemiplegia may improve gradually over a day or two but there is usually some permanent disability, a tragic happening in a child already handicapped by cyanotic congenital heart disease.

Treatment

The condition should be prevented as far as possible. Surgery should be performed whenever practicable to relieve the stimulus for a high haematocrit; iron-deficiency anaemia should be corrected. Dehydration should be prevented or treated promptly if it occurs. Anticoagulant therapy has been advocated by some but there is a danger that cerebral infarction will be converted to a cerebral haematoma. Physiotherapy for the affected limbs should be started at once.

Mural thrombosis

In conditions where there is stagnation inside the heart itself thrombosis may occur. This may be in the left ventricle in cardiomyopathy or with impaired left ventricular function complicating other lesions. It may also occur in the right atrium or in the left atrium where there are obstructive lesions. Usually the condition is silent and picked up only at autopsy or by echocardiography (Figure 17.1). Anticoagulants (heparin, followed by warfarin) should be started immediately because of the risks of embolism and the clots usually then lyse spontaneously, often remarkably

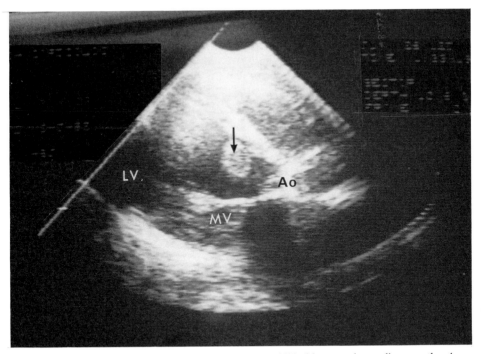

Figure 17.1 Mural thrombus (arrowed) in left ventricle in a child with congestive cardiomyopathy. Ao, aorta; LV, left ventricle; MV, mitral valve

rapidly. Long-term anticoagulant therapy is usually continued, but because of the difficulties of controlling therapy some cardiologists switch to aspirin and rely on serial echocardiograms to check for any further clot development.

Diffuse intravascular thrombosis and consumption coagulopathy

Under some circumstances, particularly when dehydration increases the haematocrit and therefore the viscosity of the blood, a few infants and children develop silent intravascular clotting. Blood-clotting factors, particularly platelets and prothrombin, are consumed to such an extent that a haemorrhagic state ensues, with haematuria, gastrointestinal bleeding and uncontrollable haemorrhage from surgical wounds. The bleeding and clotting times are prolonged, the platelet count falls to less than $10\,000/mm^3$ and the prothrombin time is greatly prolonged. Heparinization of the patient allows platelets and prothrombin to return to normal, but transfusion of platelets and other clotting factors may be necessary.

Systemic thromboembolism

The commonest cause of systemic embolism is paradoxical embolism from the systemic veins in patients with cyanotic congenital heart disease. In addition, embolism from the heart itself may occur in bacterial endocarditis, from a left atrial myxoma and from mural thrombi in primary myocardial disease. Any part of the systemic circulation may be affected by thrombosis or embolism but involvement of the cerebral circulation is much the most common. The risks are proportional both to the polycythaemia and to the degree of right-to-left shunting. Embolism is probably much more common than thrombosis *in situ* in the arterial tree but, apart from the more abrupt onset in patients with emboli, the symptoms are similar. Some idea of the degree of risk in cyanotic congenital heart disease is given by the fact that 22% of children with transposition in one series developed cerebral thromboembolism whilst waiting an average of two years for definitive surgery (Parsons and co-workers, 1971).

Cortical thrombophlebitis

Primary thrombophlebitis of cerebral veins accounts for a small percentage of patients with cerebral thrombosis. It may be precipitated by infections or follow immunization procedures. Headache and vomiting occur initially and weakness or hemiplegia with drowsiness follow.

Mesenteric artery embolism

Mesenteric artery embolism is rare in infancy and childhood. Sudden and severe abdominal pain is usually the first symptom and intestinal ileus develops quickly. There may be melaena or frank blood passed per rectum. Treatment is difficult, but a conservative approach with intravenous replacement and anticoagulants is the first choice; resection of bowel (which needs to be extensive) is reserved for patients with perforation or with no evidence of recovery after several days. With or without resection, some degree of malabsorption is common in survivors.

Mesenteric venous thrombosis

The onset of mesenteric venous thrombosis is less acute and pain is less severe but, clinically, differentiation from mesenteric arterial embolism is difficult. Conservative treatment usually results in eventual recovery.

Renal embolism

Pain in the loin and haematuria are the usual symptoms in large renal emboli, but microscopic haematuria and hypertension may occur with repeated emboli.

Renal vein thrombosis

Renal vein thrombosis causes albuminuria and a nephrotic picture. The onset is insidious and with pre-existing heart failure diagnosis may be difficult. Anticoagulant therapy is logical.

Cerebral abscess

Cerebral abscess is rare in children under 2 years of age (unlike cerebral thrombosis). Strangely enough, it is rarely associated with bacterial endocarditis even though there is a bacteraemia. Infection probably occurs in an area where there has been some previous local damage following thrombosis.

The symptoms are of malaise, fever and loss of appetite followed by headache and vomiting. There may be convulsions and visual defects. Usually pyrexia develops and headache persists. Papilloedema may be present. Hemiplegia or monoplegia may follow.

An electroencephalogram may help by localizing the lesion but if the diagnosis is still in doubt the patient should be referred to a neurologist for brain scan. The development of the CT scan has enabled abscess to be differentiated from infarct with a high degree of accuracy, and it should always be carried out if there is any doubt. Brain abscess is a treatable condition and delay in referral to a neurologist should be avoided. The abscess may rupture and cause meningitis if treatment is delayed.

Treatment

Small abscesses respond well to treatment with antibiotics. It has become clear that the organisms are often anaerobic or microaerobic and the most suitable treatment regime is flucloxacillin, netilmicin and metronidazole. A neurosurgical opinion should always be sought, first, about needling to attempt to obtain an organism and secondly regarding possible surgical drainage, which will be necessary in moderate or large size abscesses. With the routine use of computerized tomography, more appropriate antibiotic regimes and earlier surgical treatment the prognosis has improved and should be considerably better than the 40% mortality reported by Taussig in 1971 in patients with tetralogy of Fallot.

Infective endocarditis

When a child with congenital heart disease has bacterial organisms in the blood stream there is always a chance that infective endocarditis will result. It is known that lesions in which there is turbulent flow of blood onto or across the endocardium lead to platelet adherence to the endocardium. Organisms which happen to be in the bloodstream at the time can be caught with the platelets and can then multiply, separated from the natural defence mechanisms which normally destroy all but the most virulent organisms. It is this collection of organisms, platelets and fibrin which forms the vegetation.

Aetiology

The disease can occur at any age, but is uncommon below the age of 2 years. The source of infection is probably the mouth in about one-eighth of cases but nose, throat and tonsils are other common sites of entry. Sholler, Hawker and Celermajer (1986) found no history of recent (within three months) dental surgery in their series of 37 cases from Sydney. Since cardiac surgery has become more common, this has accounted for an important number of cases, about a fifth in the Sydney series having had recent surgery and one-seventh having infection on a prosthetic valve.

Streptococcus sangius (viridans) is still the commonest organism, followed by *Staphylococcus aureus,* but after surgery the non-haemolytic staphylococci (*albus* and *epidermidis*) are more common, and are usually penicillin resistant. The meningococcus, pneumococcus, proteus, haemophilus and brucella have all been reported and rarely rickettsia and fungi are seen.

The lesions most likely to develop endocarditis are ventricular septal defect, patent ductus arteriosus, coarctation of the aorta and lesions of the mitral and aortic valves – particularly when the last-named has a bicuspid valve. Isolated pulmonary stenosis is relatively immune. Small defects are more likely to develop endocarditis than large ones. It never occurs in ostium secundum atrial septal defects and when it occurs in ostium primum defect, it is the abnormal cleft mitral valve which is affected and not the atrial septal defect. The infection often develops in areas where there has been damage by a jet of blood impinging on the endocardium, so that it occurs on the right ventricular wall in ventricular septal defects and in the pulmonary artery opposite a patent ductus arteriosus. Taussig (1971) found a remarkably high incidence of subacute bacterial endocarditis (14.3%) in the long-term follow-up of 779 patients with tetralogy of Fallot. Gersony and Hayes (1977) in a series of 2420 patients with congenital heart disease found an incidence of 1.5 per thousand patient years for ventricular septal defect, 1.8 for aortic stenosis and only 0.2 for pulmonary stenosis.

Clinical presentation

Clinical presentation may be acute or subacute in onset but the symptoms and signs are essentially the same. Staphylococcal infections tend to give an acute onset but nowadays the clinical picture is often not the classic one because the patient has already been given antibiotics before referral to hospital. The initial signs are those associated with the septicaemia. There is fever, malaise, lassitude, loss of appetite and pallor due to anaemia. Clubbing of the fingers and toes may develop, the spleen is enlarged and in some patients heart failure occurs.

Emboli from the site of the endocarditis cause splinter haemorrhages, haematuria and cerebral incidents with hemiplegia or meningitis. Osler's nodes are uncommon in childhood. When the lesion is on the right side of the heart, as in pulmonary stenosis and ventricular septal defect, embolization occurs to the lungs. This may cause pleuritic pain and a cough.

If the child has been seen prior to the endocarditis, there may be a change in the cardiac signs due to involvement of a valve cusp, as for example when aortic regurgitation develops on a bicuspid aortic valve.

Diagnosis

Infective endocarditis must always be suspected when there is unexplained fever in a child with congenital heart disease. The diagnosis becomes even more likely when there is an enlarged spleen, heart failure or evidence of embolization. The following tests should be carried out immediately.

1. *Blood cultures:* Four cultures should be taken in the first 24 hours, then twice in the next 24 hours – a total of six cultures.
2. *Blood count:* This usually shows a polymorphonuclear leucocytosis but occasionally there is neutropenia. Anaemia may be severe. Erythrocyte sedimentation rate is increased as a rule but may occasionally be normal.
3. *Urine:* Microscopic examination must be carried out to look for red cells. If there is renal infection, albuminuria, casts and haematuria are found.
4. *Chest radiograph:* This may show areas of pulmonary infarction.
5. *Four-hourly temperature recordings.*

6. *Echocardiogram:* Cross-sectional echocardiography demonstrates vegetations associated with septal defects and on heart valves (Figure 17.2). It also helps to assess the extent of damage to the valves.

Ideally, it is best to know the organism involved and its sensitivity to antibiotics before beginning treatment, but positive blood cultures are not always obtained, particularly if antibiotics have been given before admission to hospital. A firm diagnosis can usually be made before the results of blood culture are available and it is often dangerous to wait for the results of these while the patient deteriorates and cardiac damage progresses. It is no light matter to embark on a six-week course of antibiotic therapy in a child, but it is preferable to withholding treatment while the child develops a cerebral embolus! The majority of patients with endocarditis can be cured today but good results depend on early diagnosis and early treatment. The motto must always be 'DO NOT DELAY'.

One presentation which has been increasingly recognized in recent years but still gives rise to problems in diagnosis is the child who develops pains in joints and a low fever. There is often a weakly positive blood rheumatoid factor, which leads to the mistaken diagnosis of rheumatoid arthritis or Still's disease. If the general rule that any child with a known heart condition developing fever and systemic symptoms has blood cultures to exclude infective endocarditis is followed, such mistakes will not be made.

Difficulties in diagnosis arise when a child with known congenital heart disease presents with pyrexia for which there is another obvious cause, such as pyelitis or cellulitis, and is then found to have positive blood cultures, which may, of course, occur in any child with these conditions. It is unreasonable to insist on a six-week course of intravenous antibiotics, but it is safest to continue on antibiotics for rather longer than usual (for example 14 days rather than 10) and to check with cross-sectional echocardiograms that there are no vegetations in the heart.

Principles of treatment

Treatment should be started as soon as possible after the initial blood cultures have been taken, with penicillin and netilmicin and modified as necessary when and if the organism has been identified. Bactericidal, not bacteriostatic, antibiotics must be used, except in the occasional chlamydia infection. The blood concentration of the antibiotic must be adjusted if necessary to give a bactericidal level against the organism in at least 1 in 8 dilution. It is best to arrange that there is a close liaison with the microbiologist with regard to results of blood cultures, advice on appropriate antibiotic regimes, arrangement of antibiotic assays and dilution studies. If aminoglycoside (netilmicin) treatment is to be continued for more than ten days, ensure that blood assays are performed more frequently (3 times weekly at least) to check for possible renal damage and drug accumulation.

Initial treatment must be for at least 2 weeks and can then sometimes be modified for a further period according to the organisms, the length of history prior to treatment and the rapidity of response to treatment.

If the part of the heart affected is one where valve perforation or other serious haemodynamic complication may arise (particularly the aortic or mitral valve) the nearest paediatric cardiac surgical centre should be notified and a plan made for emergency transfer, if necessary.

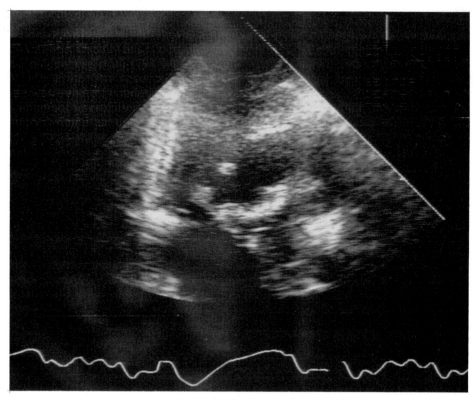

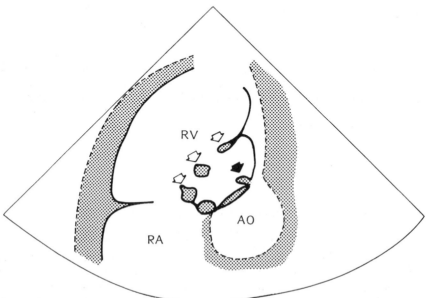

Figure 17.2 Echocardiogram showing vegetation on the tricuspid valve (open arrows) and patch closing ventricular septal defect (closed arrow). The patient had had previous repair of tetralogy of Fallot

Serial cross-sectional echocardiograms are required to check that vegetations are shrinking and no new ones developing, as well as checking generally on cardiac size and function.

Be prepared at any time to seek surgical help. Sterilization of the lesions (or indeed any antibiotic therapy) is not a prerequisite for surgery, should torrential mitral or aortic regurgitation be present or develop.

Treatment for heart failure may be required with frusemide and digoxin, but this is an indication to seek surgical help.

Treatment of individual organisms

Non- or alpha-haemolytic streptococcus
Intravenous penicillin 5–10 million units daily by continuous infusion or 6-hourly i.v. injection with netilmicin 1 mg/kg 8-hourly i.v. Adjust frequency and dose of netilmicin according to pre- and 30 min post-injection blood levels. Continue for 2 weeks and then review. If organism fully sensitive to penicillin, prompt response of temperature and no complications, change to oral penicillin or amoxycillin in full doses for further 2 weeks. Otherwise continue penicillin and netilmicin for further week and then give penicillin orally for 3 weeks.

Staphylococcal infections
Intravenous methicillin or flucloxacillin 25 mg/kg 6-hourly with netilmicin 1 mg/kg 8-hourly. If organism proves to be methicillin resistant substitute vancomycin. Continue treatment for 2 weeks, adjusting dose of netilmicin if necessary.

Streptococcus faecalis and gram-negative bacilli
Intravenous ampicillin 25 mg/kg 8-hourly with netilmicin 1 mg/kg 8-hourly for 3 or 4 weeks.

Staphylococcus albus
Intravenous penicillin and netilmicin as for *Streptococcus viridans*, provided the organism is reasonably sensitive to penicillin. If not sensitive to penicillin, other regimes, using two antibiotics from vancomycin, netilmicin and rifampicin, are required. A 6-week course is necessary. (Endocarditis with this organism is uncommon except following cardiac surgery, but the infection is difficult to eradicate.)

Prognosis

Prior to the introduction of antibiotics the condition was uniformly fatal. Now, in theory, death from infective endocarditis should be uncommon since it is almost always possible to find a combination of antibiotics to which the organism is sensitive and to repair what damage has been done surgically. The mortality is said to be still 20–25%. Reasons for the continuing high mortality include failure to diagnose the condition early, or at all, and failure to refer patients for surgery if there is evidence of deteriorating haemodynamic state. Long-term morbidity remains important with the effects of systemic embolism and valve damage being the main factors.

Care following infective endocarditis

Once the antibiotic course has been completed, and provided that there is no deterioration in the haemodynamic state which requires consideration of surgery the patient can be sent home and the temperature recorded twice daily by the child or parents.

There is really no point in keeping children in hospital to watch for a rise in temperature and the policy of taking serial cultures over the next two weeks to check that the infection is cured is also pointless when one considers that a 5-day course of oral penicillin prevents blood cultures being positive for up to 6 weeks.

Regular outpatient review with echocardiography to check for the reappearance or regrowth of vegetations is useful, although it may not be practical if the home is some way from a suitable centre.

Most children are well and walking about during the latter weeks of their treatment and if so can return to school as soon as they are discharged from hospital.

Any source of sepsis, particularly in the mouth should be dealt with as soon as the course of antibiotics is finished. Since the mouth organisms will have become resistant to penicillin and possibly other antibiotics used, it is necessary to cover the treatment with an entirely different antibiotic. If the teeth are suspect, or have not been well cared for it is important to see that a regular check is kept by the dentist. In adults one attack of infective endocarditis doubles the chance of another attack and it is wise to assume that the same applies in children.

The haemodynamic importance of the underlying condition must be reassessed. Valvar stenosis is unlikely to be worsened, but mitral and aortic regurgitation may be, and the worsening may sometimes occur some weeks after the eradication of infection. Ventricular septal defects, particularly small ones associated with pseudoaneurysm formation, may increase in size and may develop a communication into the right atrium (acquired Gerbode defect). The need for surgery must be reassessed, both from this point of view and to lessen the chances of a further attack of infective endocarditis. Occasionally, patients with tetralogy of Fallot who have had infection on the pulmonary valve actually improve as far as cyanosis is concerned, but since they will all need surgical correction anyway, the benefit is temporary only.

Prophylaxis

Surprisingly little scientific work exists on the best means of preventing infective endocarditis. The regimes advised previously have been based on the work of Durack and Petersdorf (1973) in rabbits. They showed that bactericidal drugs must be used and that there should be adequate serum levels of antibiotics both at the time of the bacteraemia and for a critical period of 6–9 hours afterwards when surviving bacteria might settle on the damaged heart and multiply. Their experiments involved producing vegetations on aortic valves by inserting catheters and introducing large doses of streptococci intravenously. Treatment was aimed at sterilizing the blood over 24 hours. In practice this may be more difficult than eliminating the transient bacteraemia which occurs after dental treatment in man, so dosage regimes based on Durack's work are likely to give a wide margin of safety.

Streptococcus sangius is the commonest organism entering the bloodstream from the mouth and this and other organisms from the upper respiratory tract are usually penicillin-sensitive. In the recent past most paediatricians have followed the recommendations of the American Heart Association (1977) and have given an oral regime using phenoxymthylpenicillin (penicillin V) or a combined parenteral and oral schedule. Unfortunately, the absorption of oral penicillin V is unpredictable so an injection regime is preferable. Since most dentists do not give intramuscular injections and an injection is difficult to organize at the appropriate time, most children are given the oral regime despite doubt about its adequacy.

Shanson, Cannon and Wilks (1978) have recently shown that in adults amoxycillin gives a higher and more sustained serum level than penicillin V and that a 3 g oral dose of amoxycillin one hour before dental treatment gives serum concentrations well above the minimal bactericidal levels for at least 10 hours – thus covering the critical period after treatment (Shanson, Ashford and Singh, 1980). Studies on oral amoxycillin in children have confirmed the same satisfactory absorption as in adults (Deasy and Bourke, 1974).

Present recommendations

All children at risk should have a high standard of oral hygiene and regular dental supervision.

Oral amoxycillin using half the adult dose for children under 10 years may be used for prophylaxis outside hospital when dental treatment is carried out without anaesthesia. If anaesthesia is required the patient should be referred to hospital and amoxycillin given parenterally.

All children at risk should be given a card to show to any doctor or dentist. A suitable format is:

'This child has a heart lesion and it is essential that he/she has prophylactic therapy against infective endocarditis before dental treatment, removal of tonsils or adenoids, or any procedure involving the upper respiratory tract. Outside hospital when anaesthesia is not required the following regime is recommended. Amoxycillin 3 g orally one hour before treatment. The dose is halved for children under 10 years.

If an anaesthetic is required the patient should be referred to hospital and amoxycillin given by i.m. injection.

If the patient is sensitive to penicillin, erythromycin 1 g orally one hour before treatment is advised, halving the dose for children under 10 years.'

In gastrointestinal and genito-urinary tract surgery, enterococci are frequently responsible for endocarditis and prophylactic therapy should be aimed at these organisms. The patient is usually in hospital and a combination of gentamicin 2 mg/kg i.m. and ampicillin 1 g i.m. (half dose under 10 years) is a suitable combination.

Patients with prosthetic heart valves have a particularly high risk of developing endocarditis and the organism may have been acquired in hospital. There is less agreement about the best prophylaxis in this group (fortunately small in children) and they should be under observation in hospital. Ampicillin 1 g i.m. and cloxacillin 1 g i.m. (half dose for children under 10 years) before treatment and repeated 8-hourly for 2 doses should suffice.

Abnormalities of acid–base balance

The acid–base status of the blood and extracellular fluid are closely linked. Hydrogen ions diffuse freely into and out of the cells so that intra- and extracellular pH are similar, but the buffering systems inside and outside the cells are different. There are three variables: the carbon dioxide tension, pH and buffer concentrations. (In the blood, bicarbonate and proteins each normally make up about a half of the buffering capacity.) If any two of the variables are known it is possible to estimate the other. In practice one of two methods is used to define the acid–base state. In the first the pH and P_{CO_2} are measured and the bicarbonate, total buffer base and base deficit or excess are calculated, or read off a nomogram. In the second, the Astrup method, the pH of the blood is measured directly and the pH is also determined after equilibration with two gases of known P_{CO_2}. From this the P_{CO_2}, total buffer base and standard bicarbonate are estimated from the Siggaard–Andersen nomogram. Results are most reliable when arterial blood is used, but by warming the foot to ensure rapid circulation, 'arterialized' capillary blood can be obtained by heel puncture which has a pH and P_{CO_2} very similar to those of arterial blood.

Metabolic acidosis

Tissue oxygenation may be impaired either by a low arterial oxygen saturation, as in cyanotic congenital heart disease, or by a reduced blood flow, as occurs with myocardial failure or with obstruction to the left heart (aortic atresia). Anaerobic metabolism results in the accumulation of lactic acid in the tissues. To some extent the kidneys compensate by excreting hydrogen ions, but, particularly in the first few weeks of life when tubular function is poor, this is usually insufficient compensation and a progressive metabolic acidosis develops. This can be demonstrated by measuring the pH and bicarbonate of the blood. The pH may fall below 7.0 and the bicarbonate below 10 mmol/l. A pH below 7.20 indicates a poor prognosis unless a palliative operation is performed.

The depressant effect of acidaemia on the myocardium is at first masked by stimulation of the sympathoadrenal system with release of catecholamines and these increase the contractile force of the ventricle. Finally, however, cardiovascular failure occurs in the presence of high catecholamines. The ventricular fibrillation threshold decreases in the presence of acidaemia.

The reduction in pH causes myocardial and central nervous system depression. The former is indicated by poor peripheral pulses and cold, blotchy extremities with poor return of capillary filling after pressure. Central nervous system depression manifests itself by absent or reduced spontaneous movements and diminished reflexes. Below a pH of 7.20 the respiratory centre is depressed, so that a respiratory element is added to the acidosis and respiratory effort becomes reduced and finally ceases.

Metabolic acidosis can be corrected temporarily by giving sodium bicarbonate. In the mild cases it can be given orally but if the pH is below 7.2 intravenous therapy is indicated. Sodium bicarbonate is a hyperosmolar solution and its administration in the acidotic and hypoxic newborn infant will result in profound vasodilatation and pooling of blood in the skeletal muscle causing severe hypotension. A solution containing 5 mmol/10 ml (0.42 g/10 ml) of sodium bicarbonate should be used in the newborn and 50 mmol/50 ml (4.2 g/50 ml) in older children. Two mmol/kg bodyweight should be given slowly and the pH measured again. Excessive sodium bicarbonate administration will produce hypernatraemia and intraventricular cerebral haemorrhage in the sick newborn. The calcium should be measured and any associated hypocalcaemia treated with calcium gluconate. Dextrose 5% should be given if there is hypoglycaemia.

The child's general condition will improve following correction of the acidosis but the acidosis recurs unless measures are taken to correct the underlying situation. Correction of the acidosis is only a means of buying time to allow cardiac catheterization or operation to take place.

Metabolic alkalosis

This rarely occurs after prolonged diuretic therapy. It may also be iatrogenic. It can be corrected by giving ammonium chloride orally.

Respiratory acidosis

Infants with reduced lung compliance due to high pulmonary blood flow or pulmonary venous congestion frequently have a mild or moderate respiratory acidosis, the P_{CO_2} rising as high as 70 mmHg. Usually there is nearly complete renal compensation with increased bicarbonate production and hydrogen ion excretion, so that the pH does not usually fall much below 7.32. Where there is superadded infection or pulmonary oedema the P_{CO_2} may rise much higher, sometimes over 100 mmHg, and, in an attempt to compensate, the bicarbonate may be increased to as high as 70 mmol/l, with a corresponding reduction in chloride. (It should be noted that if the pH is not measured this is frequently reported erroneously as a metabolic alkalosis.) A P_{CO_2} over 80 mmHg which is not corrected promptly by diuretics in the case of pulmonary oedema or by suction and antibiotics in the case of infection is an indication for artificial ventilation pending operative intervention.

Respiratory alkalosis

A respiratory alkalosis of any degree rarely occurs naturally but may be produced by over-enthusiastic artificial ventilation. The high pH may produce tetany of fits, and the kidneys excrete potassium ions in preference to hydrogen ions so that hypokalaemia results. The level of ventilation must be reduced or a 'dead space' added.

Cardiac arrest

Acid–base abnormalities must be corrected after an episode of acute cardiorespiratory failure. The administration of sodium bicarbonate is the same as described under metabolic acidosis.

Bibliography and references

Thrombosis and embolism

Johnson, C. A., Abilgaard, C. F. and Schulman, I. (1968) Absence of coagulation abnormalities in children with cyanotic congenital heart disease. *Lancet*, **2**, 660

Parsons, C. G., Astley, R., Burrows, F. G. O., *et al.* (1971) Transposition of great arteries. A study of 65 infants followed for 1 to 4 years after balloon septostomy. *British Heart Journal*, **33**, 725

Paul, M. H., Cirrimbhoy, Z., Miller, R. A, *et al.* (1961) Thrombocytopenia in cyanotic congenital heart disease. *Circulation,* **24,** 1013

Somerville, J., McDonald, L. and Edgill, M. (1965) Post-operative haemorrhage and related abnormalities of blood coagulation in cyanotic congenital heart disease. *British Heart Journal,* **27,** 440

Taussig, H. B. (1971) Long-term results of the Blalock–Taussig operation. *Johns Hopkins Medical Journal,* **129,** 243

Infective endocarditis

American Heart Association Committee Report (1977) *Circulation,* **56,** 139A

Barritt, D. W. and Gillespie, W. A. (1960) Subacute bacterial endocarditis. *British Medical Journal,* **1,** 1235

Beeson, P. B. and Ridley, M. (Eds.) (1969) *Bacterial Endocarditis.* A symposium held at the Royal College of Physicians. London: Beecham Research Laboratories

Deasy, P. F. and Bourke, M. (1974) Trial of amoxycillin in paediatrics. *Journal of the Irish Medical Association,* **67,** 463

Durack, D. T. and Petersdorf, R. G. (1973) Chemotherapy of experimental streptococcal endocarditis. I. Comparison of commonly recommended prophylactic regimes. *Journal of Clinical Investigation,* **52,** 592

Gersony, W. M. and Hayes, C. J. (1977) Bacterial endocarditis in patients with pulmonary stenosis, aortic stenosis and ventricular septal defect. *Circulation,* **56,** Suppl. 1–84

Jawetze, E. (1962) Assay of antibacterial activity in serum. *American Journal of Diseases of Children,* **103,** 81

Jordan, S. C. (1979) Dental treatment of children with heart disease. *Proceedings of the British Paedodontic Society,* **9,** 13

Keith, J. D., Rowe, R. D. and Vlad, P. (1978) *Heart Disease in Infancy and Childhood,* 3rd edn, Macmillan, New York, p. 239

Report from the Joint Study on the Natural History of Congenital Heart Defects. (1977) *Circulation,* **56,** 2, Supplement (1)

Shanson, D. C., Ashford, R. F. U. and Singh, J. (1980) High-dose oral amoxycillin for preventing endocarditis. *British Medical Journal,* **1,** 446

Shanson, D. C., Cannon, P. and Wilks, M. (1978) Amoxycillin compared with Penicillin V for prophylaxis of dental bacteraemia. *J. Antimicrobial Chemotherapy* **4,** 43

Sholler, G. F., Hawker, R. E. and Celermajer, J. M. (1986) Infective endocarditis in childhood. *Pediatric Cardiology,* **6,** 183

Abnormalities of acid-base balance

Kamath, V. R. and Jones, R. S. (1966) Acid base abnormalities in infants with congenital heart disease. *British Medical Journal,* **2,** 434

Sanyal, S. K., Ghosh, K., Bigram, R., *et al.* (1971) The biochemical aspects of congestive heart failure in children. *Journal of Pediatrics,* **79,** 250

Siggaard-Andersen, O. (1962) The pH-log P_{CO_2} blood acid-base nomogram revised. *Scandinavian Journal of Clinical and Laboratory Investigation,* **14,** 598

Chapter 18

Disorders of cardiac rhythm

Many disturbances of cardiac rhythm are of no functional significance but are problems in diagnosis when they are detected on routine examination or when an electrocardiogram is performed for some other reason. Serious cardiac dysrhythmias make up about 2% of paediatric cardiological problems but the presentation is often obscure, and in many cases the true diagnosis can only be made by careful history taking, since physical examination and special investigations may all be completely normal except during the paroxysmal dysrhythmia. A typical case is a 7-year-old boy with a long history of episodes of abdominal pain and vomiting diagnosed after various investigations as pyschosomatic. A prolonged attack led to his admission as 'acute appendicitis' when he was found to have tachycardia of 280/min and the abdominal pain was localized to the enlarged tender liver. His mother's first recorded description of the attacks included the sentence: 'The attacks upset him so much that I can see his heart beating nineteen to the dozen through his clothes'.

In the majority of children we see with arrhythmias, the heart is structurally normal and the electrocardiogram may be normal or show some abnormality of conduction, e.g. Wolff–Parkinson–White syndrome. Arrhythmias may also occur in association with congenital heart disease and the commonest are:

Atrioventricular discordance (L-transposition)
Ebstein's anomaly of the tricuspid valve
Cardiomyopathy
Mitral valve prolapse.

Nowadays an increasing number of arrhythmias are seen after surgery, particularly after Mustard's operation for transposition of the great arteries and after repair of tetralogy of Fallot. They may also be drug induced.

Normal anatomy and physiology of the conducting system

The *sinoatrial node* lies at the junction of the superior vena cava and right atrium and consists of a small crescentic mass of specially differentiated cells which possess an enhanced power of rhythmic depolarization at a rate of up to 200/min. The rate is influenced by the vagus (cardio-inhibiting) and sympathetic (cardio-stimulating) nerves. The impulse generated in the sinoatrial node spreads throughout both atria, causing depolarization and contraction of atrial muscle. Although there are 'preferential pathways' through the atria there is no specialized conducting tissue between the sinoatrial node and the *atrioventricular node*, which lies in the lower part of the right atrium, close to the tricuspid valve and coronary sinus. The atrioventricular node is histologically similar to the sinoatrial node but has two parts, the upper portion being functionally concerned with picking up the atrial depolarization and the lower portion in passing it on to the *atrioventricular bundle*, which passes through the fibrous ring separating the atrial and ventricular muscle. It then travels for a short distance in the membranous portion of the interventricular septum before dividing into right and left branches. Due to the presence of the fibrous atrioventricular ring, the atrioventricular bundle (bundle of His) is normally the *only path* by which impulses can pass between the atria and ventricles. The *right bundle branch* travels as a discrete bundle on the right ventricular aspect of the interventricular septum to the apex of the right ventricle where it divides into numerous small branches. The *left bundle branch* is a wide sheet of fibres which runs down the left ventricular aspect of the interventricular septum for a short distance before dividing into three sub-branches, the septal, anterior and inferior branches.

The atrioventricular node (and hence the ventricles) are normally controlled by the rate of the sinoatrial node; however, if the sinoatrial node ceases to function or becomes excessively slow, the intrinsic rhythmicity of the atrioventricular node takes over, but at a slower rate (normally about 50–60/min in older children but as fast as 100/min in infants). The rate is under the control of the vagus and sympathetic nerves but to a lesser extent than the sinoatrial node. If the atrioventricular node or bundle cease to conduct impulses the ventricles will produce their own idioventricular rate, usually about 30–50/min. It is thought that this impulse is generated in the conducting tissue of the ventricles rather than in the ventricular muscle.

Investigation of arrhythmias

In the past decade new techniques have become available to investigate arrhythmias. One is continuous ambulatory 24-hour monitoring of the electrocardiogram and the other is intracardiac electrocardiograms with programmed intracardiac stimulation. Exercising testing is also of value.

All these tests are not always required but their use has increased our knowledge of arrhythmias and helped us to treat them, when necessary, in the best possible way.

Twenty-four-hour continuous electrocardiographic monitoring
In the past, diagnosis of arrhythmias in childhood was made from the resting ECG taken for short periods and often depended on chance recordings. Since 24-hour electrocardiographic monitoring on magnetic tapes became available, the type, frequency and duration of any arrhythmias can usually be determined, even in newborn infants. One chest electrode is placed on the upper part of the sternum and the other in the position of the chest lead V_4. They are fixed to the skin without any air trap, taped down and connected to a battery-operated miniature analogue tape recorder. The cassette is housed in a leather bag worn around the waist, or in babies it can lie on the mattress. The children or their parents keep a diary of their activities and if they have any unusual symptoms an 'alarm' button is pressed which marks the tape so that the record at that time can be correlated with the symptoms.

For analysis an instrument is used which automatically detects changes in heart rate and rhythm from preset R–R intervals. Print-outs are made of any abnormalities and at 4-hourly intervals throughout the trace for 10-s periods even when no abnormalities are detected. The analyser is expensive but is usually available in special centres – the magnetic tapes can easily be sent to that centre for analysis. One of the problems of using these tapes is that they have been used to study the *abnormal* before the 24-hour records in *normal* healthy children have been analysed. Scott, Williams and Fiddler (1980), however, have already studied 131 boys between the ages of 10 and 13 years. They showed that:

1. The maximal heart rates during the day ranged from 100 to 200 beats/min and minimal rates from 45 to 80.
2. During sleep the maximal rates were 60–110 beats/min and the minimal rates 30–70 beats/min.
3. P waves changed in form during sleep in 15% and in 5% when awake. In 13% the abnormal 'P' waves were associated with junctional rhythm.
4. First degree heart block occurred in 8%.
5. Wenckebach phenomenon occurred in 10% mostly at night when it was associated with slow heart rates.
6. Premature ventricular beats were always single and occurred in 26%, mostly when awake but occasionally during sleep and during exercise. The number of premature beats was not greater than 4 in 24 hours except in two boys, one of whom had 35 premature beats and periods of coupling lasting for 9 seconds. The other had 27 premature beats in 24 hours.
7. Atrial premature beats occurred in 13%; they were always single and occurred during sleep and when awake. They were never more frequent than 2 in 24 hours except in one boy who had two half-hour periods of coupling during sleep.
8. Complete sinoatrial block was seen in 8% and never lasted for more than one cycle.

Some devices perform analysis of the rhythm as it is recorded and store only those portions which appear to be abnormal, usually in a solid-state memory. These can be used continuously for a week or more and clearly increase the chances of picking up a paroxysmal arrhythmia.

Patient-activated devices and transtelephonic electrocardiography
Many rhythm disturbances, particularly the common paroxysmal supraventricular tachycardia, occur too infrequently for a single 24-hour tape to record them. An alternative is to loan the family a device which will record a short strip, or several strips of the electrocardiogram, usually in solid-state memory. These records can then be played back and analysed, either by returning the device to the cardiac centre or by transmitting it over the telephone. The recording can be made by placing the device, which has two electrodes on the surface, over the chest or by holding one electrode in each hand.

Intracardiac electrophysiology
This is an invasive study in which multipolar electrode catheters are passed into the heart usually via the femoral vein. A detailed sequence of cardiac activation can be made during sinus rhythm, paced atrial and ventricular rhythms or abnormal rhythms. It can be used to localize sites of conduction delay and block. A valuable application is to delineate tachycardia circuits. Paroxysmal atrial tachycardia can be

induced and the effect of various drugs studied. Therapeutically it can be of great importance to know the exact mechanism underlying the tachycardia. The study can be done in infancy and childhood but is reserved for patients whose abnormal rhythm does not respond to standard methods of treatment.

In order to carry out such studies it is necessary to admit the patient to hospital and several days study may be necessary if different drugs have to be tried. For this reason it is reserved for the more troublesome and life-threatening rhythm disturbances.

Exercise testing
An electrocardiogram can be recorded after various measured amounts of exercise and the effect of exercise evaluated. Sometimes ectopic beats will disappear but sometimes exercise will induce some arrhythmia or aberrant conduction.

Sinus tachycardia

Infants and children have very variable pulse rates and under certain circumstances the sinoatrial node can produce a rate as high as 200/min. Such conditions include physical exercise, anxiety and pyrexia and when the sinoatrial node is freed from the inhibitory influence of the vagus by atropine. Under these circumstances the condition is harmless and no treatment is needed. Rarely, excess adrenaline secretion in thyrotoxicosis or from phaeochromocytoma may produce a prolonged tachycardia and can then be treated with beta-adrenergic blocking drugs such as propranolol, until the underlying condition can be treated. Sinus tachycardia can be differentiated from paroxysmal supraventricular tachycardia by the fact that in the former the rate varies from minute to minute and can be slowed gradually by carotid sinus pressure or, if this fails, by intravenous Tensilon.

Sinus arrhythmia

Variation in sinus rate is usual in children and normally is related to respiration, the rate increasing on inspiration and slowing on expiration. (This variation is usually absent in patients with atrial septal defects.) Occasionally the variation is so great as to simulate intermittent atrioventricular block, but the relationship to respiration nearly always allows the distinction to be made clinically.

Sinus bradycardia

A slow rate is usual in athletic children and adolescents and is not associated with any symptoms and requires no treatment. If a child has attacks of loss of consciousness associated with bradycardia, further investigations must be carried out (*see* Sinus node dysfunction, page 285).

Atrial arrhythmias

Atrial ectopic beats are not infrequently seen in newborn infants. They are usually not associated with symptoms and do not require treatment. Twenty-four-hour tapes can be used to ensure that there are no prolonged episodes of tachycardia. They are entirely benign.

Paroxysmal supraventricular tachycardia

This is the commonest arrhythmia in infancy and childhood. Approximately 70–80% of patients subject to paroxysmal supraventricular tachycardia have normal hearts, the remainder have atrial septal defects, Ebstein's anomaly, mitral prolapse or disease of the cardiac muscle. Occasionally paroxysmal atrial tachycardia occurs *in utero* and causes immediate problems at birth. Radford, Izakawa and Rowe (1976) reviewed 10 cases and concluded that cardioversion should be used promptly in severely ill patients. Fetal electrocardiography is of value in such cases. When the condition is diagnosed well before term digitalization of the mother has resulted in termination of the arrhythmia or slowing of the ventricular rate.

Pathophysiology

The majority of tachycardias in childhood are now thought to be due to re-entry tachycardias; the remainder are due to enhanced atrial or A-V nodal automaticity.
    Four abnormal pathways have been described:

1. Wolff–Parkinson–White syndrome (WPW) (Figure 18.1(c)) in which the accessory pathway goes from the left atrium to the left ventricle (Type A) or in which the accessory pathway is from the right atrium to right ventricle (Type B). When the accessory pathways are being used, the ECG shows a very short P–R interval followed by a delta wave (Figure 18.2). The appearances in Type A may be mistaken for right bundle branch block and Type B mistaken for left bundle branch block. The conduction by the accessory route may be intermittent and at times the ECG is normal. When conduction occurs in a retrograde manner in the accessory pathway there is re-entry into the chamber of origin, a circus movement is set-up and tachycardia results.
2. Lown–Ganong–Levine syndrome (Figure 18.1(d)) in which the accessory pathway bypasses the A–V node but the ventricular excitation is normal. The P–R interval is short on the ECG but there is no delta wave.
3. A type in which fibres bypass the lower part of the His bundle and enter the ventricular septum directly. This results in early and abnormal sequence of ventricular depolarization producing a delta wave, but the P–R interval is normal.
4. Intra A–V nodal pathway. The resting ECG is normal.

Clinical presentation

Paroxysms tend to occur repeatedly over several months and then frequently subside spontaneously. It is not uncommon for attacks to occur in infancy and then stop, only to recur in teenage or adult life. In infancy, brief attacks are often detected because of pallor and rapid breathing ('white attacks') or they may produce vomiting. More prolonged attacks cause cardiac failure with cough and dyspnoea due to left heart failure, and vomiting and abdominal pain due to hepatic engorgement. Older children usually, but not invariably, complain of rapid heart beating and careful questioning reveals information that attacks start suddenly: 'My heart gives a sudden thump and off it goes'. The termination may be equally sudden, but since a sinus tachycardia may persist afterwards it is not always quite as abrupt subjectively. With rapid rates there is usually faintness on standing up, breathlessness and infrequently central chest pain. Occasionally, attacks may cause sudden loss of consciousness or a major fit due to cerebral anoxia. Polyuria often occurs following an attack and is an important diagnostic pointer.

Physical signs

During an attack the patient is pale, the pulse small in volume as well as rapid. The heart rate is absolutely regular, except when there is a changing degree of block, and frequently as high as 280/min. If an attack at this high rate has lasted more than 20–30 min there will be evidence of excess catecholamine production (sweating and coldness of extremities) and the liver is enlarged.

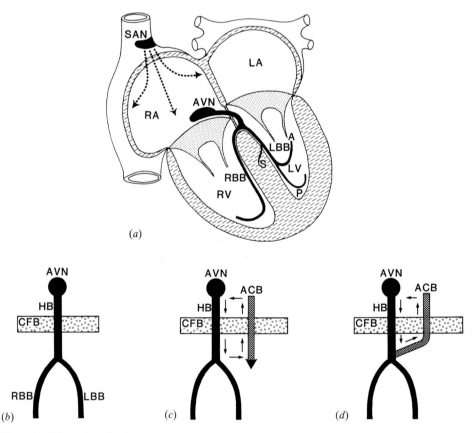

Figure 18.1 Normal conducting system of the heart (a and b) and the genesis of atrial tachycardia. (c) In the Wolff–Parkinson–White syndrome (WPW), in addition to the normal His bundle (HB) there is an accessory conducting bundle (ACB) from the atria to the ventricles. (d) In the Lown–Ganong–Levine syndrome (LGL) the accessory conducting pathway joins the His bundle. In either case a circus movement, reactivating the atrioventricular node is set up by retrograde conduction in the accessory pathway. SAN, sinoatrial node; RA, right atrium; AVN, atrioventricular node; RBB and LBB, right and left bundle branches; A and P, anterior and posterior divisions of the left bundle; S, septal branch; CFB, central fibrous body

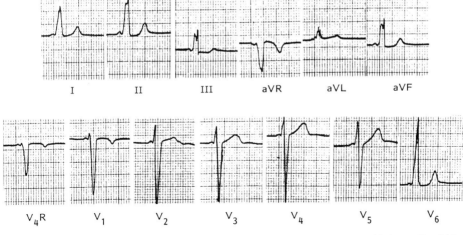

I   II   III   aVR   aVL   aVF

V$_4$R   V$_1$ V$_2$ V$_3$ V$_4$ V$_5$ V$_6$

Figure 18.2 Pre-excitation. The P wave is followed immediately by the delta wave. This is type B, which superficially resembles left bundle branch block

Examination between attacks is completely normal unless there is underlying heart disease, but clinical examination needs to be careful in order to detect associated abnormalities such as Ebstein's anomaly or atrial septal defect.

Investigation

Chest radiographs may show slight or moderate cardiac enlargement and evidence of pulmonary oedema in or following a prolonged attack.

The electrocardiogram between attacks is normal (except in patients with underlying heart disease or with the Wolff–Parkinson–White syndrome, described on page 279). Twenty-four-hour ECG tapes may show bursts of supraventricular tachycardia. Following attacks the T waves may be inverted and ST segments depressed for up to 24 hours. During attacks the electrocardiogram is characteristic and the following points are seen.

1. When P waves can be distinguished the atrial rate is completely regular at 240–300/min (often slower in older children).
2. When there is 1:1 atrioventricular conduction, the ventricular rate is also completely regular and each QRS complex has the same temporal relationship to the preceding P wave – the P–R interval is constant. When there is 2:1 or a higher degree of block the relationship of QRS to the preceding P wave is also constant (Figure 18.3).
3. The QRS complexes always have an initial rapid component. They may be identical with the patient's normal QRS complexes but occasionally there is slurring of the terminal portion due to intraventricular conduction delay.
4. Carotid sinus pressure may have no effect on the rate or produces a higher degree of block or causes return to sinus rhythm. A gradual slowing does not occur.

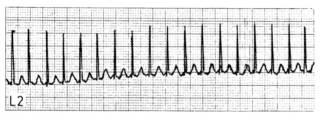

Figure 18.3 Supraventricular tachycardia

Treatment

Brief attacks with few or no symptoms require no treatment. A few patients are able to abort attacks by various manoeuvres which induce vagal stimulation, eyeball pressure, gagging, or the Valsalva manoeuvre. Carotid sinus massage will only occasionally cause reversion in a prolonged attack. Most older children find attacks revert spontaneously if they lie down for an hour or two.

Patients admitted to hospital in a prolonged attack can be treated either by electroversion or by drugs. Electroversion requires a synchronized 'defibrillator' (that is, one which can be set to deliver the direct current shock synchronous with the QRS complex to avoid the dangers of producing ventricular fibrillation) and can be performed under general anaesthesia or under sedation with intravenous diazepam. Usually sinus rhythm can be restored with a single shock varying from 5 joules (J) in an infant to 50 J in an adolescent (roughly 1 J/kg). The method has the advantage of rapidity and a limited period of monitoring and is virtually always successful, although relapse may occur. Its disadvantages are the requirements for specialized equipment and experience, and for anaesthesia (see also p. 247).

Drugs

Drug treatment to terminate an attack should always be given under continuous ECG monitoring. Digoxin is still a valuable and safe drug in infancy and should be given intramuscularly to produce a rapid effect using the schedule described in the section on heart failure (see page 251). It prolongs A–V node conduction and in addition, its inotropic effect is valuable if the child is in heart failure. Its use is not advised in Wolff–Parkinson–White syndrome (see page 283).

There is a tendency now to use drugs which act more quickly, but it is important to use one drug at a time and never give two drugs with negative inotropic action together or one after each other, such as propranolol and verapamil, because severe hypotension will result. It is, however, safe to give propranolol and digoxin together, and if digoxin has not controlled the tachycardia alone, then a combination of digoxin and propranolol may do so.

If digoxin fails to produce sinus rhythm one of the following regimes should be tried. Continuous monitoring of the electrocardiogram is required, both to indicate return to sinus rhythm and also to detect any change in the QRS complexes, such as widening, which may indicate a toxic response.

Verapamil

Intravenous injection is required and should be given through a cannula to ensure that the dose injected does enter the vein. The patient's blood pressure should be monitored manually or with an automatic external monitor such as the 'Dynamap'.

Verapamil should not be given to infants under the age of 1 year as severe and sometimes fatal hypotension may occur (Kirk *et al.*, 1987). It has been used successfully in older children in a dose of 2–3 mg from 1–5 years and 3–5 mg from 5 years upwards.

The smaller dose should be given first and a further half dose given after 10 min if not effective. The doses have to be given rapidly, over 15–20 s if they are to be effective. The injection should be stopped if there is a fall of more than 10 mmHg in systolic blood pressure or change in peripheral perfusion. Calcium chloride injection should be available to counteract any marked hypotension.

Disopyramide
This is a valuable drug for aborting attacks, but experience is mainly confined to older children. It should not be given within 30 min of injections of verapamil and very cautiously to those on beta-blockers. The dose is 2.5 mg/kg slowly over 15–20 min, and may be repeated after a further 30 min. (Intravenous disopyramide is not available in some countries, notably the USA.)

Propranolol
If possible this is best given orally, since intravenous preparations may produce severe hypotension. The dose is 1 mg/kg every 6 hours. If intravenous use is necessary due to vomiting, the dose is one-tenth the oral dose, 0.1 mg/kg.

Flecainide
This has been used to a limited extent on older children, 2 mg/kg is given as a slow infusion over 20 min (Till *et al.*, 1987). It can be given to patients on beta-blockers and digoxin. It does displace digoxin from tissues and may cause a rise in plasma digoxin levels, but this is not thought to predispose to digoxin toxicity.

Suppression of attacks

The first question which has to be asked is whether the attacks are frequent enough or disruptive of the patient's life enough to require medication. Often they are not, but it is sometimes useful to try therapy for a period as parents and patients are often happier if they know that there is a treatment which will prevent attacks if they become troublesome. A number of agents have been used, mainly on an empirical basis. Detailed electrophysiological studies to indicate which drug is most likely to be effective are required only exceptionally in patients with repetitive, life-threatening attacks which do not respond to first-line therapy.

Digoxin
This is most useful in the first year of life. Digitalization will usually have been started in an acute attack and oral maintenance treatment is continued as for heart failure, 10 µg/kg/day (see Chapter 15). If this is not effective the dose can be increased to 15 µg/kg/day.

Although in the past digoxin has been used successfully to control supraventricular tachycardia, there is a possibility in cases of pre-excitation (i.e. the Wolff–Parkinson–White syndrome) that it may shorten the anterograde refractory period of the accessory connection and make the patient susceptible to ventricular fibrillation and sudden death. Although the likelihood of this is extremely small, digoxin is no longer advised for the suppression of supraventricular tachycardia when the electrocardiogram between attacks shows pre-excitation.

Propranolol
In children over the age of a year this is usually more effective than digoxin. Usually only relatively small doses are used, 5–10 mg orally 3 times daily up to the age of 10, 10–20 mg 3 times daily over the age of 10. Owing to its short action there will be therapeutic gaps, particularly if doses are missed. Longer acting beta-blockers, such as metoprolol and atenolol can be used in older children, but there is no formulation which allows metoprolol to be given in small doses. Atenolol is now available as a liquid (5 mg/ml) and the dose is similar to propranolol, but given twice daily. Both metoprolol and atenolol are cardioselective and therefore less likely to aggravate bronchospasm in children susceptible to asthma.

Amiodarone
Amiodarone is a very effective drug for supraventricular tachycardia, but should only be used for frequently occurring attacks which do not respond to other measures as it has a number of toxic effects. These include corneal deposits, so that regular slit-lamp examination is required; photosensitivity requiring avoidance of exposure to direct sunlight; and interference with thyroid function tests, actual thyrotoxicosis or myxoedema being uncommon. On a weight-for-weight basis higher doses are tolerated than in adults, the usual starting dose being 10 mg/kg/day orally. The drug has a very long half-life (measurable amounts may still be found 3 months after stopping treatment) and may take 2 or more weeks to build up to an effective dose. Once control has been established the dose should be gradually reduced to the smallest amount that will control symptoms, usually 2–3 mg/kg/day. Amiodarone increases digoxin retention in the body and, if the two drugs are used together, the digoxin dose should be reduced by a half.

Flecainide
This drug has been used successfully in adults, but little information is available in children. It appears that higher relative doses are required to obtain satisfactory blood levels in children. Children over 10 years require 50–100 mg twice daily, from 5–10 years 25–50 mg twice daily.

Surgical treatment

In cases which prove resistant to medical therapy it may be possible to divide the accessory pathway or ablate it by cryotherapy. This requires an open-heart operation and considerable skills in mapping the conducting tissues. Most of the work has been in adults and children would normally be referred to such centres for investigation and treatment, as there are few paediatric cardiologists who have the necessary experience. An alternative approach, so far only reported in adults, is to destroy the normal atrioventricular node and bundle by the use of high-energy shocks through an electrode passed transvenously and placed over the atrioventricular node. Although in theory the accessory pathway should take over normal conduction (and not allow retrograde conduction), in practice atrioventricular conduction is not stable and permanent pacing is required.

Prognosis

When the first attack occurs during the first 3 months of life there is about a 75% chance that further attacks will not occur after the age of a year. If the resting electrocardiogram shows pre-excitation the chances of growing out of the attacks is less. Attacks may occur in groups and then be followed by a period of several years without attacks. When there has been no attack while on treatment for 6 months it is worth trying without treatment again.

Sinus node dysfunction

This is a condition in which the sinus node ceases to function and there is cardiac standstill for a few cycles after which a heart beat is initiated from an abnormal focus. Patients with this disorder frequently have syncope on exertion (Scott, Macartney and Deverall, 1976). The syndrome (also known as sick sinus syndrome) is often associated with bradycardia but at other times the patients may have tachycardia – the so-called 'brady-tachy syndrome'. Drugs which help the bradycardia may make the tachycardia worse so that drug therapy is difficult. Exercise tests may show periods of atrial arrest followed by an ectopic rhythm. The condition may be associated with sudden death and to avoid this in patients with repeated syncope, a pacemaker is required. The condition occurs after surgery for congenital heart disease (Radford and Izakawa, 1975).

Atrial flutter and fibrillation

Both atrial flutter and fibrillation are rare in childhood and almost always occur in association with severe heart disease and high left or right atrial pressures (mitral valve disease, Ebstein's anomaly) or with myocardial disease such as acute rheumatic fever or cardiomyopathy. (They may also be provoked during cardiac catheterization.) Treatment is by digitalization, or by electroversion.

Lown–Ganong–Levine syndrome

Atrial flutter and atrial fibrillation also occur in patients with an accessory conducting bundle from the atrium joining the bundle of His. The mechanism is similar to that of paroxysmal supraventricular tachycardia, the more rapid rhythm being due to the shorter pathway.

Ventricular arrhythmias

Ventricular ectopic beats

It is important to recognize that ventricular ectopic beats may occur in children whose hearts in every other respect are normal. Such ectopic beats usually occur singly, arise from the same focus and disappear on exercise. No treatment is required other than reassurance.

The situation is different if the ventricular ectopic beats:

are not abolished by exercise
are associated with heart disease
are multifocal
cause runs of coupling
are associated with a long Q–T interval on the ECG
are associated with bizarre QRS complexes on the ECG
occur more frequently than two at a time
cause syncope.

One must first make sure that the arrhythmia is primary and not secondary to hypoxia, acid–base disorder or electrolyte disturbance, particularly hypokalaemia, which may cause ectopic beats *per se* or as a result of potentiation of digitalis effects. (Hyperkalaemia occurs as a result of renal failure and the electrocardiogram shows tall T waves, atrial asystole and intraventricular block with wide QRS complexes). Drugs which cause ventricular extrasystoles include antidepressants, digitalis, and occasionally other antiarrhythmic drugs.

Investigation of malignant ventricular extrasystoles

These patients should have:

1. Twenty-four-hour electrocardiogram monitoring.
2. Exercise test.
3. Echocardiography.

If ventricular tachycardia, i.e. 3 or more successive extrasystoles with wide abnormal QRS complexes and a rate of 150–200/min, is shown or the child is symptomatic with attacks of syncope, then full investigation by cardiac catheterization, angiography and electrophysiology should be undertaken. Although ventricular arrhythmias are rare in childhood, they can cause syncope and sudden death. If ventricular tachycardia is suspected the patient must be investigated further and the aetiology of the condition determined if possible. Coronary artery abnormalities are excluded by angiocardiography. Echocardiography helps to exclude tumours, prolapse of the mitral valve and cardiomyopathy which can be further defined by ventricular angiocardiography. Twenty-four-hour monitoring may show evidence of sinus node dysfunction. Electrocardiogram may show a long Q–T interval which may be intermittent and in some of these patients syncope is provoked by exercise. Radford, Izakawa and Rowe (1977) investigated 8 children fully; only 1 patient was asymptomatic and the ventricular tachycardia was found by chance. Only 2 of these 8 cases were unexplained, the other 6 had some associated abnormality.

Treatment

Ventricular arrhythmias associated with prolapsing mitral valve are best treated by propranolol. Patients with prolonged Q–T interval may also respond to propranolol but if not they may be cured by left stellate ganglionectomy. Lignocaine 1–4 mg/kg as a bolus intravenously followed by the same dose as a slow infusion over 60 min is usually effective in controlling ventricular tachycardia. If syncope is associated with the sick sinus syndrome either because of sinus arrest or the ventricular tachycardia which may follow the sinus arrest, then a cardiac pacemaker is required.

Ventricular tachycardia associated with cyanotic congenital heart disease is probably caused by irritable foci in the myocardium secondary to ischaemia. They must be treated with propranolol or quinidine or a combination of both. Propranolol is again the drug of choice for ventricular tachycardias associated with hypertrophic obstructive cardiomyopathy.

Some patients may develop their ventricular tachycardia and syncope after exercise and in these patients a combination of propranolol and amiodarone is valuable but the possibility of corneal opacities must be remembered when the latter drug is used.

The effects of treatment as well as relieving symptoms can also be monitored by 24-hour electrocardiograms.

Both flecainide and amiodarone have proved effective in ventricular tachycardia (see under supraventricular tachycardia for doses) (Bucknall, *et al.*, 1986; Wren and Campbell, 1987). It is probably worth having treatment established in a centre with facilities for electrophysiological study, to establish both the best drug and the optimum dose.

Accidental ingestion of drugs by children

Digoxin

It is not uncommon nowadays for children to eat their grandparents' digoxin tablets. If vomiting can be induced to stop absorption, so much the better. If marked cardiac slowing occurs with heart block, cardiac pacing may be necessary. If potassium levels are low, potassium supplements should be provided (*see* page 253). Potassium should not be given without measuring the serum level as hyperkalaemia frequently occurs in severe digoxin poisoning.

There is now a specific antidote to digoxin, in the form of digoxin antibody fragments ('Digibind') which can be given intravenously and which sequestrates the digoxin. The dose is calculated on the basis of the calculated dose ingested.

Tricyclic antidepressants

These drugs cause ventricular ectopic beats with wide QRS complexes and bradycardia when taken by children. The cardiac output falls and the child loses consciousness and there is severe acidosis. Correction of this and cardiac pacing are necessary if the tablets cannot be recovered by vomiting or stomach wash-out. Unfortunately, if the myocardium is severely damaged the heart will not respond to pacing. The arrhythmias produced seem to be resistant to antiarrhythmic drugs.

Sudden infant death syndrome

The possibility of arrhythmias being associated with this syndrome has been raised. Apparently well babies have arrhythmias, some of which are associated with spells of apnoea. There is circumstantial evidence of a possible association of arrhythmias with sudden infant death syndrome but this has not so far been proved. Near-miss deaths have been known to be associated with arrhythmias (Keaton *et al.*, 1977).

Arrhythmias after surgery

Paediatricians must be informed about the possibility of arrhythmias after operations. Ventricular ectopic beats may occur after operation for ventricular septal defects and tetralogy of Fallot. They are sometimes induced by exercise. Their presence may precede episodes of ventricular tachycardia and sudden death and they must therefore be treated and suppressed – the drug of choice is propranolol. Although Mustard's operation produces very good results in the majority, some patients have symptomatic arrhythmias. The most serious is the sick sinus syndrome where there is sinus arrest and syncope. Other patients develop profound bradycardia resulting in dizziness or unconsciousness. Both conditions require cardiac pacemakers. Occasionally supraventricular tachycardia occurs – its treatment is the same for atrial tachycardias due to other causes. It is rare now to find atrial tachycardias after operation to close atrial septal defects; more care is now taken to avoid damage to the sinoatrial node. Atrial ectopic beats and atrial tachycardia occur infrequently and are treated in the same way as atrial tachycardias from other causes. Twenty-four-hour monitoring will show the frequency and duration of various arrhythmias, many of which are not associated with symptoms.

Atrioventricular block

Atrioventricular block is an interference with the normal conduction of impulses from the atria to the ventricles through the atrioventricular node. Three degrees of heart block are described.

(1) First-degree block
This is essentially an electrocardiographic diagnosis. The P–R interval is longer than it should be for the patient's age and heart rate (Figure 18.4(a)). It occurs in rheumatic carditis, diphtheria and digitalis overdosage. The most common congenital heart lesions associated with first-degree block are atrial septal defect, atrioventricular defects, Ebstein's anomaly of the tricuspid valve and L-transposition. It is also found in 8% of normal boys (Scott, Williams and Fiddler, 1980). The block itself does not cause any symptoms or require any treatment.

(2) Second-degree block
In this type some of the atrial depolarization waves are not conducted to the ventricles. This may happen irregularly, or only every second or third atrial impulse is conducted to the ventricle, giving a so-called 2:1 or 3:1 heart block (Figure 18.4(b)). Second-degree block is associated with the same heart lesions as first-degree block. There is no treatment other than for the underlying heart disease.

Sometimes there is a progressive lengthening of the P–R interval until a beat is dropped – the so-called Wenckebach phenomenon. This was found in 10% of normal boys (Scott, Williams and Fidler, 1980).

(3) Third-degree block (complete heart block)
In this type the atria and ventricles beat quite independently of each other, the atrial rate is higher than the ventricular rate (Figure 18.4(c)). It is usually

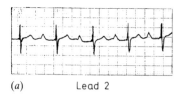

(a)   Lead 2

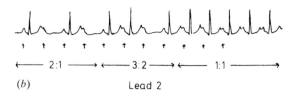

←——— 2:1 ———→ ←——— 3:2 ———→ ←——— 1:1 ———→

(b)   Lead 2

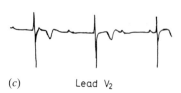

(c)   Lead V₂

Figure 18.4 Types of heart block. (a) First-degree block (lead 2). The P–R interval is 0.3 s. (b) Second-degree block (lead 2). Initially 2:1, then every third beat is dropped, and finally 1:1 conduction is restored. (c) Third degree or complete heart block (lead V₂). The atrial rate is 100/min and the ventricular rate 44/min. The QRS complexes are normal in morphology. This was a case of congenital heart block and the block is between the atria and the atrioventricular node

congenital, unassociated with any other structural heart abnormality (isolated congenital complete heart block). It may, however, be associated with L-transposition of the great arteries and may occur after operation for tetralogy of Fallot, atrioventricular defects and ventricular septal defects. If transient heart block occurs after surgery, there is a definite risk that it will recur and become permanent later in life.

In the past, congenital complete heart block was often not diagnosed until the mother was in labour. it was frequently erroneously thought to be bradycardia due to fetal distress and a Caesarean section was often performed. Nowadays if a slow fetal heart rate is noted during pregnancy, a fetal echocardiogram will show whether it is due to heart block. Indeed many cases of heart block are now diagnosed during a routine fetal scan in preganancy.

Aetiology

An interesting finding in recent years has been the occurrence of congenital complete heart block in infants of mothers who have some connective-tissue disorder, particularly systemic lupus erythematosus. In some mothers the connective tissue disorder does not develop until *after* the birth of the baby with heart block (McCue et al., 1977; Esscher and Scott, 1979). There seems no doubt that the effect on the fetus is related to the passive transfer from the mother of some auto-antibody not produced by the child. The antibody involved is anti-Ro or anti-La antibody, or one very closely related to these. The more sensitive tests for anti-Ro antibody have shown that *all* mothers of babies with isolated congenital heart block are anti-Ro or anti-La positive (Taylor et al., 1987).

If a mother has one child with isolated congenital heart block, there is a 30% risk of a subsequent child being affected (Scott and Scott, 1987). Further prospective studies are required.

All mothers of affected babies should have their serum tested for anti-Ro antibodies and should be watched for signs of a connective-tissue disorder developing (just as mothers of overweight babies are watched for diabetes). Conversely, the fetuses of mothers who have anti-Ro antibodies should be examined for the possibility of heart block; echocardiography will confirm the diagnosis. There is no known treatment at present but when the precise antibody (anti-Ro or a closely related one) is defined, it could be blocked by an appropriate monoclonal antibody.

It is not known how many anti-Ro positive mothers will subsequently become anti-Ro negative, but if they do they would be unlikely to give birth to a child with heart block.

Clinical presentation

Children with heart block have a higher ventricular rate than adults with acquired heart block; it is usually 45–60/min and may rise to 65–80/min on exercise. The pulse is of full volume because of the increased stroke output and, for the same reason, the heart is enlarged and the left ventricular beat forceful. There are large 'a' waves (Cannon waves) in the neck due to the right atrium contracting at times against a closed tricuspid valve. An ejection systolic murmur is heard at the base due to the increased stroke output. Sounds due to atrial contraction may be heard and the first sound varies in intensity depending on the closeness of atrial contraction to ventricular contraction.

Investigation

If there are no symptoms, further investigation is not required. If there are attacks of dizziness or syncope, 24-hour ambulatory monitoring should be done to assess the heart rate and look for ventricular ectopic beats and widening of the QRS factor, which are adverse factors.

Prognosis

The majority of patients with isolated complete heart block lead normal lives free of symptoms. If the heart rate is unacceptably slow, however, the patient will have dizziness or syncope and there is a risk of sudden death. The risk of death is greater if there is a low ventricular rate and frequent ventricular ectopic beats and a prolonged Q–T interval (Prinsky, Gillette and McNamara, 1979).

Treatment

None is required if there are no symptoms, but syncope or attacks of dizziness mean that a pacemaker is required. Temporary pacing can be done using a catheter until a permanent pacemaker is inserted.

Artificial pacemakers

Over the last 15 years much technical work has been carried out on the development of reliable circuitry and batteries with lives of up to 15 years. At the same time, clinical experience in the indications for pacing and the methods employed has been considerable, although most of it has been in adult patients. The paediatrician and paediatric cardiologist have benefited from this experience resulting in an increased use of pacemakers in children.

Indications for inserting a pacemaker

1. Symptoms, particularly syncope.
2. Heart failure.
3. Wide QRS complexes on the electrocardiogram.
4. Surgically-induced heart block.
5. Poor exercise tolerance in older children.

Pacing methods
Most pacing wires are inserted transvenously (subclavian, cephalic or jugular veins) and the tip positioned in the right ventricle under radiographic control (endocardial pacing). The generator is then implanted in the pectoral region. When the presence of heart block is noted at the end of an operation it may be possible to suture permanent pacing wires to the epicardium and the generator is then implanted in the abdominal wall. When there is atrial disease, it may be better to pace the right atrium, although the technical problems are greater.

Types of pacemakers
All commonly used pacemakers now have some form of lithium battery which gives an expected life, according to size and current drain, of 7–15 years. With endocardial systems the need in a growing child to replace the endocardial wire after a period of a few years makes it rather pointless to use the longest life

pacemakers, particularly as they are physically larger than those with a life of 7–10 years. Various electronic circuits are used to provide varieties of pacemaker function, but only a few are commonly used.

1. Ventricular inhibited pacemakers are 'shut off' when the patient's heart rate is higher than that of the pacemaker, thus avoiding competition between pacemaker and the patient's own rhythm.
2. Programmable ventricular pacemakers can be altered by an external device to change the pacing rate or strength of the stimulus. The increased rates available may be useful in children, and by setting the strength of the stimulus just above the minimum required, excessive drain on the battery can be avoided.
3. Atrial pacemakers are similar to ventricular pacemakers but need more sensitive circuitry to detect spontaneous atrial activity to enable them to switch off when the patient's own atrial rate is high enough.
4. Atrioventricular sequential pacemakers require a connection both to the right atrium and right ventricle. They pick up the atrial activity and generate a corresponding impulse to stimulate the ventricle so that they allow the ventricular rate to vary with exercise in a more physiological way. They are mainly used in complete atrioventricular block, but also have a regular standby mode if atrial activity ceases. Their technical problems largely outweigh the theoretical advantages.
5. Rate-responsive pacemakers. These are used to produce a rise in heart rate on exercise in patients who are not suitable for atrioventricular sequential pacing due to atrial standstill, sick sinus syndrome or unstable atrial rhythm. One form incorporates a sensor to body movement and is activated by walking or running, another uses an additional electrode to sense respiration and increases the heart rate when the respiratory rate increases with exercise and a third uses the shortening of the Q–T interval of the intracardiac electrocardiogram to initiate an increase in rate.
6. Specialized pacemakers used to interrupt tachycardias are mainly used for paroxysmal supraventricular tachycardia, which is sensed by the pacemaker and leads to a short series of impulses being delivered to the atrium, which usually abolishes the tachycardia.

Complications of pacemakers
Infection occurs in about 5–7% of all insertions or replacements, and usually requires removal of the system and reinsertion of a new one. Premature battery failure normally produces a distinct slowing of stimulus rate for some weeks before final failure, allowing a new unit to be substituted. Pacemaker generator failure due to component failure is rare with modern circuitry, but may cause slowing of pacing rate or, rarely, a speeding up. During, and immediately following insertion, ventricular ectopics and, rarely, ventricular fibrillation may occur, but these usually settle within hours or days. Wire dislodgement or breakage due to stretching from growth of the child is a real problem and frequently requires the introduction of a new system well before the generator battery fails.

Pacemaker clinics
Because of all these potential problems patients require regular follow-up at clinics where the rhythm and various pacemaker parameters can be checked. In places where patients live a long way from such a clinic it may be possible to make these checks using a special transducer with a telephone link to the pacing centre.

Bibliography and references
Supraventricular tachycardia
Kirk, C. R., Gibbs, J. L., Thomas, R., *et al.* (1987) Cardiovascular collapse after verapamil in supraventricular tachycardia. *Archives of Disease in Childhood,* **62,** 1265–1282

Radford, D. J., Izakawa, T. and Rowe, R. D. (1976) Congenital paroxysmal atrial tachycardia. *Archives of Disease in Childhood,* **51,** 613–617

Radford, D. J. and Izakawa, R. (1975) Sick sinus syndrome – symptomatic cases in children. *Archives of Disease in Childhood,* **50,** 879–885

Rowlands, D. J., Howitt, G. and Markman, P. (1965) Propranolol in disturbances of cardiac rhythm. *British Medical Journal,* **1,** 891

Scott, O., Macartney, F. J. and Deverall, P. D. (1976) The sick sinus syndrome in childhood. *Archives of Disease in Childhood,* **51,** 100

Scott, Olive, Williams, G. J. and Fiddler, G. I. (1980) Results of 24-hour ambulatory monitoring of the electrocardiogram in 131 healthy boys age 10–13 years. *British Heart Journal,* **44.3,** 304–308

Till, J. A., Rowland, E., Shinebourne, E. A., *et al.* (1987) Treatment of refractory supraventricular arrhythmias with flecainide acetate. *Archives of Disease in Childhood,* **62,** 247–252

Ventricular tachycardia
Bucknall, C. A., Keeton, B. R., Curry, P. V. L., *et al.* (1986) Intravenous and oral amiodarone for arrhythmias in children. *British Heart Journal,* **39,** 1150–1153

Canent, R. V., Spach, M. S., Morris, J. J., *et al.* (1964) Recurrent ventricular tachycardia in an infant. *Pediatrics, Springfield,* **33,** 926

Keaton, B. R., Southall, E., Rutter, N., *et al.* (1977) Cardiac conduction disorders in six infants with near-miss sudden infant deaths. *British Medical Journal,* **2,** 600–603

Radford, D. J., Izakawa, R. and Rowe, R. D. (1977) Evaluation of children with ventricular arrhythmias. *Archives of Disease in Childhood,* **52,** 345–353

Wren, C. and Campbell, R. W. F. (1987) The response of paediatric arrhythmias to intravenous and oral flecainide. *British Heart Journal,* **57,** 171–175

Heart block
Esscher, E. and Scott, J. S. (1979) Congenital heart block and maternal systemic lupus erythematosus. *British Medical Journal,* **1,** 1235–1238

Fryda, R. J., Kaplan, S. and Helmsworth, J. A. (1971) Postoperative complete heart block in children. **33,** 456

Glenn, W. W. L., de Leuchtenberg, N., von Keekeren, D. W., *et al.* (1969) Heart block in children. Treatment with a radio-frequency pacemaker. *Journal of Thoracic and Cardiovascular Surgery,* **58,** 454

Hurwitz, R. A., Riemenschneider, T. A. and Moss, A. J. (1968) Chronic postoperative heart block in children. *American Journal of Cardiology,* **21,** 185

Lev, M., Silverman, J., Fitzmaurice, F. M., *et al.* (1971) Lack of connection between the atria and more peripheral conduction system in congenital atrioventricular block. *American Journal of Cardiology,* **27,** 481

McCue, C. M., Mantakas, M. E., Tingelstad, J. B., *et al.* (1977) Congenital heart block in newborns of mothers with connective tissue disease. *Circulation,* **56,** 82–89

Mymin, D., Mathewson, F. A. L., Tate, R. B., *et al.* (1986) The natural history of first degree atrioventricular block. *New England Journal of Medicine,* **315,** 1183–1187

Prinsky, W. W., Gillette, P. C. and McNamara, D. G. (1979) Diagnosis and management of congenital complete atrioventricular block. *Paediatric Cardiology,* Abstract p. 93

Scott, O. and Scott, J. S. (1987) Immunology of congenital conduction disorders. In *Clinical Immunology and Allergy* (ed. W. A. Littler), Baillière Tindall, London, pp. 607–617

Scott, J. P. P. (1969) *Diagnosis and Treatment of Cardiac Arrhythmias.* Butterworths, London

Taylor, P. V., Scott, J. S., Gerlis, L. M., *et al.* (1986) Maternal antibodies against fetal cardiac antigens in congenital complete heart block. *New England Journal of Medicine,* **315,** 667–672

Taylor, P. V., Taylor, K. F., Norman, A., *et al.* (1988) Prevalence of maternal Ro (GSA) and La (SS-B) autoantibodies in relation to congenital heart block. *British Journal of Rheumatology,* **27,** 128–32

Chapter 19

Rheumatic fever and chorea

Rheumatic fever was always commonest in children living in poor communities with poor social conditions. Its incidence has fallen over the past 40 years so that it is now a rarity in paediatric wards in the Western world. Not only has the incidence fallen sharply but also the frequency of cardiac involvement and of recurrence is now less. Perry (1969) found that 80% of children with acute rheumatic fever seen prior to 1939 had evidence of carditis, 55% had recurrences and 71% were left with evidence of valvular disease. Between 1955 and 1962 only 55% had carditis, 9% had recurrences and 18% had permanent valvular damage.

There is little doubt that the decline in rheumatic fever is associated with socio-economic development. It began in the last century and most of the decline was achieved before prophylaxis with penicillin began (Strasser, 1978). It is difficult to assess the impact that penicillin prophylaxis has had on the incidence. The disease is still prevalent however in the less wealthy developing countries in other parts of the world. Surprisingly, when the causes of death in the age group 15–24 years were analysed in six European countries, rheumatic heart disease and rheumatic fever ranked between second and fourth commonest (Strasser, 1978). In the world as a whole, the incidence varies from 0.06/1000 (Nashville, USA) to 11/1000 in Delhi (Padmavati *et al.*, 1980). Shaper (1972) has emphasized that the occurrence of rheumatic fever in underdeveloped countries relates less to climate than to the ecology of rheumatic fever, including poverty, crowding, very poor housing and grossly inadequate health services. Climate is just one variable in which high temperatures favour the spread of pharyngeal streptococci. In other words he supports the old adage that rheumatic fever is a disease of the poor. Furthermore, the severity of the disease in such areas may well be related to the high rates of recurrent infections associated with inadequate medical care.

Aetiology

The disease is closely related to infection with group A streptococci. Kaplan (1969) reviewed the evidence and proposed the hypothesis that antibodies to the streptococcus cross-react with heart muscle in subjects whose own heart antigens resemble those of the streptococcus, causing an autoimmune reaction. In many patients a similar cross-reaction occurs with synovial tissue to produce arthritis, or with brain tissue causing chorea.

Separate cross-reactions have now been described (Kaplan, 1979) between streptococcal wall antigen and cardiac muscle antigen, heart valve fibroblast antigen and basal ganglia antigen, as well as a non-specific connective-tissue antigen. The latest work on immunological aspects of rheumatic fever has been reviewed by Gibofsky, Williams and Zabrinskie (1987).

The fact that only a small proportion of children infected with the appropriate beta-haemolytic streptococcus develop rheumatic fever, together with the tendency for the disease to be more common in certain families, has suggested that there may be a genetic predisposition. Patarroyo et al. (1979) raised an antibody to beta-cells from a patient with rheumatic fever and found an antigen which reacted to this antibody in all of 22 patients with rheumatic fever, but only 6% of controls. Relatives of the rheumatic fever patients had a higher incidence of antigen than normal controls.

Pathology

All parts of the heart are involved, that is to say there is a pancarditis. In the myocardium there is round-cell infiltration, muscle swelling and necrosis. Aschoff bodies are the scars left by areas of inflammation and consist of round cells, plasma cells and giant cells. They are more common in second and subsequent attacks than in the first. The pericardium shows swelling, infiltration and fibrinous exudate. Sometimes a small or moderate pericardial effusion occurs. The endocardium, including the valves (which are normally almost avascular), become hyperaemic, oedematous and infiltrated. Ultrasound studies have shown that, in the acute phase, the chordae tendineae become stretched, leading to mitral valve prolapse. In the chronic stages the valve cusps and chordae adhere and become thickened and fibrous, leading to predominant stenosis. These are the only changes which persist to cause clinical problems after the acute stages. The conducting tissue of the heart is also involved, leading to first-degree (and sometimes second- or third-degree) block, usually within the atrioventricular node.

Extracardiac tissues may also be involved. Erythema marginatum has no specific changes, but the rheumatic nodules show similar appearances to Aschoff nodules with giant cells, round cells and fibroblasts, often with central necrosis. Occasionally the lungs are involved producing a patchy infiltration, and the progression of these changes is thought to lead to pulmonary ossific nodules which are seen in adult patients with mitral stenosis.

The changes in the central nervous system in patients with chorea are entirely non-specific and do not resemble the features of rheumatic disease elsewhere in the body. There is perivascular infiltration and some swelling of neurones and glial tissue. The changes are not confined to the basal ganglia, but occur throughout the cerebrum and cerebellum.

Clinical presentation

The condition is rare before the age of 3 years and symptoms occur between 10 and 21 days after a streptococcal infection, usually a sore throat. The onset is insidious and arthritis is usually the first manifestation; the large joints are affected and the pain moves from one joint to another. The child is pale and often sweats freely and is pyrexial. The joints are swollen and warm, and movement is painful. The severity of the arthritis bears no relation to the severity of the carditis and indeed about 15% of patients have carditis without any joint manifestations. They present with fever, cough and dyspnoea. Skin rashes often occur, particularly erythema marginatum and occasionally erythema nodosum. About 10% of patients have rheumatic nodules, either over the occiput or on the extensor surfaces of elbows, wrists and fingers.

In patients with arthritis it may be difficult to be certain whether there is cardiac involvement and the following points are helpful.

1. *Heart murmur.* A blowing, high-pitched systolic murmur is heard at the cardiac apex and is conducted to the axilla and back. It is evidence of mitral insufficiency due to stretching of the chordae. A mid-diastolic mitral murmur may be heard (the Carey Coombes murmur due to swelling of mitral valve leaflets). Aortic incompetence may occur and causes a high-pitched diastolic murmur immediately after the second sound. It is best heard down the left sternal edge when the patient sits up, leans forward and holds his breath in expiration.

2. *Cardiac enlargement.* Increasing size of the heart is good evidence of carditis and this may be detected clinically or radiographically. It is important, however, to make sure that the radiograph is a good inspiratory one with correct tube distance, otherwise apparent enlargement may be misinterpreted.

3. *Pericarditis.* A pericardial friction rub is evidence of cardiac involvement.

4. *Heart failure* occurs in severe cases and is often preceded by vomiting and abdominal pain.

Investigations show a raised erythrocyte sedimentation rate and a leucocytosis but these are non-specific. A rising antistreptolysin O titre is good evidence of previous streptococcal infection even when the organism cannot be cultured. The absence of a rising titre, however, does not rule out streptococcal infection because a few organisms do not produce streptolysin, or antibiotics may have suppressed the antistreptolysin O response. The presence of C-reactive protein in the serum of patients with rheumatic fever indicates a pathological state and suggests rheumatic activity. C-reactive protein is not present in normal blood but may be present in acute nephritis, malignant tumours and rheumatoid arthritis as well as rheumatic fever. Prolongation of the P–R interval (greater than 0.2 s) on the electrocardiogram is good evidence of rheumatic infection. Flattening of T waves, Q–T prolongation and ventricular ectopic beats are less specific. Typical changes of pericarditis may be seen. Jones (1944) enumerated the various criteria necessary to diagnose rheumatic fever. These were modified by the American Heart Association in 1955.

The chest radiograph shows only mild cardiac enlargement unless there is a pericardial effusion or mitral regurgitation, but sometimes shows interstitial oedema.

Echocardiography is useful, showing lengthening of the chordae of the mitral valve in patients with acute mitral regurgitation. Some reduction in contractility with dilatation of the left ventricle may be seen. A small pericardial effusion may be detected, even in the absence of clinical evidence of active pericarditis.

Chorea

Sydenham's, or rheumatic, chorea consists of jerky, repetitive movements, particularly of the hands and face. They may continue during sleep. There is also severe hypotonia which allows over-extension of joints. A request to hold the hands out in front with the palms down results in a 'dinner-fork' position, with the wrists flexed but the metacarpophalangeal joints overextended. A request to put the arms above the head results in the palms facing outward (supinator sign). Mood changes, with inattention and easily induced crying, are almost always present and may precede the chorea. This, with the tendency to drop objects (due to the hypotonicity) frequently leads to troubles at school. Cardiac involvement is only about half as common in chorea as it is in rheumatic fever, and is more common in girls, whereas rheumatic fever is more common in boys.

Treatment

Patients with typical joint involvement are usually more comfortable in bed. Although strict bed rest used to be enforced for patients with cardiac involvement during and for several weeks after the acute phase, this has been shown not to affect the development of chronic rheumatic heart disease (Simon, Mack and Rosenblum, 1952; Lendrum, Simon and Mack, 1959). However, the presence of mitral regurgitation, implying stretching of chordae, or ventricular dilatation, suggests that excessive activity may be detrimental. The usual compromise is to keep the child in bed or in a chair, but allow visits to bathroom and toilet and games and study in bed or at a table.

Adequate antibiotic therapy should be given to eradicate the streptococcal infection. Intramuscular penicillin should be used initially and throat swabs taken to make sure that the organism is no longer present. Benzathine penicillin G 600 000–1 200 000 units is given once intramuscularly or oral treatment with 240–500 mg penicillin at 8-hourly intervals is given for 10 days. If the patient is sensitive to penicillin, erythromycin should be used. Salicylates are specific in relieving the joint pains and this is a good diagnostic test. A dose of 120 mg/kg/day is given up to a maximum of 8 g/day. The full dose should be continued for two weeks and then halved until the signs of rheumatic activity have disappeared. If the dose is too great, salicylism will occur; tinnitus, deafness, vomiting, hyperpnoea and headache should be looked for when salicylates are being given so that if necessary the drug can be withdrawn or the dose reduced.

Doctors may worry about the use of salicylates with the possible association with Reye's syndrome, but there is nothing to suggest that salicylates are dangerous in the absence of a viral infection.

There is no conclusive evidence that any drugs, salicylates, cortisone or ACTH influence the long-term course of the disease. Some workers believe that steroids should be given when carditis is present but there is insufficient evidence to support this. When there are acute, life-threatening complications of heart failure or complete heart block, steroids may induce a temporary remission although a 'spring-back' usually occurs following their withdrawal.

In general, heart surgery should be avoided in childhood because of the presence of rheumatic activity in the heart. There are now reports, however, of valve replacement in children who were unresponsive to conservative therapy (see Chapter 5).

Prevention

Rheumatic fever can be prevented if an infection with group A β-haemolytic streptococcus is diagnosed early and adequately treated. The beta-haemolytic streptococcus is unlikely ever to be eradicated because it is so prevalent and there are high carrier rates. If recurrences, however, can be prevented in susceptible individuals then the secondary effects of the disease on the heart will be lessened. Supervision is essential to ensure that prophylactic penicillin continues to be taken. Also the relatives of children who have had rheumatic fever should be closely watched, as children having oral penicillin for prevention may have masked infections which may spread to their siblings.

The control of rheumatic fever in developing countries is difficult. The cost of its prevention has to be assessed with other priorities; there may be a scarcity of trained personnel and scattered populations making surveillance impossible. It is hoped that there will be a decline in the disease with improved socio-economic conditions but meanwhile streptococcal infections must be controlled. This may be accomplished by:

1. Early and adequate treatment of streptococcal infections when they occur.
2. Prevention of repeated streptococcal infections.

Treatment of streptococcal infection

This must be given early and adequately. It is wise to give crystalline penicillin by injection for 48 hours and then follow this with oral treatment for 8 days to ensure that the infection is completely eradicated. Alternatively, an injection of a long-lasting penicillin such as benzathine penicillin G may be used. If the patient is sensitive to penicillin, cephalexin should be used.

Prevention of repeated streptococcal infections

The Rheumatic Fever Committee of the Council on Rheumatic Fever and Congenital Heart Disease of the American Heart Association (1971) recommends the following programme.

Prophylaxis should be continued indefinitely:

1.   Benzathine Penicillin G i.m. is best
      Dosage: 1 200 000 units/month
or 2. Penicillin G orally
      Dosage: 200 000 units b.d. ½ hour before a meal
or 3. Sulphadiazine
      Dosage: 1 g/day if the patient is over 60 lb weight
                0.5 g/day if the patient is under 60 lb weight
or 4. If the patient is sensitive to penicillin and sulphadiazine use erythromycin 250 mg b.d.

Tetracyclines should not be used because there is a high prevalence of strains resistant to this antibiotic.

Convalescence

As the disease has become less severe and cardiac involvement less common the restrictions enforced in previous years have been generally relaxed. If there has been no clinical or electrocardiographic evidence of cardiac involvement the patient is allowed up one week after arthritis has disappeared. If carditis is suspected bed rest is usually continued until the sedimentation rate has returned to near normal levels (below 20 mm) although sometimes a compromise has to be reached when the sedimentation rate stays high but the patient is well. Return to school can be allowed from 2–4 weeks later, but organized games are advised against for six months if there has been evidence of carditis.

Continued follow-up is important for two reasons: first to ensure that prophylactic penicillin is taken regularly and secondly to detect evidence of established rheumatic valvular disease. Mild mitral regurgitation particularly may only become apparent when the patient increases his activities. Increasing signs of valve damage or persistent or increasing heart size on radiography should be regarded as evidence of active rheumatism.

If there has been evidence of carditis, even though the heart is subsequently normal clinically, there is a risk of bacterial endocarditis and antibiotic prophylaxis is indicated for at least two years if the patient requires dental extractions. Since the patient will already be taking penicillin, another antibiotic must be used. The best choice at the moment is cephaloridine or erythromycin. Purely bacteriostatic antibiotics, such as tetracycline, are useless.

Bibliography and references

American Heart Association (1971) Rheumatic Fever Committee of the Council on Rheumatic Fever and Congenital Heart Disease. Prevention of rheumatic fever. *Circulation,* **43,** 983

American Heart Association (1977) Rheumatic Fever Committee of the Council on Rheumatic Fever and Congenital Heart Disease. Prevention of rheumatic fever. *Circulation,* **55,** 1–4

Gibofsky, A., Williams, R. C. and Zabrinskie, J. B. (1987) Immunological aspects of acute rheumatic fever. *Ballière's Clinical Immunology and Allergy,* **1,** 577–590

Jones, T. D. (1944) The diagnosis of rheumatic fever. *Journal of the American Medical Association,* **126,** 481

Kaplan, M. E. (1969) The cross-reaction of group A streptococci with heart tissue and its relation to induced autoimmunity in rheumatic fever. *Bulletin on the Rheumatic Diseases,* **19,** 560

Kaplan, M. H. (1979) Rheumatic fever, rheumatic heart disease and the streptococcal connection: the role of streptococcal antigens cross reactive with heart tissue. *Review of Infectious Diseases,* **1,** 988–996

Kinsley, R. H., Girdwood, R. W. and Milner, S. (1981) Surgical treatment during the acute phase of rheumatic carditis. *Surgery Annual,* **13,** 299–323

Lendrum, B. L., Simon, A. J. and Mack, I. (1959) Relation of duration of bed rest in acute rheumatic fever to heart disease present 2 to 14 years later. *Pediatrics, Springfield,* **24,** 389–394

Padmavati, S., Sreshta, N. K., Vijayan, N. K., *et al.* (1980) Secondary prophylaxis of rheumatic heart disease in Delhi. Abstract. World Congress on Paediatric Cardiology

Patarroyo, M. E., Winchester, R., Vejerano, A., *et al.* (1979) Association of B-Cell alloantigen with susceptibility to rheumatic fever. *Nature,* **278,** 173

Perry, C. B. (1969) The natural history of acute rheumatism. *Annals of the Rheumatic Diseases,* **28,** 471

Shaper, A. G. (1972) Cardiovascular disease in the tropics. *British Medical Journal,* **3,** 683

Simon, A. J., Mack, I. and Rosenblum, P. (1952) Accelerated rehabilitation in rheumatic fever. *American Journal of Diseases in Children,* **83,** 454–462

Strasser, T. (1978) Rheumatic fever and rheumatic heart disease in the 1970s. *W.H.O. Chronicle,* **32,** 18–25

United Kingdom and United States Joint Report (1955) 1: The treatment of acute rheumatic fever in children: a co-operative clinical trial of ACTH, cortisone and aspirin. *Circulation,* **11,** 343–371

Wilson, M. G., Schweitzer, M. D. and Lubschez, R. (1943) The familial epidemiology of rheumatic fever. *Journal of Pediatrics,* **22,** 468

Chapter 20

Myocardial and pericardial disease

Endomyocardial diseases

This is a group of diseases in which the heart muscle, or the endocardium, or both, are involved in a degenerative or inflammatory disease. Three of them, acute myocarditis, congestive cardiomyopathy and endocardial fibroelastosis are linked clinically and probably aetiologically.

Acute myocarditis

Inflammation of the heart muscle occurs particularly in association with infection with enteroviruses. Both Coxsackie (particularly types B1–5 in infants and A4–5 in older children) and ECHO viruses have been implicated, but in only about a third of cases has the virus been isolated from the stools, urine or sputum during the acute attack. The histological findings in patients who have died or been submitted to endocardial biopsy are initially swelling of muscle fibres, increase in interstitial fluid and infiltration with both polymorphonuclear and mononuclear white cells. Later there are shrinkage of cell nuclei, lysis and disappearance of muscle fibres and lymphocyte and histiocyte infiltration. Late findings include fibrous replacement of groups of muscle fibres and sometimes calcification.

Clinical presentation
Infants usually present with a prodromal phase of vomiting and lethargy, older children with malaise, myalgia and diarrhoea. This is followed after 2–3 days by the cardiac symptoms which may be either breathlessness or sudden collapse with cardiogenic shock. Examination reveals evidence of cardiac failure with a large liver, tachycardia and often a prominent third heart sound, although the significance of this will be doubtful in association with a tachycardia.

Investigation
The electrocardiogram shows low-voltage QRS complexes, flat T waves and prolongation of Q–T. P waves are often enlarged or widened, indicating left atrial dilatation. Pathological Q waves indicating selective areas of severe damage are seen in about 20% of the more severe cases. Chest radiographs show mild cardiomegaly but obvious pulmonary venous congestion and frequently interstitial oedema.

The echocardiogram is the most useful investigation. The heart is usually mildly enlarged, and this is most apparent in the left ventricle, but the most conclusive finding is impaired left ventricular contractility with the ejection fraction reduced to 40% or less. Thickening of the ventricular wall is not seen, and such a finding would lead to the conclusion that there was a more chronic condition, or some other cause for the cardiac failure.

Cultures of stool, urine and sputum for viruses should be taken, and blood for antibody titres, although neither will provide an answer within the acute period of the disease. Blood urea or creatinine may be raised due to poor renal perfusion. Cardiac enzymes are raised, the lactic dehydrogenase and the more selective alpha-hydroxybutyrate dehydrogenase are often two or three times the upper limit of normal in the acute stage and may take up to four weeks to fall to normal (Joffe, 1986). Myocardial biopsy has been advocated as a means of making the diagnosis, but is not without risk and does not influence the child's treatment.

Treatment
Diuretics should be given to relieve pulmonary venous congestion and hepatomegaly. If there is cardiogenic shock or oliguria, or a poor response to diuretics, a dopamine infusion (5 µg/kg/min) should be started. Digoxin is probably not useful in the acute stages, but should be given in patients who show evidence of continuing impairment of left ventricular contractility after the acute phase (usually regarded as about two weeks).

Natural history
About one-third of diagnosed cases with cardiogenic shock or obvious cardiac failure die in the acute stage, or over the next year, one-sixth remain with chronic impairment of left ventricular function and half make a complete clinical recovery, with normal left ventricular function on echocardiography. Clearly there will be children with subclinical cardiac involvement (mild electrocardiographic changes or mild reduction in left ventricular function on echocardiography) who may be detected during non-specific viral infections, and these will be expected to have a much better prognosis.

Acute influenzal myocarditis

In some epidemics of influenza, cardiac involvement (shown by minor electrocardiographic abnormalities) has been reported in up to half of adults, and it is likely that children are similarly involved. Occasionally, more severe and protracted cardiac involvement occurs. This often resolves rapidly with a short course of prednisolone, which has led to the suggestion that there may be an autoimmune element.

Other forms of myocarditis

Besides the viruses noted above, a number of other pathogens may cause acute myocarditis. Usually this is part of a specific illness. (A comprehensive list is given in Brandenburg *et al.* (1987).) Conditions where it may be important in children include acute streptococcal infections, meningococcal septicaemia, typhoid, psittacosis and, of course, rheumatic fever.

Immunocompromised patients may suffer from myocardial infiltration by a number of unusual organisms, including fungi.

Congestive cardiomyopathy and endocardial fibroelastosis

These two conditions have a number of similarities, and are regarded by many cardiologists as identical in aetiology. Clinically they are also strongly related to viral myocarditis, since patients who have had acute myocarditis and show long-term impairment are clinically and pathologically indistinguishable. Both congestive (or dilated) cardiomyopathy and endocardial fibroelastosis show a severely dilated left ventricle with impaired contractility, the difference being that in patients with endocardial fibroelastosis there is a complete or patchy white lining to the left ventricle which consists histologically of fibrous tissue, extending into the inner layers of the myocardium. In both conditions the myocardium itself is abnormal, showing hypertrophy of the remaining myocardial fibres with increase in interstitial collagen. Infants presenting in the first few months of life are most likely to have endocardial fibroelastosis, and it is almost invariable in those detected prenatally.

It is now accepted that most, if not all, cases of endocardial fibroelastosis and congestive cardiomyopathy result from previous virus infection. It is uncertain whether the conditions are the straightforward result of virus infection or whether there is an autoimmune element in addition. The strongest evidence for a virus aetiology comes from two sources. First, epidemics of viral myocarditis are followed, after 3–6 months, by an increased incidence of cardiomyopathy and endocardial fibroelastosis. Secondly, although it is rare to find actual viruses in the myocardium, Bowles et al. (1986) have found coxsackie B virus-specific RNA sequences in the muscle of patients with congestive cardiomyopathy. Lowry and Littler (1987) have reviewed the possible immunological aspects of cardiomyopathy in adults. Anti-heart muscle antibodies are found in 10–50% of cardiomyopathy patients, and it has been suggested that these patients have impaired suppressor T lymphocyte function which encourages the development of anti-heart muscle antibodies.

Clinical presentation
The highest incidence of endocardial fibroelastosis is seen at about 6 months of age, with most patients below 2 years. A small number are seen at birth or are detected by antenatal echocardiography, and these must represent prenatal infection. Patients presenting beyond two years rarely have the marked degree of endocardial thickening seen in infants, and are more correctly called congestive cardio-myopathy, although the clinical presentation is the same. Breathlessness and tachypnoea are the commonest presenting symptoms, and frequently the infant comes to attention with an intercurrent respiratory infection. Clinical examination reveals enlargement of the liver and displacement of the cardiac impulse into the anterior axillary line. There is a third heart sound and sometimes an apical pansystolic murmur, due to functional mitral regurgitation.

Investigations
Chest radiographs show a greatly dilated heart, with a smooth, sharp outline, due to the relative lack of movement during the period of exposure of the film (Figure 20.1). A lateral view shows that the enlargement is in the left ventricle and left atrium. The pulmonary veins are dilated and there may be interstitial oedema. The electrocardiogram is typical and shows the pattern of severe left ventricular hypertrophy (Figure 20.2), often with left atrial hypertrophy in addition.

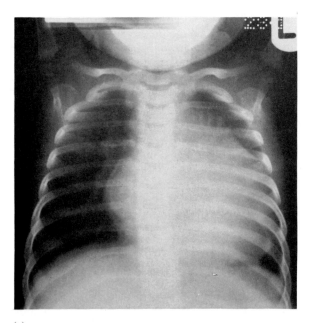

(a)

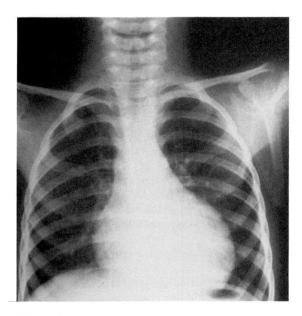

(b)

Figure 20.1 Endocardial fibroelastosis. There is marked cardiac enlargement at 10 months (a) and decrease in heart size by 3 years (b)

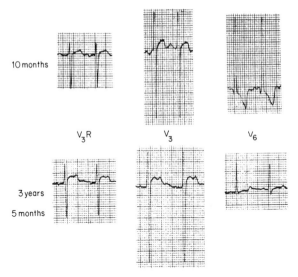

Figure 20.2 Endocardial fibroelastosis. ECG shows severe left ventricular hypertrophy in a 10-month-old child (upper trace) and slight left ventricular hypertrophy by 3 years (lower trace) – the T waves are now upright

Two-dimensional echocardiography is the most helpful investigation (Figure 20.3). The left ventricle is dilated, often to twice the normal diameter, and contraction is very poor, the ejection fraction being 20% or less, compared with the normal value in children of 60% or greater. Endocardial fibroelastosis, when present, can be seen as increased density of the echoes from the endocardium. The mitral valve looks anatomically normal, but it may be apparent that the annulus is stretched and the cusps barely meet, allowing functional regurgitation, which can also be picked up by the Doppler technique. The flow pattern through the mitral valve is also abnormal, the greatest flow being during atrial systole rather than, as normally, in early diastole.

Diagnosis
The diagnosis of endomyocardial fibroelastosis or congestive cardiomyopathy is made from the presence of a dilated left ventricle and the absence of any other cause for this, such as aortic stenosis or hypertension. When the onset is relatively acute it may be difficult to distinguish from acute myocarditis, but the presence of a very dilated heart and an electrocardiogram showing the pattern of severe left ventricular hypertrophy make the diagnosis of acute myocarditis very unlikely. Endomyocardial biopsy has been used to distinguish the two conditions, but involves some risks and does not materially affect the treatment. The only real need for such an investigation is the possibility of a specific myocardial abnormality for which there is a particular treatment, but such conditions are exceedingly rare.

Treatment
Digoxin and frusemide should be given, and continued even when there is no overt heart failure, as long as there is echocardiographic evidence of impaired left ventricular contractility. This often means for several years, but it is generally

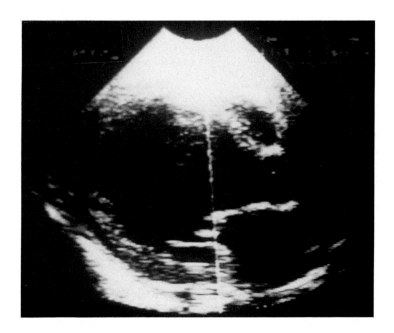

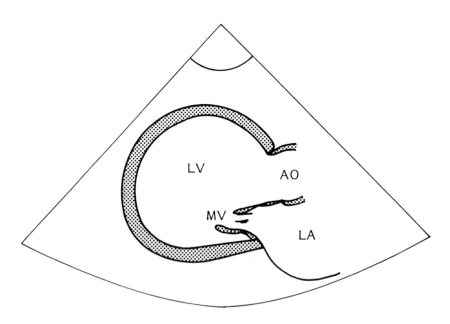

Figure 20.3 Congestive cardiomyopathy. Echocardiogram (systolic frame, long-axis view) showing globular left ventricle over 5 cm in diameter. (Normal 1.5–2 cm for age)

accepted that such treatment improves the chances of eventual recovery, as well as making the child less at risk from a recurrence of heart failure from intercurrent infections. In those who remain severely handicapped by symptoms and show no evidence of spontaneous improvement, heart transplantation may be considered, but the difficulties in knowing that the child definitely will not survive more than a matter of months, together with the difficulty in obtaining a donor heart at short notice when it is clear that deterioration is inevitable, usually make it impracticable.

Natural history

Many of the severe cases die within months of presentation, despite treatment. Others show marked improvement with treatment and gradually, over months or years, the cardiomegaly and electrocardiographic abnormalities regress. Echocardiography is invaluable in following the progress. Eventual recovery is more likely when the diagnosis is made within the first year of life. A further group follow an intermediate course, with initial improvement, but the heart remaining large. Joffe (1981) reported a series of patients from Cape Town with a clinical diagnosis of endocardial fibroelastosis in whom about one-third died within the first year from diagnosis, mainly within the first 3 months. Very few patients who survived the first year subsequently died, and electrocardiographic evidence of left ventricular hypertrophy had disappeared by a year in over 75% of survivors. It should be noted that the survival curves for acute myocarditis and endocardial fibroelastosis were similar over the first year from diagnosis, although rather fewer myocarditis patients died. The clinical implication is that any child presenting with heart failure due to myocardial disease has a similar prognosis whether the clinical diagnosis is acute myocarditis or endocardial fibroelastosis and the treatment is basically the same.

Contracted endocardial fibroelastosis

Edwards (1960) divided fibroelastosis into dilated and contracted forms. The descriptions given so far refer to the dilated form. The contracted form occurs in two clinical situations.

First, newborn infants may present with the hypoplastic left heart syndrome and either have no aortic or mitral lesion, or mild valvular disease, but still have a small left ventricular cavity with a thick endocardial lining. It is thought that this results from an early intrauterine infection, and that the endomyocardial disease prevents adequate flow of blood through the left heart *in utero*, stopping its growth. As with other forms of hypoplastic left heart, no treatment is possible.

The second group are children who present with heart failure with no clinical cause and are found to have a normal-sized heart radiologically and on echocardiography, but left ventricular function is impaired both in terms of contractility and diastolic filling. Treatment with diuretics produces improvement, but the condition is usually progressive. The clinical picture is similar to endomyocardial fibrosis and the hypereosinophilic cardiomyopathy seen in adults, but eosinophilia is not a feature.

Secondary endocardial fibroelastosis

Lesions which cause obstruction to the left heart (coarctation and aortic stenosis) frequently show some degree of endocardial fibroelastosis and some patients, particularly those with coarctation of the aorta, have abnormal myocardial function as shown by an unusual degree of cardiac enlargement which is not reversed by operation. Patients with hypoplasia of the left heart due to coarctation, aortic atresia or severe aortic stenosis usually show endocardial fibroelastosis, sometimes described as the contracted type. A few patients with ventricular septal defects also have myocardial disease with or without endocardial fibroelastosis and are more ill and have larger hearts than those with uncomplicated ventricular septal defects. When myocardial disease is associated with an atrial septal defect the raised left atrial pressure increases the left-to-right shunting and severe heart failure occurs. Indeed, when heart failure is diagnosed in childhood or infancy as due to an atrial septal defect it is likely that there is an associated obstructive lesion or myocardial disease on the left side of the heart.

Right heart endocardial fibroelastosis

The occurrence of endocardial fibroelastosis in the right side is seen in association with pulmonary atresia and hypoplastic right ventricle and with Ebstein's anomaly of the tricuspid valve, when both atrium and ventricle are involved.

Endomyocardial fibrosis

A condition in which there is extensive overgrowth of the endocardium with fibrous tissue has been extensively reported from Central and East Africa, and later from South America. Davies (1948) first drew attention to the condition in Uganda as accounting for about 10% of all cases of heart failure in that country. He also noted that some of his patients, particularly those with evidence of systemic illness, also had eosinophilia. The condition was not seen in very young children and had its greatest incidence in late childhood and early adult life. Gerbaux et al. (1956) drew attention to the similarity with Loeffler's eosinophilic endocarditis, which had been described twenty years previously, and Brockington and Olsen (1973) reported that histologically the two conditions were indistinguishable. This suggested that both conditions were caused by eosinophil overactivity, the tropical form being related to intestinal infestation with parasites, particularly microfilaria.

Pathology and physiology
In the acute inflammatory stage there is infiltration of the myocardium with round cells and eosinophils, and the muscle cells themselves show the same changes as in viral myocarditis, swelling, shrinkage of nuclei and necrosis. The endocardium becomes partly covered in mural thrombus and this thrombus, together with the endocardium itself, becomes infiltrated with fibroblasts which result in the production of collagen. In the chronic stages this fibrous tissue becomes more hyaline and further thrombus is laid down, particularly at the apices of the ventricles. The fibrous process involves both ventricles, the left usually predominating, and extends onto the mitral and tricuspid valves via the papillary muscles, so that the parts of the cusps closest to the valve rings are least affected. The aortic and pulmonary valves may also be affected but less often than the atrioventricular valves. The process of thrombosis and fibrosis continues and the whole of the apical parts of either or both ventricles become obliterated. This is

particularly the case in the right ventricle where shrinkage of the apical part of the heart, with the inflow and outflow portions of the ventricle relatively less affected, leads to a sulcus around the mid-ventricular region resulting in the appropriately named 'map of Africa' shape. Internally the extent of the endocardial involvement is often clearly delineated, with the inflow and outflow portions of both ventricles spared. Even in the chronic stages there is usually extensive clot around the undersides of mitral and tricuspid valves.

The endocardial thickening and cavity obliteration impair ventricular filling and involvement of the mitral and tricuspid valves prevents the cusps closing and causes regurgitation.

Clinical presentation
Patients may present during the phase of acute illness with fever and eosinophilia, or without these manifestations. Right and left heart failure occur, usually together, but one or other form may predominate. Peripheral and pulmonary embolism occur, the latter leading to pulmonary hypertension.

Investigations
The electrocardiogram generally shows small voltage QRS complexes but relatively or absolutely increased P waves. T waves are generally flat, but may be inverted in left or right ventricular leads. Atrioventricular block and atrial fibrillation have been described, mainly in adults. The heart is little, if at all, enlarged on chest radiography. Echocardiography shows the cavity obliteration and valve regurgitation. Conventional measurements of contractility are usually not impaired in the chronic stages, but may be reduced in the acute phase. According to the side of the heart most affected, the left or right atrium is usually enlarged.

Treatment
Diuretics, used with caution, relieve oedema and ascites, but overuse leads quickly to a low-output state, as a high filling pressure is required by the stiff ventricle. Digoxin is not regarded as useful, since the main problem is not impaired contractility and atrial fibrillation is uncommon in childhood. (Slowing the ventricular rate, which is generally beneficial, may be harmful when stroke output is low and fixed.) Anticoagulants to prevent peripheral and pulmonary embolism and operations to remove the thickened endocardium ('freeing the ventricle') or replace mitral or tricuspid valves have all proved beneficial, but are impractical in many of the areas where the condition is most prevalent.

In patients seen during the acute stages it seems logical to take steps to eliminate the cause of the eosinophilia by treating parasitic infestation, but there is no evidence yet that this affects the outlook. Public health measures along the same lines could be expected to control the incidence of the disease.

Prognosis
The most severely affected cases usually die within a few years of diagnosis, but some, like patients with chronic rheumatic heart disease, continue for up to twenty years. Sudden death, presumably from arrhythmia, is the final event in about 10%. Patients with predominant left-sided involvement live only about half as long as those with mainly right-sided disease, who may remain with oedema and ascites for several years.

Hypertrophic obstructive cardiomyopathy (HOCM)

Hypertrophic obstructive cardiomyopathy is a disease of children, adolescents and young adults which has been described under various names, starting as 'asymmetric cardiac hypertrophy'. It was first diagnosed at autopsy in patients dying suddenly without previous symptoms of heart disease.

Incidence and aetiology

Although rare, recognition of the condition has led to the diagnosis being made in a greater number of patients. It is now known that the condition is passed on with a Mendelian dominant form of inheritance with incomplete penetrance. The evidence for this comes from echocardiographic studies on relatives of patients with the clinical condition, in which 50% were shown to have an interventricular septum 30% or more thicker than the left ventricular free wall (Clark, Henry and Epstein, 1973). One or other parent, where both could be tested, showed such a thickening. In most cases these relatives had no clinical or electrocardiographic abnormalities but a small proportion had clinical features to suggest HOCM.

Follow-up studies by Maron *et al.* (1986) have shown that the condition progresses with age, so that some children with only mild septal hypertrophy when first studied by echocardiography go on to develop the full pattern of the disease several years later. In our experience the condition is seen commonly in patients with the Ullrich–Noonan syndrome. Lentiginosis is another associated condition. The cause of the abnormality is unknown. Theories included a hamartomatous overgrowth of muscle, increased sensitivity to sympathetic stimulation and abnormal distribution of muscle bundles increasing the work of the ventricle and producing secondary hypertrophy. An alternative theory is that the muscle fibres are initially normal but the septum has an abnormal curvature in its long axis, convex towards the left ventricle, which results in longitudinal and circumferential fibres acting against each other when they contract, so that the septum hypertrophies from excessive tension built up by isometric contraction.

A striking histological feature is the 'myocardial disarray' pattern, in which the normal pattern of muscle fibres all running in the same direction in any part of the septum is replaced by a more random arrangement of fibres running in different directions. This suggests that the fibres may 'pull against each other' thus performing isometric work under unusual tension, and that this is responsible for the hypertrophy.

Clinical presentation

Many children are referred because of a systolic murmur and are asymptomatic. Breathlessness, ischaemic cardiac pain and syncope are common in adolescence and adult life. Sudden death occurs in this condition in about 15% of patients who have been previously diagnosed, but a similar number of patients come to autopsy having died suddenly, not always upon exertion, when the disease has not been suspected in life. Supraventricular and ventricular tachycardias, and ventricular extrasystoles are experienced by a few.

The clinical signs are characteristic and in many cases allow a diagnosis to be made. The pulse is unusually jerky, due to rapid ventricular ejection, and may give a double spike. The left ventricle is forceful and usually shows a double impulse.

Forceful atrial contraction may produce a palpable fourth heart sound so that the impulse becomes triple. An early systolic murmur at the left sternal edge is conducted into the aortic area. Aortic closure is delayed so that splitting of the second heart sound becomes absent or reversed. About one-quarter of patients have an apical systolic murmur due to mitral regurgitation.

Radiology and electrocardiography

Chest radiographs in the early stages may be normal, but later the left ventricle is enlarged and in symptomatic patients the left atrium is prominent. Pulmonary venous congestion and frank oedema occur as the disease progresses. The electrocardiogram is usually abnormal. Most patients, even without symptoms, show advanced left ventricular hypertrophy but about 20% show abnormal Q waves in many leads, simulating infarction but probably due to the septal hypertrophy (Figure 20.4).

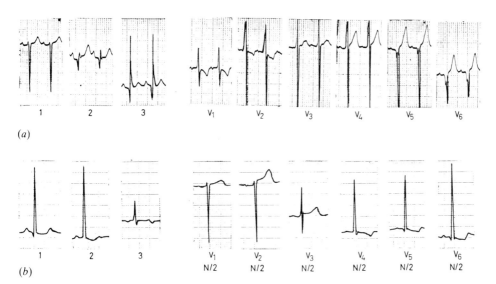

Figure 20.4 The electrocardiogram in hypertrophic obstructive cardiomyopathy. (*a*) From a 3-month-old boy, showing Q waves in leads 2, 3, and V_{5-6}. (*b*) From a 12-year-old girl, showing marked left ventricular hypertrophy. Note that leads V_{1-5} are recorded at half sensitivity

Echocardiography

The diagnosis can nearly always be established by echocardiography (Figure 20.5), which is more reliable than cardiac catheterization. The most constant finding is gross thickening of the interventricular septum – often to twice or more the normal for age. The left ventricular free wall is also thickened but to a lesser degree. The mitral valve echo shows a characteristic pattern of apparent systolic anterior movement of the mitral valve (Figure 20.6). In fact this echo has been shown by two-dimensional studies to be due to greatly hypertrophied papillary muscles.

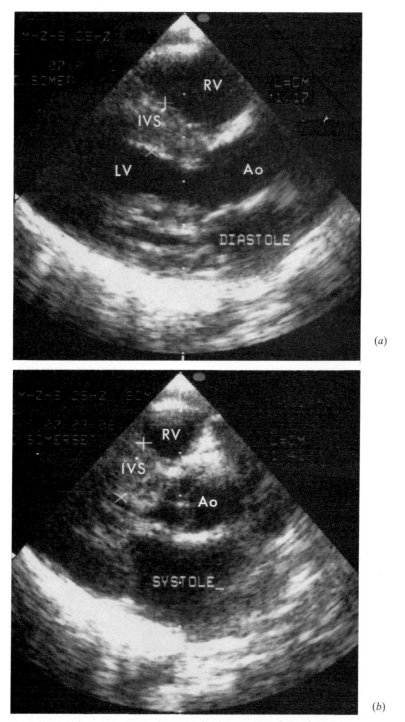

(a)

(b)

Figure 20.5 Hypertrophic cardiomyopathy (18-month-old girl) (a) Diastole. The thickness of the interventricular septum (+ . . . ×) is 1.17 cm which is over twice the normal for age. The free wall of left ventricle is only slightly thickened. (b) In systole the cavity of the left ventricle is almost completely obliterated. Ao, aorta; IVS, interventricular septum; LV, left ventricle; RV, right ventricle

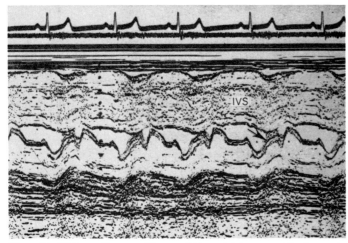

Figure 20.6 Echocardiogram of 7-year-old boy with hypertrophic obstructive cardiomyopathy. Note the greatly thickened interventricular septum (IVS) −4.5 cm and apparent systolic anterior movement of mitral valve due to hypertrophied papillary muscle

Because the ejection from the left ventricle is completed early in systole the aortic valve cusps show premature closure, although this is a less rapid movement than is seen in discrete subaortic stenosis.

Treatment

Beta-blocking drugs are currently the mainstay of treatment, although the calcium antagonists verapamil and nifedipine have also been used. Fairly high doses need to be given, usually 1 mg/kg of propranolol 4 times daily. Atenolol is now available in the form of a syrup which allows better dosage than the tablets available and can be given twice daily in a dose of 1.5 mg/kg. In adults verapamil has been associated with increase in symptoms and possible arrhythmias and is now seldom used. Since almost all patients with the clinical picture of hypertrophic cardiomyopathy have had beta-blocking drugs, it has been difficult to show any clear influence on the incidence of sudden death, but symptoms are relieved in the minority of children who have chest pain or breathlessness. The most striking support for their routine use has been the demonstration that the septal hypertrophy can regress if treatment is started early enough in infancy, and not progress in older children. In addition, infants who present with cardiac failure improve rapidly following administration of beta-blocker drugs, whereas digoxin usually makes them worse.

Surgical resection of the hypertrophied muscle has been used in adults to relieve symptoms, but there are no reports of surgery in children.

Natural history

The condition has a wide spectrum of severity and symptomatic and asymptomatic patients are frequently diagnosed for the first time in the sixth to ninth decades of life, so that overall survival figures have little meaning. In Bristol, of 44 children diagnosed in life as having the condition, 5 died suddenly (3 in one family which had also had a previously undiagnosed child die) during childhood. Two infants died of congestive cardiac failure; 7 other children during this period were only diagnosed at autopsy. None of the children who died was receiving beta-blocker therapy at the time of death.

Counselling

The demonstration of the beneficial effects of beta blockade has made the job of counselling children and their parents both easier and harder. It had not been our policy to stress the risks of sudden death, but the protective effect of treatment means that the reason for giving treatment to asymptomatic children must be mentioned. However, it can be stressed that, provided treatment is continued the risks are low. Hypertrophic cardiomyopathy is one of the few conditions where strenuous physical exercise may be dangerous, although it is uncertain whether sudden deaths are due to arrhythmias or to sudden hypotension due to a restricted cardiac output. We ban all exercise and competitive sports. Regular 24-hour monitoring for arrhythmias has been advocated in adults, but has not revealed such abnormalities in asymptomatic children, in our experience.

Cardiac tumours

Primary cardiac tumours are rare, but four types have been described.

Rhabdomyomas

Rhabdomyomas (tumours of cardiac muscle) present with systolic murmurs due to obstruction to right or left ventricular outflow. They can be demonstrated by echocardiography (Figure 20.7). If managed conservatively they will often disappear; surgery should be avoided if possible. They occur with epiloia.

Fibromas

Fibromas present in a similar way to rhabdomyomas but may also give rise to ventricular tachycardia. Surgical removal has been reported.

Teratomas

Teratomas are usually outward growing and produce cystic tumours within the pericardium. Cardiac compression or unexplained cardiomegaly are the presenting features. Operation is possible without cardiopulmonary bypass and is usually successful.

Myxomas

Myxomas occur most commonly in the left atrium, attached to the interatrial septum. Rarely, they are found in the ventricles or right atrium. They produce systemic effects, malaise, weight loss and low-grade fever with high sedimentation rate and abnormal serum proteins, and also give rise to emboli, as well as producing local effects. Left atrial myxomas may simulate mitral stenosis and the combination of mitral murmurs (frequently variable) and low-grade fever suggests rheumatic

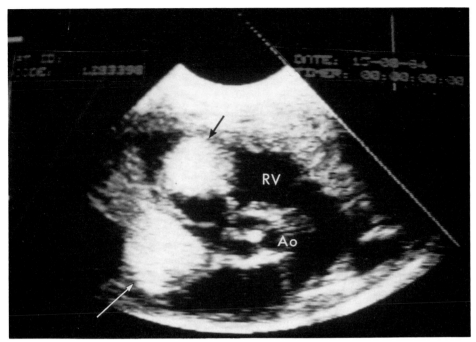

Figure 20.7 Multiple rhabdomyosarcomas, one in the right ventricle (black arrow) and one in the right atrium (white arrow) from a 4-hour-old baby presenting with perinatal arrhythmias. Ao, aorta; RV, right ventricle

carditis. The systemic emboli raise the possibility of bacterial endocarditis. Diagnosis is now made by echocardiography.

Right-sided myxomas usually produce embolic pulmonary hypertension.

Surgical removal, using cardiopulmonary bypass, is indicated urgently as soon as the diagnosis is made since the risks of catastrophic embolism are high and the possibility exists of the tumour completely obstructing the circulation. Regrowth has only occasionally been reported.

Pericardial diseases

Acute pericarditis

Bacterial infection of the pericardial cavity occurs occasionally by spread from the lungs, or as a result of septicaemia – particularly with staphylococci, less often with pneumococci or other organisms. Tuberculous pericarditis may present as an acute infection. Virus pericarditis, due mainly to Coxsackie B virus, is probably the commonest form of so-called benign acute pericarditis. The disease is rare in infants and young children but occurs in adolescents, sometimes in mild epidemics. There is usually a prodromal period with malaise and fever, and the presenting symptom of the pericarditis is central chest pain which may be constant or accentuated by changes in posture, respiration or coughing. It is sometimes felt mainly in the epigastrium. The characteristic sign is the pericardial rub, and the electrocardiogram shows changes illustrated in Figure 20.8.

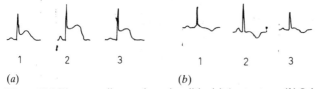

(a)   (b)

Figure 20.8 Electrocardiogram in pericarditis. (*a*) Acute stage. (*b*) Subacute stage. Note that in the acute stage there is ST elevation in all the standard leads

Despite the term 'benign', serious complications occur in half the patients. Atrial and ventricular tachycardias occur and tamponade may develop. Relapses after weeks or months are not uncommon.

Rest and mild analgesics are all that is required in mild cases. Corticosteroids will suppress the disease but make relapse rather more common.

Apart from virus infection, pericarditis may occur in rheumatoid disease, disseminated lupus erythematosus and leukaemic infiltration of the heart.

Pericardial effusion

Small effusions within the pericardial cavity are common in patients with cardiac failure, and a small serous effusion frequently occurs in acute pericarditis. An effusion large enough to cause interference with cardiac function is rare in childhood but may occur in the course of benign pericarditis, as a complication of rheumatoid disease, following cardiac surgery (postpericardiotomy syndrome) and in malignant disease, including leukaemia. A syndrome of chronic pericardial effusion with constriction, possibly postviral, has been reported (Jordan and Haycock, 1979).

Presentation
The clinical picture varies according to the rapidity with which the effusion gathers. With rapid accumulation of fluid, children experience dyspnoea, cough and abdominal pain due to hepatic engorgement. With subacute effusions symptoms are more vague and consist of tiredness, mild breathlessness and swelling of the abdomen due to ascites. Physical signs are characteristic. The pulse has a small volume and is reduced or disappears on inspiration. The venous pressure is often so high that the upper limit of filling is above the angle of the jaw; the liver is enlarged. The cardiac impulse is impalpable, cardiac dullness is increased and the heart sounds are very soft.

The chest radiograph shows enlargement of the cardiac silhouette which is sharply defined and in children and infants it is often possible, especially on screening, to see the heart as a separate shadow within (Figure 20.9). The electrocardiogram shows low-voltage complexes and usually widespread T wave inversion. Echocardiography is diagnostic showing the effusion separating the pericardium from the cardiac surface (Figure 20.10) Angiocardiography is no longer necessary. Albuminuria, severe enough to simulate the nephrotic syndrome, and malabsorption, have been reported as complications.

Treatment
Digitalis is contraindicated, because slowing of the heart rate reduces cardiac output when the stroke volume is fixed. Diuretics should be given with caution as

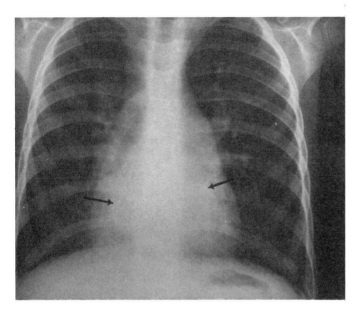

Figure 20.9 Pericardial effusion with constriction. There is a slight increase in the size of the cardiac shadow and a faint inner shadow due to the heart within the effusion. In this case there is little enlargement of the cardiac shadow because the pericardium was thickened and causing constriction

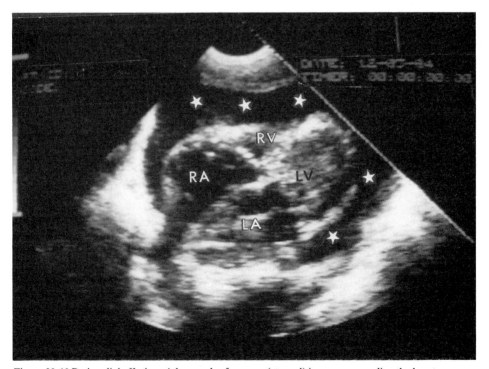

Figure 20.10 Pericardial effusion. A large echo-free area (starred) is seen surrounding the heart (subcostal 4-chamber view). LA, left atrium; LV, left ventricle; RA, right atrium; RV, right ventricle

too great a reduction in venous pressure may further lower the cardiac output. Aspiration of the effusion is indicated if there is rapid accumulation or very high venous pressure, and is carried out either in the fourth left interspace inside the midclavicular line (through the portion of the pericardium not covered by lung) or from below, immediately lateral to the xiphisternum. Facilities for monitoring and cardioversion should be available because ventricular fibrillation is a complication of pericardial aspiration. If the fluid reaccumulates, partial pericardiectomy is indicated.

Constrictive pericarditis

Tuberculosis is still the commonest cause of constrictive pericarditis in children in most countries, but occasional cases complicating rheumatoid disease or other collagen diseases are seen. Constriction due to a combination of effusion and pericardial thickening is seen in rheumatoid disease.

Presentation
Lassitude, abdominal pain and swelling of the abdomen are usual, while breathlessness and oedema are uncommon. There is sometimes atrial fibrillation, especially in older children; the pulse is of small volume and shows a reduction in volume on inspiration. The jugular venous pressure is high and shows a rapid descent at the beginning of ventricular diastole. Coincident with this there is a clearly audible early diastolic sound, often as loud as the heart sounds, due to rapid filling of the ventricle. There is no murmur. The liver is enlarged and ascites is frequently present.

Investigations
Chest radiographs show the heart to be normal or small in size, except where there is an associated effusion, and screening shows poor pulsation. Pericardial calcification occurs in about half of tuberculous cases. The electrocardiogram shows widespread T wave inversion.

Treatment
As with pericardial effusion, digitalis is contraindicated and diuretics must be used with care. Pericardiectomy is indicated if the venous pressure is more than slightly raised. Antituberculous therapy is indicated if there is any reason to suspect active infection.

Bibliography and references

Endomyocardial diseases
Ainger, L. E. (1964) Acute aseptic myocarditis: corticosteroid therapy. *Journal of Pediatrics*, **64,** 716
Brandenburg, R. O., Fuster, V., Guiliani, E. R. *et al.* (1987) *Cardiology: Fundamentals and Practice,* Year Book Medical Publishers Inc. Chicago, pp. 1564–1565
Brockington, I. F. and Olsen, E. G. J. (1973) Loeffler's endocarditis and Davies' endomyocardial fibrosis. *American Heart Journal*, **85,** 308–322
Bowles, N. E., Richardson, P. J., Olsen, E. G. J. *et al.* (1986) Detection of Coxsackie-B virus-specific RNA sequences in myocardial biopsy samples from patients with myocarditis and dilated cardiomyopathy. *Lancet*, **i,** 1120
Edwards, J. E. (1960) Congenital malformations. Malformations of endocardium and pericardium. In *Pathology of the Heart*, 2nd edn, (ed. S. E. Gould), Charles C. Thomas, Springfield, Illinois

Gerbaux, A., Ben Naceur, M., de Brux, J., *et al.* (1956) Contribution a l'etude de l'endocardite parietale fibroplastique avec eosinophilie sanguine (endocardite de Loeffler). *Archives des Maladies du Couer et des Vaisseaux,* **49,** 689–715

Grist, N. R. and Bell, E. J. (1969) Coxsackie virus and the heart. *American Heart Journal,* **77,** 295

Harris, L. C., Rodin, A. E. and Nghiem, Q. X. (1968) Idiopathic non-obstructive cardiomyopathy in children. *American Journal of Cardiology,* **21,** 153

Hastrecter, A. R. (1968) Endocardial fibroelastosis. In *Heart Disease in Infants, Children and Adolescents.* (eds. A. J. Moss and F. H. Adams), Williams and Wilkins, Baltimore, Maryland

Joffe (1981) The role of viruses in heart disease in infants and children. In *Paediatric Cardiology,* Vol. 4. (ed. M. J. Godman), Churchill Livingstone, Edinburgh

Joffe (1986) Myocardiopathy: Clinical picture and prognosis. In *Paediatric Cardiology* (Proceedings of Second World Congress) (eds. E. F. Doyle, M. A. Engle, W. M. Gersony, *et al.*) Springer-Verlag, New York

Kibrick, S. (1966) In *Year Book of Paediatrics 1965–1966,* Year Book Medical Publishers, Chicago, p. 262

Lowry, P. and Littler, W. A. (1987) The immunology of cardiomyopathies. In *Clinical Immunology and Allergy,* Vol 1, no. 3. Baillière Tindall, London, pp. 531–536

Noren, G. R., Adams, P. Jr and Anderson, R. C. (1963) Positive skin reactivity to mumps viral antigen in endocardial fibroelastosis. *Journal of Pediatrics,* **62,** 604

Rosenberg, H. S. and McNamara, D. G. (1964) Acute myocarditis in infancy and childhood. *Progress in Cardiovascular Diseases,* **7,** 179

Endomyocardial fibrosis

Abrahams, D. G. (1962) Endomyocardial fibrosis of the right ventricle. *Quarterly Journal of Medicine,* **31,** 1

D'Arbela, P. G., Mutazindwa, T., Patel, A. K. *et al.* (1972) Survival after first presentation with endomyocardial fibrosis. *British Heart Journal,* **34,** 403

Davies, J. N. P. (1948) Endocardial fibrosis in Africans. *East Africa Medical Journal,* **125,** 10–14

Parry, E. H. O. (1964) Endomyocardial fibrosis. In *Cardiomyopathies,* Ciba Symposium. London, Churchill

Shillingford, J. P. and Somers, K. (1960) Clinical and haemodynamic patterns in endomyocardial fibrosis. *British Heart Journal,* **22,** 546

Hypertrophic cardiomyopathy

Clark, C. E., Henry, W. L. and Epstein, S. E. (1973) Familial prevalence and genetic transmission of idiopathic hypertrophic subaortic stenosis. *New England Journal of Medicine,* **289,** 709

Hopf, R., Kober, G., Bussmann, W. D., *et al.* (1980) Treatment of hypertrophic obstructive cardiomyopathy with verapamil. *British Heart Journal,* **42,** 35

Maron, B. J., Spirito, P., Wesley, Y., *et al.* (1986) Development and progression of left ventricular hypertrophy in children with hypertrophic cardiomyopathy. *New England Journal of Medicine,* **315,** 610–614

Rossen, R. M., Goodman, D. J., Ingham, R. E., *et al.* (1974) Echocardiographic criteria in the diagnosis of idiopathic hypertrophic subaortic stenosis. *Circulation,* **50,** 747

Shand, D. G., Sell, C. G. and Oates, J. A. (1971) Hypertrophic obstructive cardiomyopathy in an infant. Propranolol therapy for 3 years. *New England Journal of Medicine,* **285,** 843

Swan, D. A., Bell, B., Oakley, C. M., *et al.* (1971) Analysis of symptomatic course and prognosis and treatment of hypertrophic obstructive cardiomyopathy. *British Heart Journal,* **33,** 671

Cardiac tumours

Simcha, A., Wells, B. G., Tynan, M. J., *et al.* (1971) Primary cardiac tumours in childhood. *Archives of Disease in Childhood,* **46,** 508

Van der Hanwaert, L. G. (1971) Cardiac tumours in infancy and childhood. *British Heart Journal,* **33,** 125

Pericardial diseases

Cayler, G. G., Taybi, H., Riley, H. D. Jr, *et al.* (1963) Pericarditis with effusion in infants and children. *Journal of Pediatrics,* **63,** 264

Jordan, S. C. and Haycock, G. B. (1979) Chronic pericardial constriction with effusion in childhood. *Archives of Disease in Childhood,* **54,** 11

Plouth, W. H. Jr, Waldman, R. A., Wachner, R. A., *et al.* (1964) Protein losing enteropathy secondary to constrictive pericarditis in children. *Pediatrics, Springfield,* **34,** 634

Simcha, A. and Taylor, J. F. N. (1971) Constrictive pericarditis in childhood. *Archives of Disease in Childhood,* **46,** 515

Chapter 21

Cardiac abnormalities associated with systemic diseases or syndromes

Systemic hypertension in infants and children

Measurement of the blood pressure (BP) should be part of the routine examination in every infant and child. Details of the precise method of measuring BP are given in Chapter 3.

Before hypertension can be diagnosed we must have data from normal infants and children related to age, sex, height and weight. The Brompton study by de Swiet, Fayers and Shinebourne (1980) showed that on the second day of life the mean *systolic* pressure is 70 mmHg and then rises gradually over the next six weeks to a level of 93 mmHg. Thereafter the pressure remains remarkably level at 95 mmHg until 2 years of age. The Second Task Force on Blood Pressure Control in Children has now issued its 1987 report. They have computed data from nine different sources and prepared BP distribution curves related to age, sex, height and weight. Their tables show that the BP gradually rises from the age of 1 year to 13 years. On the 50th percentile the BP rises from 90/56 to 110/68 mmHg. A normal BP is regarded as one that is less than the 90th percentile, i.e. 105/69 at 1 year rising to 125/78 at 13 years. Significant hypertension is diagnosed when the reading is equal to or above the 95th percentile. Table 21.1 summarizes the recommendations of the Task Force. It is emphasized that repeated BP measurements are necessary to show that the rise in BP is sustained. The high BP recorded in obese children is probably related to their excessive weight and loss of weight causes a fall in BP (Rames, Clarke and Connor, 1978).

Table 21.1

Age	Significant hypertension when BP ≥ figures below (mmHg)	Age	Significant hypertension when BP ≥ figures below (mmHg)
Newborn	Systolic 96	6–9 years	122/78
7 days	Systolic 104	10–12 years	126/82
Infant (<2 yrs)	112/74	13–15 years	
3–5 years	116/76		

Causes of hypertension

Some conditions are more common at different ages and it is useful to consider the causes in relation to age. In the newborn infant coarctation of the aorta, renal artery stenosis and thrombosis, and congenital renal abnormalities are most common; bronchopulmonary dysplasia has been found to be associated with hypertension. In children between infancy and 6 years, coarctation and renal artery stenosis are still common causes; structural and inflammatory lesions of the kidneys and renal tumours occur. The same causes persist up to adolescence but there is an increasing incidence of primary essential hypertension.

It is useful also to consider the causes of hypertension in different systems:

Renal   Acute glomerulonephritis
            Chronic glomerulonephritis
            Chronic pyelonephritis
            Polycystic kidneys
            Wilms' tumour
            Hypoplastic kidney
            Collagen diseases such as polyarteritis nodosa and systemic lupus
            erythematosus
Vascular   Coarctation of the aorta
            Abnormalities of the renal artery
            Thrombosis of the renal artery or vein
Endocrine Phaeochromocytoma
            Neuroblastoma
            Adrenogenital syndrome
            Cushing's disease
            Primary aldosteronism
Drugs   Cortisone ACTH
            Antidepressants

Diagnostic evaluation

The most important aspects of diagnosis are to take a good medical history, a detailed family history and then do a thorough clinical examination. Infants who have had umbilical artery catheterization have an increased risk of renal hypertension. Some tumours (e.g. phaeochromocytoma) and some forms of renal disease (e.g. polycystic kidneys) are familial. There may be a family history of hypertension and coronary artery disease.

Clinical presentation

Hypertension may be discovered on routine examination and be symptomless. When symptoms occur they are essentially due to complications of the disease. Headache and vomiting, the most constant symptoms, are due to cerebral oedema and raised intracranial pressure, which may also cause fits, hemiplegia, ophthalmoplegia, visual defects and clouding of consciousness. Breathlessness on exertion and cough or breathlessness at night are due to left ventricular failure. Nocturia and polyuria or oliguria are due to renal involvement. Cerebral or subarachnoid haemorrhage may occur catastrophically, as may dissecting aneurysm of the aorta.

Examination of the ocular fundi is important prognostically. The first signs are narrowing and irregularity of the arterioles with decreased arteriovenous diameter ratio. Haemorrhages, exudates and papilloedema indicate a poor prognosis, likely to be measured in weeks or months.

The cardiac impulse will usually show some degree of left ventricular enlargement and either the third or the fourth heart sound is accentuated. The former sound suggests left ventricular failure and the latter left atrial hypertrophy occurring when the disease has been present for several months at least. Normal splitting of the second heart sound is lost in the presence of left ventricular failure and may be replaced by 'reversed' splitting – left ventricular ejection may delay aortic closure beyond pulmonary closure so that splitting is heard on expiration.

Examination of the abdomen should include palpation of kidney size and gentle palpation for the presence of adrenal or other tumour. (Pressure on a phaeochromocytoma may precipitate a hypertensive episode.) Auscultation over the kidneys both at the front and at the back should be performed. A single arterial stenosis frequently causes a bruit.

After physical examination the patient's urine should be examined. Acute nephritis may present with hypertension rather than oliguria and haematuria, but examination of the urine for albumin, red cells and casts will confirm the diagnosis. In chronic glomerulonephritis and chronic pyelonephritis (particularly if there has been no acute episode) hypertension is frequently the finding which leads to the detection of the disease, and in renovascular disease hypertension is virtually the only indication. Hypertension may occur in polycystic renal disease before there is obvious renal involvement and in childhood and adolescence is frequently asymptomatic.

Systemic hypertension complicating intracranial lesions usually only occurs when there is raised intracranial pressure and other symptoms will precede it, but difficulties may arise in differentiating this situation from cerebral symptoms of encephalopathy resulting from severe hypertension.

An adrenaline- or noradrenaline-secreting adrenal medullary tumour (phaeochromocytoma) may present with fixed or spasmodic hypertension. In the latter instance, hypertensive attacks may be accompanied by pallor, sweating, tachycardia, chest pain, abdominal pain and headache. Older children complain of a feeling of tension or anxiety and there may be diarrhoea and vomiting. Differentiation of these symptoms from functional disturbances is made by the absence of precipitating emotional cause and the intense sweating. About 20% of the tumours occur outside the adrenal glands, in proximity to the aorta, bladder, heart or base of the skull. Hyperglycaemia and glycosuria occur when the tumour secretes a high proportion of adrenaline.

The features of Cushing's syndrome are obvious and hypertension is mild. Conn's syndrome is excessively rare and hypertension is again mild. The diagnosis is usually suspected from the low serum potassium (below 3.0 mmol/l) and raised sodium (over 143 mmol/l).

Investigation

Hypertension in the presence of symptoms or of advanced retinopathy should be regarded as a medical emergency and investigation planned and started at once. Since essential hypertension is uncommon and the prognosis poor unless a treatable condition is detected, no effort should be spared to find a cause.

Urine examination
Proteinuria and small numbers of red cells may result from renal damage due to the hypertension as well as from intrinsic renal disease. Heavy proteinuria with cellular and granular casts favour chronic glomerulonephritis. Numerous white cells, pus cells and bacteria suggest chronic pyelonephritis, but even in their absence the urine should be cultured. In addition a 24-hour collection of urine for catecholamine estimation should be made as soon as possible since treatment (particularly with methyldopa) interferes with the test. Different measurements are used in some centres but the most widely used estimation is that of vanillyl mandelic acid (VMA). In the presence of a phaeochromocytoma the results are usually excessively high but since catecholamine excretion may be irregular two or more estimations may be required.

Electrocardiography
Even when the hypertension is of recent origin the electrocardiogram usually shows an increase in R wave voltage in left ventricular leads, and when left ventricular failure occurs as a complication there is ST segment depression or, less frequently, T wave inversion in these leads.

Chest radiography
Chest radiography is useful in determining heart size and indicating pulmonary venous hypertension.

Echocardiography
This will establish a base-line of the left ventricular mass and can be repeated after treatment to look for improvement.

Blood urea
Blood urea estimation is useful as a prognostic guide. In severe hypertension the blood urea is often slightly or moderately raised, but a value over 120 mg/100 ml (20 mmol/l) is suggestive of primary renal disease.

Blood creatinine
This is probably a better measurement than blood urea because it is less related to protein intake.

Blood electrolytes
A low serum potassium (under 3.2 mmol/l) and a raised serum sodium are suggestive of hyperaldosteronism, but may occur as a secondary finding in renal hypertension. Aldosterone antagonists (spironolactone) correct both the electrolyte abnormalities and the hypertension in primary aldosteronism, but have no effect on the hypertension of secondary aldosteronism.

Corticosteroid estimations
Corticosteroid estimations in urine and blood are only indicated where there are clinical findings suggestive of Cushing's syndrome.

Renal ultrasonography
This helps to demonstrate renal abnormalities, e.g. whether one kidney is smaller than the other (which may be congenital, or the result of infection or some vascular

abnormality). Hydronephrosis, cysts and tumours can also be identified. Renal artery stenosis may also be seen.

Intravenous pyelography
Unilateral renal artery stenosis produces a characteristic triad of delayed excretion, higher density (due to increased water reabsorption) and a smaller capacity renal pelvis compared with the normal side.

Aortography
Renal artery stenosis is demonstrated and, in addition, a phaeochromocytoma in or near the adrenals is demonstrated by a 'blush' of increased vessels. Some care is required in interpreting apparent arterial stenoses when these are mild, since they may not be functionally important.

Renography
The renogram is the pattern of excretion of radioactive substances, usually ^{131}I Hippuran, by the kidney. Counters are placed over both kidneys and counting performed following intravenous injection of the tracer. There is normally a rapid increase in counting rate to a maximum at about 5 min and then a gradual decay over 30–40 min. Renal artery stenosis produces a delayed peak and a slow fall.

Scintillation renography
Scintillation renography is performed using a gamma camera or similar scanning device over the renal area following the injection of a tracer (technetium-99) which is taken up in the renal tubules. Functional defects (for example, tumours, cysts or areas served by an obstructed arterial branch) give a lower count than the normal kidney.

Renal biopsy
Renal biopsy is probably the most sensitive way of detecting glomerulonephritis and may also be helpful in detecting systemic diseases such as disseminated lupus erythematosus. In many cases it will be necesary to biopsy both kidneys, particularly if nephrectomy is contemplated.

Treatment

Where a definite underlying cause is found, it should be treated medically or surgically.

If no cause is found and a diagnosis of primary hypertension is made, management depends on the degree of hypertension. If it is mild, attention should be given to weight reduction, exercise and diet (particularly sodium restriction) and this often achieves a fall in BP.

If the hypertension is moderate or severe, then drug therapy is considered. In children the risks of using these drugs must be balanced against their benefits, although most of the established forms of therapy are safe.

Where no underlying cause is found, the majority of patients respond well to treatment with hypotensive drugs.

Drugs
A stepped approach to treatment is recommended. First a thiazide diuretic such as chlorothiazide (10 mg/kg twice daily) is given. This will not be effective in chronic

renal failure when a loop diuretic such as frusemide (1–5 mg/kg/day) is advised. If the hypertension is not controlled by this, then a beta-blocker such as propranolol is added (0.5–1.0 mg/kg three times a day, increasing the dose to 2.0 mg/kg as necessary). Children have few side-effects from this drug but irritability is sometimes observed. If the child is prone to bronchospasm, metoprolol (25–100 mg/kg twice daily) which is relatively cardioselective is given instead of propranolol. The third step if the blood pressure is still not controlled is to give a vasodilator such as hydralazine (0.5 mg/kg three times daily). Some patients are sensitive to this drug and a test dose should always be given to avoid severe hypotension developing.

The angiotensin-converting enzyme inhibitor, captopril (0.5–2 mg/kg 12-hourly) is valuable in cases of renal hypertension. Its effect is increased by the addition of a diuretic.

Hypertensive crises
Prompt treatment is necessary in children with hypertensive encephalopathy. An intravenous line should be inserted so that fluid balance can easily be maintained and the BP must be continuously monitored. Sodium nitroprusside which is short acting should be given as an intravenous infusion 0.5–1 µg/kg/min. Alternatively, frusemide 2–5 mg/kg i.v. can be used.

Prognosis

When a correctable lesion, such as phaeochromocytoma or unilateral renal disease, is detected and removed prior to the development of complications the prognosis is excellent. If delay occurs, hypertensive changes in the kidneys may result in the postoperative BP not returning to normal. In hypertension complicating advanced bilateral renal disease or systemic disease the hypertension can usually be controlled and the prognosis is that of the underlying disease.

Hyperkinetic circulatory states

There is a group of conditions in which the cardiac output is increased by a tachycardia and a raised venous filling pressure. There is dilatation of the skin and muscle vessels. The arterial pulse is collapsing and capillary pulsation may be seen. In children, anaemia is the commonest and most important cause of such a high cardiac output, but it may also occur in association with arteriovenous aneurysms and shunts, and in thyrotoxicosis.

Anaemia

Heart failure does not usually occur until the haemoglobin in the blood falls below 6.0 g% (g/100 ml), but in children who already have heart failure due to a congenital heart lesion, a milder degree of anaemia may make the heart failure worse and such children improve considerably when the anaemia is corrected.

In severe chronic anaemia from any cause the circulation is hyperkinetic. The patient has bounding pulses with a high pulse pressure and warm extremities. The heart is increased in size with a forceful left ventricle and the neck veins are distended. A basal ejection systolic murmur due to an increased flow through the pulmonary and aortic valves is heard. Congestive heart failure may follow with oedema and enlargement of the liver.

The cause of the anaemia should be determined first, but if it is causing heart failure, blood transfusion is usually necessary. A transfusion of packed red cells (20 ml/kg) should be given over a period of 8 hours. Intravenous frusemide should be given at the start of the transfusion and th epatient carefully observed. If there is any evidence of pulmonary oedema developing (as shown by a rise in respiratory rate, cough or restlessness) then a further dose of frusemide should be given. Further transfusion of the same amount of blood may be given over the next 8 hours if indicated.

Arteriovenous aneurysm

In a congenital cirsoid aneurysm, arteries and veins are in direct communication with one another. An impressive continuous machinery murmur may be heard over the aneurysm and will disappear if the arteries supplying it can be compressed. When the aneurysm is in the cerebral circulation a murmur can be heard by listening over the eyeball or over the skull. If the aneurysm is in a limb, the affected limb will be larger and the skin feel warmer than the normal one. When the aneurysm is large, all the pulses are collapsing, the heart is enlarged and a systolic ejection murmur is audible at the base of the heart. Heart failure may occur and it is important to appreciate that there is an extracardiac cause for the heart failure in these patients, otherwise unnecessary cardiac investigations may be carried out. The heart failure resolves when the aneurysm has been treated.

Hyperthyroidism

Hyperthyroidism is rare in childhood. There is a high cardiac output with tachycardia, bounding pulses and an increased pulse pressure. The heart gradually enlarges and a systolic murmur is audible at the cardiac apex or in the pulmonary area.

The thyrotoxicosis should be controlled by drug therapy and the cardiac state then improves. If heart failure is present when the patient is first seen, then digoxin should also be given to control this. Newborn infants of mothers with thyrotoxicosis may develop heart failure and require treatment with digoxin as well as drugs to control the hyperthyroidism.

Hypothyroidism

Cretinism and juvenile hypothyroidism are both rare. In the cretin, symptoms begin after the second week of life, the infant feeds poorly, is inactive and constipated and later appears apathetic. As the child grows it is noticed that the eyelids are prominent, the tongue is large and the skin dry and wrinkled. In the older child with juvenile myxoedema there is apathy, dullness and growth retardation. The skin is dry and there is an increase in subcutaneous fat.

There may be no cardiac symptoms but the heart action is quiet and slow. In severe cases heart failure occurs. The radiograph shows a normal or slightly enlarged heart. The electrocardiogram shows distinctive changes (Figure 21.1).

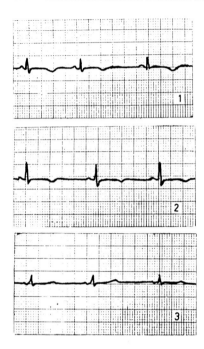

Figure 21.1 Hypothyroidism. Electrocardiogram of an 8-year-old girl. There is slow sinus rhythm (56 per minute in lead 2), inverted T waves and a prolonged (0.5 second) Q–T interval

There is slow sinus rhythm, the P–R interval is often prolonged, QRS complexes are of low voltage and the T waves are flattened or inverted. The Q–T interval is prolonged. The electrocardiogram is of value in making the diagnosis; if it is normal, cretinism or myxoedema is unlikely. After treatment with thyroid, the electrocardiogram returns to normal and changes in the electrocardiogram may be used to assess the adequacy of the dose of thyroid being given.

Noonan's syndrome

This is an autosomal dominant syndrome in which there is a high incidence of congenital heart abnormalities. The children have the facial and skeletal features seen in Turner's syndrome but the chromosomes are normal. Most have a normal intelligence but some are mentally retarded.

The commonest cardiac lesion is pulmonary valve stenosis and the valve is usually dysplastic. It is interesting that one often sees children with widely separated down-sloping eyes without other features of Noonan's syndrome who also have dysplastic pulmonary valves. Indeed the possibility of the valve being dysplastic should always be considered in such children. Such valves are not amenable to treatment by valvuloplasty (see Chapter 8). Obstructive cardiomyopathy of the left ventricle, either alone or with pulmonary stenosis, is another common finding and should always be looked for at echocardiography. The electrocardiogram in patients with pulmonary stenosis associated with Noonan's syndrome is unusual in that is shows left axis deviation instead of right.

Turner's syndrome

Patients with Turner's syndrome are short of stature, have webbing of the neck, a low hairline, cubitus valgus, a broad chest with wide apart nipples and sexual infantilism. Pitting oedema of the hands and feet is often present in infancy and then gradually disappears. Chromosomal studies have shown that there is a deficiency of a sex chromosome. A single X is present.

Coarctation of the aorta is the commonest cardiovascular lesion but aortic stenosis is also frequently found. Ventricular septal defect has also been observed.

The management of the cardiac lesions is the same as in normal patients.

Lentiginosis

A high incidence of hypertrophic cardiomyopathy has been reported. There appears to be some overlap with Noonan's syndrome as some of the reported cases have had similar skeletal abnormalities. Cardiac tumours, including myxoma, have also been reported.

Gargoylism

Gargoylism is an inherited disorder of connective tissue in which the mucopolysaccharide metabolism is abnormal.

The facies are grotesque, the head is large with hypertelorism and the nasal bridge is depressed. The mouth is held open and the tongue protrudes. There is kyphosis and a broad chest. The hands are held in a claw-like position. Corneal opacities may be present.

The cardiac disorders involve the valves of the heart and the coronary arteries. The valves have shiny nodules along their free margins and the chordae tendineae are shortened. This results in valvar incompetence. The mitral and tricuspid valves are most commonly affected. There is thickening of the intima of the coronary arteries, causing narrowing.

Friedreich's ataxia

Friedreich's ataxia is a rare, familial, inherited disease in which there is degeneration of the posterior columns and the spinocerebellar and pyramidal tracts of the spinal cord.

Symptoms are usually present by 10 years of age. The gait is broad based, there is incoordination of movement and speech is impaired. Knee and ankle jerks are lost and there is loss of vibration and position sense but pain and temperature sensation remain.

Cardiac abnormalities are present in the majority of patients. The heart is normal in size or moderately enlarged and there may be no murmurs or soft systolic murmurs which are of no help in diagnosis. The electrocardiogram shows inverted T waves in leads aVF, V_5 and V_6. Dysrhythmias are common as the condition progresses. Patients may die from heart failure in adult life or suddenly, presumably from dysrhythmias. The cause of death is usually cardiac.

Treatment

There is no specific treatment and the heart failure and dysrhythmias should be treated in the usual way.

Down's syndrome

This is the commonest chromosomal abnormality. At least 40% of patients have some congenital heart defect (Greenwood and Nadas, 1976); atrioventricular defect is the commonest lesion and occurs in more than 40% (Park, Mathews and Zuberbuhler, 1977). Ventricular septal defect is found in about one-third of patients, and tetralogy of Fallot and patent ductus arteriosus occur less commonly. More patients with Down's syndrome are now referred to paediatric cardiology centres to determine whether a cardiac lesion is present and it may be, now that echocardiography can make a firm diagnosis, that the incidence of heart disease is higher than previously recorded.

Prior to surgery, patients with Down's syndrome frequently died from their heart defects. Although surgery ought now to be possible in these children, the problem of pulmonary hypertension is an important one in children with atrioventricular defects and ventricular septal defects. It has been observed for many years that children with Down's syndrome develop pulmonary vascular obstructive diseases much earlier in life than normal children. Indeed, pulmonary vascular disease has been observed and reported in Down's syndrome *without* heart disease (Wilson, Hutchins and Neill, 1979; Levine and Simpser, 1982). There is no doubt that chronic upper airways obstruction causes pulmonary hypertension (Macartney, Panday and Scott, 1969); this may be due to enlarged tonsils and adenoids, laryngomalacia, obstructive sleep apnoea and enlarged tongue. All these factors may operate in children with Down's syndrome. There is also some evidence that the lungs themselves may be abnormal, having a decreased number of alveoli and therefore a decreased alveolar surface area.

In the past, many children were inoperable when first seen because of pulmonary vascular disease. This is less likely now because children are referred so much earlier in life. Nevertheless they need to be operated on at an earlier age than other children to prevent pulmonary vascular obstructive disease developing. This means that they will be smaller and the risks of operating on atrioventricular defects, which have a high mortality and morbidity in normal children, will be further increased.

Patients with tetralogy of Fallot, ventricular septal defect and patent ductus can be managed in the same way as normal children. Careful consideration must be given to the management of a child with Down's syndrome and complete atrioventricular defect. There must be full discussion of the risks and imponderables with the parents. Bull, Rigby and Shinebourne (1985) reviewed 75 patients with Down's syndrome and complete atrioventricular defect. The results of those with and without surgery were compared and also compared with the outcome in patients with Down's syndrome without a cardiac defect. They concluded that survival in childhood was better with medical than surgical treatment; without surgery there will be deterioration in late teens and early 20's and death from pulmonary vascular disease will occur between 20 and 30 years of age; early surgery is the only chance of preventing pulmonary vascular disease but the risks are in the region of 30% and furthermore the life expectancy will not be normal but will be that of Down's syndrome; residual cardiac abnormalities after surgery will also shorten the lives of some children. The choice really is between the probability of survival in childhood with death in early adult life or a high risk of death in early life but the possibility, if the child survives surgery, of a life carrying the same outlook as that of a patient with Down's syndrome and no cardiac defect. It must be stated quite clearly that operation on heart defects will not influence the other features of Down's syndrome.

Glycogen storage disease affecting the heart

There are eight groups of inherited abnormalities in glycogen metabolism which result in excessive glycogen storage. Type II (Pompe's disease) seriously affects the heart. It is an autosomal recessive cardiomyopathy and is very rare. There may be a family history of the disorder and amniocytes may show the enzyme deficiency. Glycogen accumulates in the heart muscle and also in skeletal muscle (especially the tongue and diaphragm) and in the liver.

Symptoms begin early in life. There is lethargy, hypotonia, a feeble cry, a large tongue, difficulty in sucking and a poor weight gain. The heart enlarges as the glycogen is deposited in the ventricular muscle and the liver enlarges as heart failure develops. Arrhythmias frequently occur and there is tachycardia. The disease is progressive and few patients survive the first year of life.

Electrocardiogram

This shows a short P–R interval, a high QRS voltage with wide complexes. There is left ventricular hypertrophy often with a strain pattern. Sometimes biventricular hypertrophy occurs.

Radiography

The heart is enlarged and globular and the lungs are congested.

Echocardiography

This is the most useful cardiac investigation. The ventricular walls are thickened often to twice the predicted ventricular mass. The contractility is normal initially (unlike hypertrophic obstructive cardiomyopathy). In four cases reported by Lubbers, Naeff and Losekoot (1985) the echocardiograph and electrocardiogram findings were non-specific in the first week but in the following months concentric left ventricular hypertrophy developed and was present in all four cases. There was no left ventricular outflow obstruction seen.

Diagnosis

The definitive diagnosis is made by the finding of deficiency of lysosomal alpha-1, 4 glucosidase in fibroblasts grown from a skin biopsy. A blood film shows vacuolated lymphocytes and the white blood cells show an increased amount of glycogen. These tests, together with the clinical picture and findings at echocardiography, confirm the diagnosis.

Treatment

This is supportive only. Diuretics are used when there is heart failure. Digoxin is best avoided because it may provoke arrhythmias.

Marfan's syndrome

Marfan's syndrome is an inherited disorder in which the dominant gene is transmitted by either sex. There is a widespread disorder of connective tissue, the exact nature of which is not understood.

Severe cases may be suspected at birth, the infant being particularly long and thin with poor musculature. The child is slow to thrive and is easily tired and complains of vague pains in the limbs. The pubis-to-sole measurement is greater than the pubis-to-vertex measurement. The arm span is greater than the height. There is hypermobility of the joints. The palate is high and arched, the skull is dolichocephalic and there is pectus excavatum. The eyesight is poor, there being a high degree of myopia associated with dislocation of the lenses.

Cardiovascular manifestations

The majority of deaths in Marfan's syndrome are due to cardiovascular abnormalities. Since mitral valve prolapse has been recognized and can be diagnosed by echocardiography, its incidence in Marfan's syndrome has been reported to be as high as 91% (Brown et al., 1975). On clinical examination there is a midsystolic click which may be accompanied by a late systolic murmur or pansystolic murmur. The findings vary with the patient's position as in idiopathic mitral valve prolapse. Mitral regurgitation occurs and gradually worsens in some patients. Aortic root dilatation has been found in 60% of patients (Brown et al., 1975). Again echocardiography is the most sensitive indicator of this dilatation and its progress can be monitored; it gradually worsens with the passage of time. In patients with severe scoliosis echocardiography may be difficult and CT scanning or magnetic resonance imaging may be necessary to get a complete picture of the ascending aorta. The sinuses of Valsalva dilate in the region of the commissure attachment and aortic regurgitation results. The degree of regurgitation worsens and can do so rapidly causing left ventricular failure.

Aortic dissection which usually occurs in the ascending aorta may occur acutely and the patient presents with chest pain and aortic regurgitation. In other patients there is gradual increasing size of the aorta over a matter of months. Aortic dissection should always be suspected and looked for. It may not be diagnosed by echocardiography and magnetic resonance imaging or digital subtraction angiography may be required to confirm the diagnosis.

Management

Patients can now be monitored by echocardiography as well as clinically and an annual review is advised. If the aortic root is dilated, patients should not take part in recreational exercise or competitive sports. Antibiotic prophylaxis for dental or surgical procedures is advised. The mortality of operative procedures in Marfan's syndrome has been high and operation is not usually advised if the patient is free of symptoms. If, however, symptoms occur it is wise to consider surgery before the patient deteriorates further and there is left ventricular dysfunction. Some workers advise surgery if the aortic root diameter is twice that of a normal aorta, i.e. about 5.0 cm. A composite graft consisting of a prosthetic valve in a woven conduit is inserted into the proximal aorta. Urgent operation is required if aortic dissection or rupture occurs. If there is severe mitral regurgitation, mitral valve replacement is necessary but the widespread abnormality of the tissues in this condition increases the risks of any surgery.

Kawasaki syndrome (also called muco-cutaneous lymph node syndrome (MCLS))

This condition was described by Kawasaki in Japan in 1967 but it is identical in presentation to the case described by Scott and Rotondo in 1944 when it was called infantile periarteritis nodosa. The cause is unknown; the diagnosis is made from the characteristic clinical features. There is no specific diagnostic test but the diagnosis must always be considered when a child presents with fever of unknown aetiology and is under the age of 5 years.

The principal symptoms are fever, congestion of the conjunctivae, dry, red and fissured lips, protuberance of the papillae of the tongue (strawberry tongue); redness of the oral and pharyngeal mucosa; redness of the palms and soles of the feet with indurative oedema which is followed by desquamation of fingers and toes. There is a generalized morbilliform rash and non-purulent swelling of the cervical lymph nodes. Arthritis, aseptic meningitis, abdominal pain and diarrhoea all occur. There may be hepatitis and acute hydrops of the gallbladder (which can be seen on echocardiography).

The most important laboratory findings are of a raised erythrocyte sedimentation rate (often 80–120 mm in the first hour) and thrombocythaemia. There is also a neutrophil leucocytosis with a shift to the left and a fall in the red cell count and haemoglobin.

About one-fifth of the patients have cardiac involvement. Any part of the heart may be involved – the myocardium, pericardium, endocardium and conducting tissue. Pericardial effusion, mitral regurgitation and arrhythmias are relatively common but the most serious complication is the development of an arteritis which results in coronary artery aneurysms. These may present as early as the fourth week of the disease. Death in the acute phase is mainly due to myocarditis but in later weeks may be due to myocardial ischaemia and ruptured coronary aneurysms. Late deaths are due to ischaemic heart disease.

The electrocardiogram may show ST–T wave changes, prolonged P–R interval and Q–T intervals. It may, however, be quite normal in the presence of extensive coronary artery aneurysms.

Echocardiography is valuable in the first 2 or 3 weeks in showing whether there is any pericardial effusion and in assessing myocardial function and any mitral regurgitation. Later, at 4 weeks, coronary artery aneurysms can be looked for. There is a lot of evidence that if no aneurysms are seen at the commencement of the coronary arteries (which is all one can see on echocardiography), then distal aneurysms are unlikely. Some aneurysms resolve but others persist and may rupture and cause death.

If there is a lot of cardiac involvement with pericarditis, mitral regurgitation, an ischaemic electrocardiogram and aneurysms in the peripheral arteries, then coronary angiography is advised to assess the extent of the involvement.

Treatment

The aetiology is unknown and drugs used are employed for their anticoagulant and anti-inflammatory actions. When the disease is suspected, aspirin 30–100 mg/kg/day should be given until 2 months after the fever subsides. If there is no evidence of coronary involvement the dose can be reduced to 10 mg/kg/day and discontinued after 2 years if there is no relapse and no complications. If there is coronary involvement the drug should be continued indefinitely in a small dose of 3–5 mg/kg/day to reduce thrombotic complications.

The long-term effects of this disease are still unknown and follow-up of patients is important.

Williams' syndrome

In 1961 Williams, Barratt-Boyes and Lowe, described 4 cases of supravalve aortic stenosis in children who had a curious facial appearance and resembled each other and who were mentally retarded. Shortly afterwards Beuren et al. (1962) reported further cases. In 1964 Beuren reported 10 cases in all of whom there was peripheral pulmonary stenosis as well as supravalve aortic stenosis and mental retardation. In 1963 Black and Bonham-Carter reported 5 cases with a similar appearance and signs of aortic stenosis; they regarded their facial appearance as resembling that of patients with hypercalcaemia and called the facies 'hypercalcaemic facies'. In fact none of their cases had calcium levels measured and there is no evidence that the cases described by Williams and Beuren had hypercalcaemia. It is better therefore

Table 21.2 Williams' syndrome

Genetic aspects	Family history in about 25%
Facies	Epicanthic folds
	Hypertelorism
	Snub nose
	Carp mouth
	Low-set ears
Dental	Hypoplastic primary dentition
	Serrated secondary dentition
	Missing first premolars
Neurological	Mental retardation
	Ataxia
	Personality defect
Hypercalcaemia	Clinical
	Biochemical
	Latent
Cardiac	Supra-aortic stenosis
	Aortic valve stenosis
	Peripheral pulmonary artery stenoses
	Coarctation of aorta
	Atrial septal defect
	Peripheral arterial stenoses
	Ventricular septal defect
	Mitral regurgitation
	Hypertension

to use the term Williams' syndrome. Most cases are sporadic but Cortada, Taysi and Hartmann (1980) reported pedigrees compatible with autosomal dominant inheritance. The possible components of this syndrome are given in Table 21.2.

The personalities of these children are similar and help to make the diagnosis. They are affectionate and compassionate and are continuously chattering and restless. They continually interrupt and seek attention. They are a great strain on their parents and disrupt family life. The presentation and management of supra-aortic stenosis is described in Chapter 7.

Peripheral pulmonary artery stenosis

This occurs in Williams' syndrome and is also found in some patients with the rubella syndrome. It is also seen occasionally associated with tetralogy of Fallot.

The lesions are multiple and give rise to loud systolic murmurs extending into diastole and best heard over the lungs. When the stenoses are severe there is right ventricular hypertrophy and the pulmonary element of the second sound is loud.

Chest radiographs may show variation in vascularity in different parts of the lung. Electrocardiograms show mild or moderate right ventricular hypertrophy, depending on the severity of the stenoses. Gradients of 10–80 mmHg have been recorded across the stenoses and the lesions can be demonstrated by angiography (Figure 21.2).

In the past no treatment was possible but now attempts are being made to dilate these stenoses with balloon catheters. About half of them have been successfully dilated (Ring *et al.*, 1985).

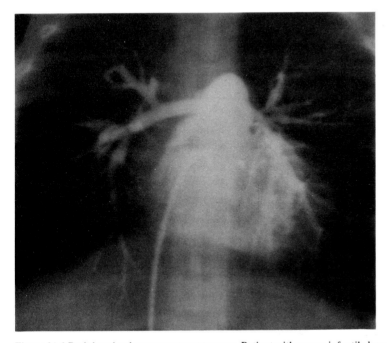

Figure 21.2 Peripheral pulmonary artery stenoses. Patient with severe infantile hypercalcaemia and typical facies. There are narrowings on the origins of all branches of the right pulmonary artery, with poststenotic dilation. Coarctation was also present

Bibliography and references

Systemic hypertension in infants and children

de Swiet, M., Fayers, P. and Shinebourne, E. A. (1980) Value of repeated blood pressure measurements in children – the Brompton study. *British Medical Journal*, **280**, 1567–1569

Rames, L. K., Clarke, W. R. and Connor, W. E. (1978) Normal blood pressure and the evaluation of sustained blood pressure elevation in childhood. The Muscatine study. *Pediatrics, Springfield*, **61**, 254–251

Report of the Second Task Force on Blood Pressure Control in Children (1987) (From the National Heart Lung and Blood Institute, Bethesda, Maryland). *Pediatrics, Springfield*, **79**, 1–25

Down's syndrome

Bull, C., Rigby, M. L. and Shinebourne, E. A. (1985) Should management of complete atrioventricular canal defect be influenced by co-existent Down syndrome? *Lancet*, **1**, 1147–1149

Greenwood, R. D. and Nadas, A. S. (1976) The clinical course of cardiac disease in Down syndrome. *Pediatrics, Springfield*, **58**, 893–897

Levine, O. R. and Simpser, M. (1982) Alveolar hypoventilation and cor pulmonale associated with chronic airway obstruction in infants with Down syndrome. *Clinical Paediatrics*, **21**, 25–29

Macartney, F. J., Panday, J. and Scott, O. (1969) Cor pulmonale as a result of chronic naso-pharyngeal obstruction due to hypertrophied tonsils and adenoids. *Archives of Disease in Childhood*, **44**, 585–592

Park, S. C., Mathews, R. A. and Zuberbuhler, J. R. (1977) Down syndrome with congenital heart malformation. *American Journal of Diseases in Children*, **131**, 29–33

Wilson, S. K., Hutchins, G. N. and Neill, C. A. (1979) Hypertensive pulmonary vascular disease in Down syndrome. *Journal of Paediatrics*, **95**, 722–726

Glycogen storage disease affecting the heart

Lubbers, L. J., Naeff, M. D. and Losekoot, M. D. (1985) Glycogen storage disease Type II (Pompe's disease). Electrocardiographic and echocardiographic features. *Abstracts Second World Congress of Paediatric Cardiology*, Springer-Verlag, New York, p. 43

Marfan's syndrome

Brown, O. R., De Mots, H., Kloster, F. E., *et al*. (1975) Aortic root dilatation and mitral valve prolapse in Marfan's syndrome. *Circulation*, **52**, 651–657

Kawasaki syndrome

Kawasaki, T. (1967) Acute febrile mucocutaneous syndrome with lymphoid involvement with specific desquamation of the fingers and toes. *Japanese Journal of Allergy*, **16**, 178–222

Scott, E. P. and Rotando, C. C. (1944) Periarteritis nodosa; report of two cases, one complicated by intrapericardial haemorrhage. *Journal of Pediatrics*, **25**, 306–310

Williams' syndrome

Beuren, A. J., Apitz, J. and Harmjanz, D. (1962) Supravalvular aortic stenosis in association with mental retardation and a certain facial appearance. *Circulation*, **26**, 1235–1239

Beuren, A. J., Schulz, C., Eberle, P., *et al*. (1964) The syndrome of supravalvular aortic stenosis, peripheral pulmonary stenosis, mental retardation and similar facial appearance. *American Journal of Cardiology*, **13**, 471–483

Black, J. A. and Bonham-Carter, R. E. (1963) Association between aortic stenosis and facies of severe infantile hypercalcaemia. *Lancet*, **2**, 745–749

Cortada, X., Taysi, K. and Hartmann, A. F. (1980) Familial Williams' syndrome. *Clinical Genetics*, **18**, 173–176

Ring, J. C., Bass, J. L., Marvin, W., *et al*. (1985) Management of congenital stenosis of a branch pulmonary artery with balloon dilatation angioplasty: report of 52 procedures. *Journal of Thoracic and Cardiovascular Surgery*, **90**, 35–44

Williams, J. C. P., Barratt-Boyes, B. G. and Lowe, J. B. (1961) Supravalvular aortic stenosis. *Circulation*, **24**, 1311–1317

Chapter 22

Psychosocial and primary care problems of congenital heart disease

There have been tremendous advances in the diagnosis and treatment of congenital heart disease over the past 20 years. Investigation is less traumatic and the results of surgery have continued to improve. Treatment is given whenever possible before the child reaches school age and many can now enjoy a normal school life. Problems remain for children whose condition cannot be cured or who, after palliative surgery, still have symptoms or who are at risk from some complication which has followed surgery. It is part of the paediatric cardiologist's job to ensure that such children are managed in the best possible way so that they lead as full and happy a life as possible yet are protected from taking unnecessary risks. On the other hand, it must be ensured that children with mild forms of heart disease who do not need treatment are not restricted unnecessarily. There is no doubt that in order to achieve the best management of each and every child, there must be good communication and cooperation between all the people involved in their care – parents, nurses, doctors, social workers, teachers, school doctors and general practitioners. When the child reaches adolescence careers officers, employers, insurance doctors and gynaecologists are all involved.

Information about the particular heart lesion

When a mother is first told that a child has heart disease, she is in a state of shock and has difficulty in listening to what the doctor is saying and in understanding it. A further visit with both parents present is of great value and should be arranged whenever possible. The doctor must speak in simple terms; a parent often does not realize that a heart murmur which has been heard is actually caused by abnormal flow of blood related to the defect present. Written information with diagrams of the heart has proved to be of great value; parents should be told only about their own child's problem so that they are not confused. Such information sheets can be updated appropriately when investigation or treatment changes, e.g. there is now a need for more information about echocardiography and a description of how stenotic valves can be treated by balloon valvuloplasty. The parents can read the information in a more relaxed and receptive way and ask any questions subsequently. It is important to stress that children can have the same heart lesion but in one it may be severe and require treatment whereas in another the lesion is mild and the child needs no restrictions or treatment.

Genetic counselling

We all look for an explanation when some disaster happens; parents want to know why their particular child has been born with a heart lesion. It is important to emphasize that it is not the fault of either parent. The paediatric cardiologist can give some information about the aetiology of heart disease (as described in Chapter 1) but parents should be given the opportunity of seeing a genetic counsellor if they wish.

Effect on the family

When a child is severely handicapped there is a great strain on the parents, particularly the mother, who will often opt out of all social life and feel she can never leave her child in anyone else's care. Parents' sleep is frequently disturbed and they become exhausted in trying to look after the sick child and meet the demands of other healthy siblings. Such families need help from relatives, social workers and medical and nursing staff in order to avoid complete disruption of the family.

Financial help

The burden of these families can be greatly eased by financial support so that they do not need to worry about money as well as everything else. Trusts and Charities help greatly by supplying telephones (so that help can be summoned as required) and washing machines and holidays to make life easier for the mother. Parents should be made aware of sources of help and encouraged to use them early rather than late.

Growth and development

Patients with acyanotic obstructive lesions who do not have left-to-right shunts, grow and gain weight normally. Cyanotic patients and patients with shunts, however, fail to grow and gain weight at the normal rate although height is less affected than weight. The delay in weight and height maturation in patients with shunts is proportional to the size of the shunt (Suoninen, 1971); in cyanotic patients the growth failure is related to particular lesions and aggravated by heart failure (Linde, Dunn and Schireson, 1967). As well as the abnormal haemodynamic situation in children with shunts, they are too breathless and exhausted to finish their feeds and they also suffer from frequent infections. There is a higher metabolic rate in such patients so they require a greater calorific intake in order to gain weight, yet are incapable of taking it. Mothers become very depressed by the poor weight-gain, particularly in infancy. The babies can often be helped by being given high calorie feeds and smaller feeds more frequently.

Mothers can be assured, however, that when a corrective operation is possible, the child will catch up with growth after surgery and the earlier surgery is carried out (preferably before the age of 2 years) the more beneficial will it be (Suoninen, 1971).

Children with shunts and with cyanosis show some delay in motor skills. Cyanotic children tend to have lower I.Q.s than normal children. The study of Newburger, Gilbert and Buckley (1984) showed that the earlier the operation for transposition of the great arteries was carried out, the greater the improvement in intellectual and gross motor skills. A study by Aisenberg, Rosenthal and Nadas (1982) found that congestive heart failure may be a more important cause of delayed mental development than cyanosis. Nevertheless, many cyanosed children have a normal I.Q. and do well at school, given the necessary stimulation and encouragement.

Infection

Children with left-to-right shunts are particularly prone to respiratory infections which further impair any ventilation-perfusion problem and make hypoxaemia worse. It is important always to maintain fluid balance in patients receiving digoxin and diuretics. Alteration in cardiac medication may be necessary during intercurrent illnesses. A child's condition can deteriorate rapidly due to electrolytic disturbances during gastroenteritis and these must always be corrected. Hypokalaemia and impaired renal function can lead to digoxin toxicity. If the patient is cyanosed and polycythaemic, then a fall in intravascular volume predisposes to thrombosis, so such patients must always be kept well hydrated. Swabs should be taken to try to find the causative organism in chest infections and antibiotics should be given promptly.

Immunization

There are no contraindications to carrying out immunization in children with heart disease. It should be done at the appropriate time as in normal children. Parents, however, often have great difficulty in persuading clinic doctors and general practitioners to do them. In fact children with heart disease who develop measles or pertussis become extremely ill. It must be emphasized that *congenital heart disease is not a contraindication to giving immunizations*.

Dental care

This is fully discussed in Chapter 7 and the recomendations given must be followed.

Education

Fortunately it is now the trend to allow as many handicapped children as possible to attend ordinary schools. This demands a good liaison between all the staff involved. There should be clear instructions as to what the child can and cannot do and most of these instructions relate to exercise (see below). This varies so much with individual patients that each patient must be catered for separately. If a patient is likely to remain handicapped it is important that he has as good an education as possible so that he is capable of obtaining a sedentary job.

Exercise

Most children nowadays who have operable heart disease will have had their operation before starting school. There is a tendency for teachers to restrict such children when they realize they have had heart surgery but it must be emphasized that the scar is there because the heart has been made normal. Except for a few, who may have some complication, such children can lead normal lives at school and exercise normally. Also, nowadays echocardiography and Doppler echocardiography can confirm the clinician's diagnosis of a lesion being a mild one and he can quite confidently advise full activity and exercise.

In the series of Lambert, Menon and Wagner (1974) in which 254 cases of sudden death were analysed, the commonest four lesions were:

1. Aortic stenosis   18%
2. Eisenmenger's syndrome   15%
3. Cyanotic heart disease   10%
4. Hypertrophic obstructive cardiomyopathy   9%

These are the four most worrying lesions, although only 10% of them were engaged in active sport when they died. Children with obstructive lesions on the left side of the heart cannot maintain their cardiac output during exercise and syncope results. Patients with moderate aortic stenosis should not be allowed to exercise competitively and must be kept under routine surveillance at the clinic where repeat Doppler echocardiography can be done to measure the gradient across the valve. If symptoms occur or the gradient is increasing, operation is indicated. The problem with hypertrophic obstructive cardiomyopathy is that the lesion may not have been diagnosed because the patient has not had symptoms and there are often no murmurs. The first attack of syncope may be the last. Patients who have dizziness or syncope should always be referred to hospital because obstructive cariomyopathy can be confirmed or excluded by echocardiography.

Patients with tetralogy of Fallot became increasingly blue on exercise but will usually restrict themselves. They should always be allowed to stop any physical activity when they wish. In patients with pulmonary vascular disease there is resistance to blood flowing into the arteries in the lungs and they cannot increase their cardiac output. Such patients may lose consciousness and die. Patients who have primary pulmonary hypertension increase their pulmonary artery pressure with exercise and acute right ventricular failure may develop with myocardial ischaemia, arrhythmias and death.

Children with left-to-right shunts usually tolerate exercise well; they may become more breathless than normal children but they restrict themselves by slowing down or resting.

If there is disease of the heart muscle such as myocarditis or dilated cardiomyopathy (which may follow treatment with adriamycin), then exercise should be restricted. Such children may be comfortable at rest but cannot increase their cardiac output with exercise.

Children with congenital heart block who have an adequate heart rate at rest usually do well on moderate exercise but may develop symptoms of breathlessness and dizziness on the more severe exercise. Supraventricular tachycardias usually occur unrelated to exercise but some patients can induce attacks on exercise. Abnormal heart rhythms which follow heart surgery require careful monitoring and if a child known to have abnormal rhythms develops symptoms then 24-hour Holter monitoring should be carried out and medical treatment or a pacemaker, or both, prescribed as indicated. Doctors and teachers should not delay in referring such children back to their paediatric cardiologist.

It must be appreciated that there is a great variation in the energy expended in different sports. Long-distance swimming and cross-country running require peak performance throughout whereas netball or tennis allow periods of rest after short bursts of activity. Golf, bowling and horse-riding require little increase in metabolic activity. Competitive sports require periods of training with maximum stress and emotional involvement and children with moderate and severe heart disease must be excluded from these.

It is difficult then to decide what each individual child should be allowed to do. Exercise testing on a bicycle or treadmill will help in evaluating the child's response to exercise. The electrocardiogram is monitored and the heart rate response to exercise and any ischaemic changes noted. The blood pressure is monitored before, during and after exercise and any hypertension recorded. If hypotension occurs then it is an indication of poor cardiac reserve and exercise should be avoided.

Advice is given as follows related to whether the heart disease is trivial, mild, moderate or severe and then consult with teachers and school doctors as to what an individual child may do. It is important that children are not forced to carry on doing exercise if they complain of tiredness or breathlessness.

1. Trivial heart disease – no restrictions in recreational exercise or competitive sports

This includes patients with small patent ductus, small ventricular septal defect and small atrial septal defects, or patients who have had these defects satisfactorily closed. Mild pulmonary stenosis with a gradient less than 30 mmHg, mild aortic stenosis with a gradient less than 20 mmHg, coarctation of the aorta which has been repaired and with a resting gradient of less than 10 mmHg. Trivial degress of aortic and mitral regurgitation.

2. Mild heart disease – no restrictions in recreational exercise but restriction of strenuous competitive sports

This includes patients with patent ductus, ventricular septal defect and atrial septal defect in whom there is some pulmonary hypertension, but less than half the systemic pressure. Pulmonary stenosis with a gradient between 20 and 60 mmHg, coarctation of the aorta with a gradient of 10–20 mmHg; mild mitral regurgitation and aortic regurgitation where the electrocardiogram remains normal.

3. Moderate heart disease – moderately strenuous recreational exercise allowed but no competitive sports

This includes aortic stenosis with a gradient of 20–50 mmHg, moderate aortic and mitral regurgitation with changes on the electrocardiogram but no ischaemic changes; postoperative tetralogy of Fallot and other cyanotic heart disease; prosthetic valve replacement; Marfan's disease with normal aortic root; prolonged Q–T syndrome.

4. Severe heart disease – no recreational exercise allowed, no competitive sports

This includes the four conditions where the risk of sudden death is greatest – aortic stenosis with a gradient greater than 50 mmHg; hypertrophic obstructive cardiomyopathy; pulmonary vascular disease; cyanotic congenital heart disease (unoperated on); Marfan's disease with dilated aortic root.

It must be remembered that the severity of a child's heart lesion may increase with growth and advice about exercise must be continually reviewed.

Travel

Patients should be discouraged from going to hot climates because they may become dehydrated and have a diminished cardiac output which may cause syncope. In cyanosed and polycythaemic patients dehydration may predispose to thromboembolic complications. Commonsense should dictate the length and type of journey so that the patient is not exhausted. The patient should carry a letter with the diagnosis, name of the hospital and consultant who is looking after him, medications and any special problems which may occur. Nowadays paediatric cardiologists usually know a colleague whom the patient could reach in an emergency, e.g. the Association of European Paediatric Cardiologists has a list of names and hospitals of their members to whom a patient could go if on holiday in Europe. It is useful for a child to wear a metal disc with a telephone number where information about him may be obtained.

The main problem of the actual travel is advisability of going by air. Patients with moderate cyanosis, moderate or severe pulmonary hypertension or congestive heart failure should only fly if arrangements are made for supplementary oxygen to be available during the flight. Airlines will provide this if asked in advance.

Driving licence

The ability to drive gives a patient with symptomatic heart disease great independence and allows him to go to and from work without a tiring journey by public transport. Only patients who are at risk from syncope need be banned from holding a licence.

Careers

Most teachers and school medical officers have become accustomed to looking after children with heart disease. Careers officers, however, have no experience and the majority find that the easiest decision is to deny them employment. This happens when the child has a scar on his chest despite the heart having been satisfactorily repaired. Competent doctors will often refuse entry of a girl to a career in nursing because she has a chest scar. It seems best to tell the child and her parents at an early age to ask careers officers or doctors to contact the paediatric cardiologist concerned so that every possible help is given and information is sent to the appropriate person. If the patient is handicapped, he sometimes fares better if he is listed on the Disabled Persons' Register. He is more likely to get a job and to be able to keep it. This is a difficult time in the patient's life when he may be leaving a children's clinic and trying to cope without the advice of his parents. Fortunately, adolescent units are now being set up where all possible advice is available for such patients. A good liaison between doctors is essential.

Contraception and pregnancy

This must be discussed with teenagers who would be at risk during a pregnancy; in some, pregnancy is life-threatening. Oral contraceptive pills are contraindicated in patients with pulmonary hypertension, cyanotic congenital heart disease and patients with prosthetic valves, because of the risks of thrombosis. An intra-uterine device is a possible source of infection which may predispose to infective endocarditis. The remaining possibilities are abstinence, a diaphragm or a condom. The latter two are not completely reliable so the remaining measure is tubal ligation unless the male partner is willing to have a vasectomy.

The risk of congenital heart disease occurring in the fetus must be discussed (see Chapter 1) and fetal echocardiogrpahy advised. If pregnancy occurs and the mother is not fit to tolerate a pregnancy, then termination is advised. If the mother is fit to tolerate a pregnancy she must be advised to stop smoking or taking alcohol and to avoid drugs such as amphetamine, thalidomide and propranolol, thus excluding as many environmental factors involved in the aetiology of congenital heart disease as possible.

The management of non-cardiac surgery

The two main problems for patients with heart disease undergoing non-cardiac operations are the anaesthetic and the necessity for prophylaxis against infective endocarditis. There is no worry about surgery for the patients who are asymptomatic and acyanotic. On the other hand, if there is pulmonary hypertension, cyanosis, congestive heart failure or the risk of arrhythmias, then there is a greater risk. As long as all the information about the patient is available and the anaesthetist is aware of the haemodynamic situation, then most surgery has a satisfactory outcome. The anaesthetist can discuss the management of possible complications in advance and the patient's electrocardiogram and blood pressure should be monitored throughout the operation. Patients who are polycythaemic should be given intravenous maintenance fluids to avoid thrombotic complications. The arterial Po_2 should be monitored as well as the pH. Any acidosis which develops must be corrected.

If the patient has heart failure the fluid balance must be carefully assessed and electrolytes measured and corrected. Alterations in the electrolytes and an increased digoxin concentration can precipitate arrhythmias. Patients with pacemakers should not have diathermy during surgery.

If there is a risk of serious arrhythmias, or severe hypoxaemia or severe outflow tract obstruction, then it is wise to arrange surgery at a centre with the appropriate cardiological services.

All patients should have prophylaxis against endocarditis as outlined in Chapter 17.

Parents' associations

In the past ten years parents of children with heart disease have formed Associations in most big centres in order to help their children in the best possible way. They have, quite rightly, demanded more information about their children's defects. Parents of children with the same lesions can meet and discuss their problems and this can be therapeutic. Parents play an increasing role in looking after their children in hospital and if there is a good relationship with the nursing staff, this can be of benefit to everyone concerned. More parents want to stay near the hospitals and they have helped to provide or equip rooms for accommodation.

Parents can help in liaising between doctors and teachers so that their children have the best possible education and school-life and later can ensure they are not denied suitable employment.

Adolescent units

By the time they reach adolescence most patients want to be told everything themselves and want their parents to stay in the background. Doctors must be sympathetic to this and, arrange accommodation on adult wards if admission to hospital is necessary. Patients fare best if they are in a hospital where paediatric and adult cardiac units are in close proximity.

Doctors must also speak frankly to girls about contraception and pregnancy so that there are no misunderstandings. Doctors can also help in directing patients to the best form of employment and ensure that they remain under medical supervision if they move from one town to another. They should always be given written information about their medical problem so that it is immediately available to any doctor being called to see them.

Insurance

Parents are anxious to know not only about the employability of their child but also whether he will be able to take out life insurance. A guide to the problem has been produced by Brackenridge (1985). Understandably, insurers tend to be cautious. When operation has been carried out they tend to wait for a year before giving an opinion. They also appreciate that the earlier in life surgery is performed, the less will be the secondary effects of the lesion on the function of the heart muscle. When operations are done early in life many years will pass before the patient asks for life insurance and the insurer can be more certain of the prognosis.

In the past it was unjustifiable to repeat invasive investigations specially for life insurance and the insurers were usually dependent on clinical assessment, a radiograph and electrocardiogram. Now, however, the patient can have an up-to-date assessment of the form and function of the heart by echocardiography and Doppler echo. Some insurers in the past have not given standard insurance to individuals with innocent murmurs but one hopes they would now do so when the echo and Doppler echo are completely normal.

The decision about insurance will tend to vary from one company to another and each patient must be assessed individually as there is a great variation in the severity in each lesion and in the surgical results. The reader is referred to Brackenridge's paper but a summary of the situation in common lesions is given below.

Untreated cyanosed patients will not be given insurance.

Atrial septal defect (secundum)
Tiny isolated defects in which surgery is not considered necessary, are likely to be given standard insurance. Moderate and large defects will be loaded, the loading depending on the size and secondary effects of the shunt.

After closure surgically – the younger the patient at surgery and the longer the time between surgery and the application for insurance, the better the risk and when a single defect is closed in childhood and examination in adult life is normal, standard insurance is given. A loading is imposed, however, when operation is done later in life and there is only a short interval between surgery and the application.

Complicated atrioventricular defects are not insurable.

Ventricular septal defect
If a small defect is confirmed at investigation and surgery not warranted, standard insurance may be given. Large defects, however, would be heavily loaded.

After closure surgically – defects closed by direct suture are deemed to have a normal life expectancy; when a synthetic patch is used, however, a risk factor is introduced in the rating. Also, the loading will be increased if there is residual cardiac enlargement.

Patent ductus arteriosus
Insurance is unlikely to be given in unoperated ducts.

After closure surgically – as in atrial septal defects if operation is satisfactory and the form and function of the heart are normal, standard insurance is given. If there is cardiac enlargement remaining, a loading is given.

Pulmonary stenosis
Standard insurance is given when the lesion is mild, but moderate lesions will carry an appropriate loading and severe stenosis will be uninsurable.

After surgery – standard insurance may be given but a loading made if there is residual cardiac enlargement or right ventricular hypertrophy.

Aortic stenosis
Standard insurance is not given in aortic stenosis whether valvar or subvalvar. Children who have had surgery in childhood are considered to be unacceptable insurance risks.

Coarctation of aorta
Applicants for life insurance in unoperated cases would usually be refused.

After surgical treatment – if investigation shows an excellent result and there are no associated lesions, standard insurance may be given. If there is residual hypertension, left ventricular hypertrophy or associated lesions, a loading is made.

Tetralogy of Fallot
Unoperated cases are uninsurable.

After surgical treatment – the most favourable terms will be given to patients who have no residual gradient across the right ventricular outflow tract, no pulmonary incompetence, no selective enlargement on the chest radiograph and normal lung vascularity.

Transposition of the great arteries
There is insufficient follow-up into adult life at present for insurers to make a decision. The problem of arrhythmias after the Mustard operation and the possibility that the right ventricle cannot function at systemic pressure for a normal lifespan are adverse factors.

Bibliography and references

Aisenberg, R. B., Rosenthal, A. and Nadas, A. S. (1982) Developmental delay in infants with congenital heart disease. *Paediatric Cardiology*, **3**, 133–137

Brackenridge, R. D. C. (1985) *Medical Selection of Life Risks*, Macmillan, Journals Division, London, pp. 241–261

Lambert, E. C., Menon, V. A. and Wagner, H. R. (1974) Sudden unexpected death from cardiovascular disease in children. A co-operative international study. *American Journal of Cardiology,* **34,** 89–96

Linde, L. M., Dunn, O. J. and Schireson, R. (1967) Growth in children with congenital heart disease. *Journal of Pediatrics,* **70,** 413–419

Newburger, J. W., Silbert, A. R. and Buckley, L. P. (1984) Cognitive function and age at repair of transposition of the great arteries in children. *New England Journal of Medicine,* **310,** 1495–1499

Suoninen, P. (1971) Physical growth of children with congenital heart disease. Pre- and post-operative study of 355 cases. *Acta Paediatrica Scandinavica,* (Suppl.), **225,** 1–45

Chapter 23

Preventive cardiology

While great advances have been made in the treatment of heart disease in children over the past 25 years, the prevention of such disease has remained a rather remote ideal for most paediatricians and cardiologists. Two small, but important, successes are the detection of thalidomide as a cause (over 60% of infants with the embryopathy had cardiac malformations), and the virtual abolition of rubella in pregnancy by immunization of non-immune teenage girls. Understandably, with congenital heart disease the most common problem in the Western World, it is this which has most occupied the minds of paediatric cardiologists but in other parts of the world rheumatic heart disease remains the dominant problem. Furthermore, the possibility of starting measures in childhood which would reduce the enormous mortality and morbidity for coronary heart disease in adult life should occupy a greater place in paediatrics than it currently does. Myocardial disease due to viruses and iatrogenic heart disease provides relatively small numbers of cases, but their treatment is unsatisfactory, compared with structural abnormalities so that prevention becomes relatively more important.

Congenital heart disease

Thanks to detailed studies of the aetiology of cardiac abnormalities we have a clear view of the predisposing factors, including genetic influences (mainly multifactorial inheritance), maternal illness (diabetes) and drugs taken during pregnancy (see Chapter 1). Unfortunately children with recognizable risk factors comprise only a small proportion of those with congenital heart disease, at most 8%, and, with very few exceptions, the risk factors only increase the actual chances of any pregnancy producing an infant with an abnormal heart from the usual 0.8% to something like 4%, which is only marginally greater than the normal risk of producing an infant with some form of cardiac or non-cardiac abnormality (usually given as 3.5%). Although this additional risk may sway some parents away from further pregnancies, the numbers will be small. Genetic counselling on its own could only reduce the incidence of congenital heart disease by 4%, even assuming that all mothers with a family history of the condition elected to have no further family.

Fetal echocardiography is now an accepted and reliable technique for determining major cardiac abnormalities from a gestational age of 17 weeks onwards. Obstetricians, radiologists and radiographers can be taught to look for and record the presence of two ventricles of comparable size and two atrioventricular valves, and thereby exclude the occurrence of primitive ventricle and hypoplastic left and right hearts, the commonest uncorrectable abnormalities. With a little more experience it is possible to check that there are two semilunar valves and two great arteries, correctly connected, thus excluding truncus arteriosus, pulmonary atresia and transposition. In most centres it is usual to refer any woman in whom the scan does not allow identification of the basic cardiac structures to a specialist in antenatal cardiac diagnosis, usually a paediatric cardiologist or a radiologist working with cardiologists. When a hypoplastic left heart is confirmed before 20 weeks it is likely that the mother will opt for termination and many will do so for single ventricle. The decision is obviously much less clear for conditions such as transposition and tetralogy of Fallot where surgical treatment is generally possible with a low risk and good subsequent outlook.

Atrioventricular septal defects can be diagnosed, particularly if they are the complete variety. Many of these will be in a fetus with Down's syndrome and may strengthen the case for termination of pregnancy.

Isolated ventricular and atrial septal defects will probably not be detected if small (the normal foramen ovale looks like an atrial septal defect in early pregnancy) and, if apparently large are not normally regarded as indicating termination, but their detection may cause distress to the parents, with the implication of surgery. We do not understand enough about the behaviour of such defects during the second half of pregnancy to know how likely they are to close.

Currently, specific ultrasound examination of the fetal heart is only offered to mothers at higher-than-average risk of producing an infant with congenital heart disease. The full list of aetiological factors is given in Chapter 1, but briefly this includes those with a family history of congenital heart disease (themselves, in the father or in a previous child), those with diabetes, phenylketonuria or other conditions increasing the risk and those mothers on drugs with a teratogenic potential (alcohol, lithium, amphetamines, anticonvulsants and progestins). These comprise only about 8% of pregnant mothers, and they can be expected to produce an abnormal 17-week scan in only about 3%. In addition there will be mothers who have had a routine scan and a possible fetal abnormality is found. This may be either an intrinsic cardiac abnormality or an extracardiac abnormality known to be associated with a high incidence of cardiac anomalies, such as oesophageal atresia or diaphragmatic hernia. In our experience, roughly equal numbers of referrals come from the high-risk group and those with a chance finding of possible fetal abnormality, but the latter group, of course have a higher incidence of confirmed cardiac abnormality.

Overall, the present policy of selective fetal cardiac ultrasound scanning will therefore only detect about 4% of all cardiac abnormalities and its potential for a major reduction in the incidence of congenital heart disease is small. If all pregnancies were studied at 17–20 weeks specifically to check for the presence of two atria, two normally contracting ventricles of roughly equal size with atrioventricular valves, two great arteries and the absence of an atrioventricular septal defect, we could potentially prevent a further 6%, but this would include most of the conditions which are most difficult to treat, namely hypoplastic left and right heart syndromes, primitive ventricle, truncus arteriosus and atrioventricular septal defect, together with some occurrences of endocardial fibroelastosis. Such a level of diagnosis is achievable by any experienced ultrasound operator and this should be the aim for the next few years. Detection of transposition, tetralogy and abnormalities of systemic and pulmonary venous drainage require an experienced cardiac specialist, but these are conditions which are generally treatable with good results so that termination of pregnancy will rarely be recommended, and measures to ensure their detection not routinely indicated.

Until we know more of the factors causing congenital heart disease, other methods of prevention are restricted to those which are normally recommended generally during pregnancy, avoidance of all but the most essential medications, not smoking or drinking alcohol, eating a sensible diet and optimal control of any maternal illness such as diabetes. From the little we know, it seems that the widespread acceptance of these principles would have at least as much impact on the incidence of congenital heart disease as routine scanning in pregnancy.

Rheumatic heart disease

Acute rheumatism has shown a steady fall in incidence over the first half of the century and Glover in 1930 predicted that it would ultimately disappear altogether. It has, in fact, all but disappeared from affluent countries before its aetiology was fully understood, and the countries in which it is still prevalent do not have the resources to study it in detail. It is generally accepted that the decline in incidence had more to do with improvement in housing and other social conditions and possibly a natural decline in virulence of the beta-haemolytic streptococcus than to the coming of sulphonamides and penicillin.

Prevention will therefore involve different strategies according to whether one looks at a socially developed country or an undeveloped one. In developed countries secondary prevention, i.e. prevention of recurrences of rheumatic fever, is more important, although some attention to primary prevention is appropriate.

Primary prevention (Table 23.1) consists of limiting the spread of the beta-haemolytic streptococcus and treating infections promptly before the immune mechanism, which is thought to underly the pathological abnormalities, can start to work. Unfortunately there are other, commoner, causes of a sore throat, particularly viruses of the common cold, influenza and infectious mononucleosis, so that the ideal of taking a throat swab on all children and adolescents with a sore throat is hardly achievable. However, a sore throat with marked injection of the pharynx, particularly with exudate, and absence of nasal congestion should warrant a throat swab and a course of oral phenoxymethylpenicillin. (Amoxycillin is best avoided, particularly in adolescents, in view of the rash which occurs with infective mononucleosis and other virus infections.) If a beta-haemolytic streptococcus grows on culture the oral penicillin should be continued for at least ten days or an injection of benzathine penicillin given (see below for doses). When cultures are positive it should also be policy to treat other children in the family. When there is a known allergy to penicillin, erythromycin should be given.

Secondary prevention (Table 23.1) consists of long-term administration of penicillin or sulphadiazine to prevent recurrent infection with the streptococcus. Patients with acute rheumatic fever should be given a therapeutic course of penicillin to eradicate any existing infection, even if the organism has not been grown from throat swabs and should then be started immediately on long-term treatment. Penicillin is the most common agent, either as phenoxymethylpenicillin or monthly injection of benzathine penicillin. The latter has been recommended for areas where non-compliance is likely, although it is arguable whether a painful injection is more or less likely to be acceptable than the need to take tablets daily. It is probably better to allow the patient and the parents the initial choice and be prepared to change over if the first route seems not to be acceptable. Penicillin is often denied to patients on the basis of supposed or possible allergic reactions. Many 'penicillin allergies' turn out, on questioning, to be a rash from ampicillin or amoxycillin, which does not occur with penicillin itself. If the reaction has occurred to penicillin it is still worth while carrying out testing and an attempt at desensitization, in hospital, to allow penicillin to be used. Fears are also expressed that the large amount given in a single injection of benzathine penicillin may provoke a catastrophic sensitivity reaction. In practice this does not occur, and in any case, sensitivity reactions are not directly dose related.

Sulphonamides are equally effective in preventing recurrent attacks and are much cheaper. There is no greater risk of sensitivity reactions and, in the doses used, renal precipitation does not occur. There is a very small incidence of granulocytopenia, but this is less than 0.01% and does not warrant routine haematological monitoring. Nevertheless it is the usual reason given for preferring penicillin. The use of sulphonamides does have one bonus and that is the avoidance of penicillin-resistant alpha-haemolytic streptococci in the mouth so that it is still possible to use penicillin prophylaxis against infective endocarditis to cover dental extractions, whereas patients on long-term penicillin require admission to hospital for intravenous gentamicin or vancomycin.

As used in developed countries, long-term prophylaxis gives about 80% protection against further attacks of rheumatic fever. It is uncertain whether the remaining 20% are those who seldom took their treatment or whether some other mechanism underlies recurrent attacks. It is certainly uncommon to grow streptococci from the throat in such patients, but the culture rate generally is lower in recurrent attacks.

Table 23.1 Primary prevention: treatment of streptococcal pharyngitis or initial treatment in acute rheumatic fever

	Age	Dose	Frequency/Duration
Primary prevention			
Phenoxymethylpenicillin	1–5	125 mg	
(Penicillin V)	6–12	250 mg	8-hourly 10 days orally
(or Penicillin G)	12+	500 mg	
Benzathine Penicillin	1–5	0.4 M Unit	
	6–12	0.8 M Unit	Intramuscular, one dose
	12+	1.2 M Unit	
Secondary prevention			
Phenoxymethylpenicillin	1–5	62.5 mg	
(or Penicillin G)	5+	125 mg	twice daily
Benzathine Penicillin	1–5	0.4 M Unit	Monthly intramuscular
	6–12	0.8 M Unit	
	12+	1.2 M Unit	
Sulphadiazine	1–8	0.5 g	
	8+	1.0 g	Orally daily

The duration of treatment is still controversial. Some cardiologists feel that it should be lifelong, and that is probably wise in countries where the disease is rife and in any patient having an apparently first attack in adolescence or adult life. When the first attack occurs before the age of 10, the treatment must be continued for 10 years, or until the child leaves school or college, in the belief that such institutions have a high potential for transmitting streptococci.

Some cardiologists also differentiate between patients who have had evidence of carditis in their first attack of rheumatic fever and those who have not. This follows the observation that, in any one individual, the pattern of attacks is similar, that is to say that a first attack without carditis is unlikely to be followed by a second attack with carditis. This view is not universally held and, since rheumatic fever, even without carditis, is an unpleasant, painful disease it seems reasonable to make every attempt to prevent recurrences.

The doses given in Table 23.1 are about twice those originally shown to prevent recurrent streptococcal infections, but allow for continuous prophylaxis if the occasional dose is missed. This scheme differs from that originally suggested by the American Heart Association in 1971, which was directed largely at adults and older children. Since, in the countries where rheumatic fever is prevalent, the disease is often seen below the age of 5, we have felt it advisable to include some recommendation for younger children.

Myocardial disease

The chronic myocardial, or endomyocardial diseases comprise a group of conditions of varying clinical presentation and aetiology. The commonest form seen in temperate zones causes dilatation of the left ventricle and poor contractility and is accompanied in many cases by thickening of the endocardium to produce the pathological syndrome of endocardial fibroelastosis. More common in subtropical zones is a similar condition where gross fibrosis obliterates ventricular cavities and impairs valve function, known as endomyocardial fibrosis. Neither of these conditions is aetiologically defined, but infection by one or more agents, together with altered immune response, is generally regarded as the cause.

The progression of virus myocarditis (particularly from coxsackie virus) to dilated cardiomyopathy is well authenticated in adults and probably occurs in children. An infectious-autoimmune combination is suggested by the finding of high viral titres together with immunofluorescence to human IgM in affected myocardial nuclei. Antiviral agents against coxsackie virus are in the process of development and may prove to be of clinical benefit, although the detection of acute viral myocarditis is not easy. An alternative suggestion, not yet tried, is to give steroid drugs once the acute stage has subsided (during the acute phase it is thought that they may worsen myocardial damage) in the hope of preventing the autoimmune part of the process. It seems likely that myocardial biopsy would be necessary both for diagnosis and controlling treatment.

Prospects for control and prevention of endomyocardial fibrosis (restrictive or obliterative cardiomyopathy) are even less promising. The eosinophilic form is usually rapidly progressive and does not appear to respond to drugs directed against eosinophils themselves (prednisolone and hydroxyurea). Clearly our ability to prevent or arrest the condition is unlikely to improve until the aetiology is more clearly understood. At the moment, with the view emerging that parasitic (particularly microfilarial) infestation causes the eosinophilia which produces the endomyocardial damage, the best hope lies with improved sanitation and living conditions, since drug treatment of the parasites produces only temporary benefit when reinfestation occurs almost immediately.

The myocardium is involved in a number of generalized degenerative diseases, notably Hurler's syndrome and Friedreich's ataxia. Hurler's syndrome can now be treated by bone marrow transplantation to provide the necessary missing enzymes and such treatment appears to prevent the cardiological deterioration. It seems likely that genetic engineering of this type may provide relief in other conditions.

Myocardial damage may be produced by drugs and the most important ones are adriamycin and daunorubicin. It was felt that there was a threshold of cumulative dose which had to be reached, but serial studies of contractility during treatment show that there is a progressive fall as the cumulative dose increases. Monitoring by echocardiography or other non-invasive means of measuring contractility is important and allows the drug to be withdrawn before left ventricular function falls below the normal limits.

Hypertrophic cardiomyopathy is frequently transmitted as a dominant condition, although the degree of clinical penetrance varies widely. Demonstration of the gene responsible has been suggested by experimental work and is likely to become a clinical possibility very soon (Matsumori et al., 1981). Detection of the disease is an indication to screen all first-degree relatives, and many cases are now coming to attention in this way. In families with a high incidence of symptomatic or clinically apparent disease there is a need for genetic counselling. The condition can be detected prenatally by echocardiography, but the absence of obvious disease does not mean that the fetus will not develop the disease. Now that early treatment with beta-blocking drugs has been shown to prevent progression and cause regression, early diagnosis has become more important, fully justifying the effort of echocardiography in first-degree relatives of a proven case.

Coronary heart disease

While only about 5 in 1000 children will require surgical treatment and 1 in 1000 die from congenital heart disease, about 40% will ultimately die from coronary heart disease (atheroma). Only rarely does classical coronary atheroma occur in childhood and such cases are confined to individuals homozygous for the familial hypercholesterolaemia gene. This gene occurs in heterozygous form in about 1 in 500 of the population so that a marriage between such heterozygotes occurs once in 125 000 marriages and 1 in 4 of their offspring will be homozygous, an incidence of 2 per million live births. Although the condition is an intriguing one paediatricians need to take a broader outlook on the overall problem of coronary heart disease.

The aetiological factors are now well known. Smoking is a risk factor which operates from an age well within the paediatric range. (In Great Britain 1 child in 8 is already addicted to smoking before teenage and a further 30% acquire the habit before leaving school. Girls are currently more likely to be smokers than boys.) Education from parents and teachers and avoidance of advertising directed specifically against the young have already been shown to affect boys' smoking habits, and girls appear to follow the boys' example, but more slowly. Paediatricians have many opportunities to give advice, both to individuals and families and to schools and other institutions, as well as making their views known nationally. Smoking has the great advantage as a target that there are no contraindications to not smoking.

The second risk factor for coronary heart disease is the level of cholesterol in the blood. In affluent societies this rises steadily throughout life up to the age of 70 years, but it appears that levels up to about 4.5 mmol/l are not atherogenic. Very few children, other than those with familial hypercholesterolaemia, achieve such levels, irrespective of their diet, so that the aim is more to educate children about healthy diets and to establish habits for healthy eating than to lower the current levels of cholesterol. At the same time it is important to detect children who carry the hypercholesterolaemia gene. Random testing for an occurrence of 1 in 500 is clearly not indicated, but paediatricians should look out for children in whom one or other parent has shown a suggestive history. Basically this means a coronary (or other atheromatous) history in a father or grandfather of under 55 or mother or grandmother under 60, particularly if the sufferer was not a heavy smoker. Children in such families should have an estimation of blood lipids. Interpretation of the results is also important. Laboratories commonly do not give age-related normal values and never give values for children. Nelson gives the following ranges for American children:

Newborn	1.37–1.35 mmol/l
Under 1 year	1.81–4.53
1 year to 12	3.11–5.18
12–18	3.11–5.44
(Adult	3.63–8.03)

These are not ideal levels, and the upper limits could be improved with dietary adjustment.

Generally those children with familial hypercholesterolaemia will be some 50% above the upper limit of normal for age, typically between 6.5 and 10 mmol/l. These are the patients who should receive continuous monitoring and dietary advice. Only a small proportion will require lipid-lowering agents during childhood, but these may be required if the cholesterol level remains above 6.5 mmol/l. If the result of the estimation is equivocal, a low fat diet should be recommended and the investigation repeated. A level at the upper limit of normal does not require any treatment but should be repeated after an interval of 3 years. Generally cholesterol levels show evidence of 'tracking' throughout childhood, but the level found clearly indicates not only the genetic aspect but also the current dietary practice. Some help can be obtained in separating non-affected from affected siblings if the levels of affected members of the family are known as these are often remarkably similar.

Recently attention has been focused on the separation of total cholesterol into high-density lipoprotein bound cholesterol, which is generally protective, and medium-density lipoprotein cholesterol, which is positively correlated with risk of coronary heart disease. However, those who have high total cholesterol levels generally have low levels of high-density cholesterol and vice versa, so that determination of the various fractions does little to improve the predictive value of the measurement.

Details of low animal fat diet are beyond the scope of this review, but are well known to dietitians, whose help should be encouraged at an early stage. A number of teenagers adopt a vegetarian diet for reasons other than prevention of atherosclerosis. Unfortunately, these usually rely heavily on dairy produce to provide protein and calories and these are no better than a normal mixed diet for reducing cholesterol levels. Vegan diets, with no animal produce, do achieve substantial reductions in cholesterol, but diets in which fish, particularly oily fish, are substituted for meat are as good and do not run the risk of vitamin lack or excess weight loss.

In the severer forms of hyperlipidaemia, lipid-lowering agents may be required and this always applies in homozygous hypercholesterolaemia. The most effective are the resins cholestyramine and colestipol, but they are unpleasant to take. They act within the gut to sequestrate bile salts and reduce the cholesterol pool. Supplements of fat-soluble vitamins and folic acid are usually required as these substances are also sequestrated. Fibrate drugs, clofibrate and bezafibrate, reduce the production of cholesterol in the liver. They have rather little effect on their own but a greater effect when given with sequestrating agents.

Patients who are homozygous for the hypercholesterolaemia gene have cholesterol levels in the region of 20 mmol/l and usually do not respond adequately to dietary and drug treatments. Recently, removal of cholesterol by repeated plasmapheresis has produced satisfactory reductions in serum cholesterol and regression of xanthomata.

There is at the moment no way of detecting familial hypercholesterolaemia prenatally, although attempts have been made to sample the blood from the umbilical cord. Genetic counselling would clearly be appropriate for any couple who both have heterozygous familial hypercholesterolaemia since any of their offspring would have a 50% chance of heterozygous disease, a 25% chance of homozygous disease and only a 25% chance of normal serum lipids.

The third important risk factor for coronary heart disease is hypertension. Detection of children with a tendency to raised blood pressure is easy if the blood pressure is taken at routine examinations. Tracking is established from about 7 years onwards and enables those with a higher than normal risk of established hypertension in adult life to be detected. Unfortunately, there is little that can be done to prevent the rise entirely, but counselling with regard to maintaining ideal weight, reducing salt intake and limiting alcohol intake is sensible. The main reason for detection, however, is to establish a pattern for monitoring blood pressure throughout adult life and establishing suitable drug therapy when this becomes indicated. Drug treatment for hypertension is now effective and palatable. The problems arise from failure to diagnose it at an early enough stage to prevent complications such as coronary artery disease.

There are a number of minor risk factors which are worth considering but have little practicable value in prevention. Body weight has some predictive value and keeping weight near the ideal does no harm. Exercise has a protective effect in adults but it is not certain whether children who undertake vigorous exercise are directly affecting their chances of coronary disease or establishing patterns for the future which could be important. Personality is important as coronary heart disease is almost twice as common in Type A personality (driving personalities, unhappy with present achievements and feeling oppressed by colleagues) as in Type B, who have a generally more 'laid-back' approach to life.

Bibliography and references

General

Nora, J. J. and Nora, A. H. (1983) Genetic aspects of preventive cardiology. In *Preventive Cardiology* (ed. D. G. Julian and J. O'N. Humphries), Butterworths, London

Congenital heart disease

Allan, L. D., Crawford, D. C., Anderson, R. H., *et al.* (1985) Spectrum of congenital heart disease detected echocardiographically in prenatal life. *British Heart Journal,* **54,** 523–526

Allan, L. D., Crawford, D. C., Chita, S. K., *et al.* (1986) Prenatal screening for congenital heart disease. *British Medical Journal,* **292,** 1717–1719

Nora, J. J. and Nora, A. H. (1983) Prevention of congenital heart disease. In *Preventive Cardiology* (ed. D. G. Julian and J. O'N. Humphries), Butterworths, London

Nora, J. J. and Nora, A. H. (1978) The evolution of specific genetic and environmental counselling in congenital heart disease. *Circulation,* **57,** 205–213

Rheumatic heart disease

Markowitz, M. (1983) Prevention of acute rheuamtic fever and rheumatic heart disease. In *Preventive Cardiology* (ed. D. G. Julian and J. O'N. Humphries), Butterworths, London

Myocardial disease

Maron, B. J., Nichols, P. F., Pickle, L. W., *et al.* (1984) Patterns of inheritance in hypertrophic cardiomyopathy. Assessment by M-mode and two-dimensional echocardiography. *American Journal of Cardiology,* **53,** 1087–1094

Matsumori, A., Kawai, C., Wakabayashi, A., *et al.* (1981) HLA–DRW4 antigen linkage in patients with hypertrophic obstructive cardiomyopathy. *American Heart Journal,* **101,** 14–16

Atherosclerosis and coronary heart disease

Nora, J. J. (1983) Primary prevention of atherosclerosis. In *Preventive Cardiology* (ed. D. G. Julian and J. O'N. Humphries), Butterworths, London

Index